W9-CEQ-628

SPORTS INJURIES

Diagnosis and Management

SPORTS INJURIES

Diagnosis and Management

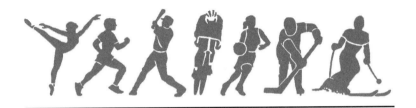

SECOND EDITION

JAMES G. GARRICK, MD
Director, Center for Sports Medicine
Saint Francis Memorial Hospital
San Francisco, California

DAVID R. WEBB, MD
Co-Director, St. Mary's/Duluth Clinic Sports Medicine Network
Duluth, Minnesota

W.B. SAUNDERS COMPANY
A Division of Harcourt Brace & Company
Philadelphia   London   Toronto   Montreal   Sydney   Tokyo

W.B. SAUNDERS COMPANY
A Division of Harcourt Brace & Company

The Curtis Center
Independence Square West
Philadelphia, Pennsylvania 19106

Library of Congress Cataloging-in-Publication Data

Garrick, James G.
Sports injuries: diagnosis and management / James G. Garrick, David R.
Webb.—2nd ed.

p.   cm.

Includes bibliographical references and index.

ISBN 0–7216–4434–1

1. Sports injuries.   I. Webb, David R. (David Ray)   II. Title.

[DNLM: 1. Athletic Injuries—diagnosis. 2. Athletic Injuries—therapy.
QT 260G241s 1999]
RD97.G373 1999

617.1′027—dc21

DNLM/DLC   98-28594

Sports Injuries: Diagnosis and Management, 2nd Edition   ISBN 0–7216–4434–1

Printed in the United States of America.

Last digit is the print number: 9   8   7   6   5   4   3   2   1

Preface

The preface to the first edition applies equally now as it did then. The book remains directed at those who provide the primary care for sports-related musculoskeletal injuries and conditions. By providing all of the material in the book ourselves, we have tried to maintain a consistent format and philosophy.

We have tried to make decision-making easier by introducing each chapter with a triage section that provides guidelines for making referral decisions and obtaining radiographs. We have also tried to place in perspective the use of rapidly expanding imaging technology.

While the principles of diagnosis and management of sports injuries remain unchanged, both the patient population and the providers have undergone some alterations. An increasingly active aging population makes it necessary to consider activities and injuries well beyond those seen in school-based, team sport participants. For instance, common problems such as meniscus injuries are managed differently in older athletes, and we have tried to address these issues.

We have also tried to enhance the ability of the practitioner to manage injuries in a relative vacuum, given the difficulty (impossibility?) of obtaining authorization to refer in many managed care environments. We have also endeavored to provide the information necessary to initiate treatment and rehabilitation programs without outside help at the time of the initial visit.

Caring for the athletically inclined continues to reward us with an upbeat, motivated patient population presenting with a seemingly endless array of fascinating sports-related problems. We hope that the information provided in this book will help you achieve similar rewards.

JAMES G. GARRICK
DAVID R. WEBB

Acknowledgments

We gratefully acknowledge the personal and professional contributions of Ms. Ariel Bleth, Mr. Thomas Buck, Ms. Betsy Cook, Dr. Steven Crane, Mr. Peter Dumas, Mr. Jeff Frey, Mr. J.C. Garrick, Mr. Chris Gebeck, Ms. Judith Gentry, Mr. Rick Kollath, Ms. Karla Kukowski, Mr. Jacob Marxhausen, Ms. Michelle O'Neal, Mr. Ralph Requa, Mr. Thomas Segal, Mr. Drew Van Brunt, Ms. Annika Viragh, Ms. Arielle Webb, Mr. Dennis Wiseman, Ms. Jamie Zimmerman, our families, and the Saint Francis Foundation, whose talents, hard work, encouragement, constructive criticism, and financial support helped make this book possible.

JAMES G. GARRICK
DAVID R. WEBB

Contents

Chapter 5

Chapter 6

Chapter 7

Chapter 8

Approach to the Injured Athlete

There are few injuries unique to the sports environment. Although we speak of jumper's knee, tennis elbow, or runner's heel, these same injuries are frequently seen in a nonathletic environment. Indeed, some sports injuries are more common in industry than they are in athletics. Yet treating an "athletic injury" is different. Failure to recognize this difference results in frustration for the physician, dissatisfaction for the athlete, and inappropriate medical care.

Physicians unaccustomed to dealing with athletes are often uncomfortable when attempting to manage a sports injury. A great deal of this discomfort stems from the incessant questions posed by the athlete/patient. Although most medical professionals agree that patients have a right to be informed about their condition, most patients fail to exercise this right. On the contrary, many patients do not want to know very much about their injuries or illnesses—they simply want to be made well. Athletes, on the other hand, want to know not only exactly what is wrong, but also why it happened and precisely how soon they will be well again. Thus the first major difference in treating injured athletes is *a need for greater communication and patient education*.

The second difference is in the quantity of treatment. Interestingly, the *quality* of treatment—namely surgical intervention—receives the most attention in the media and often *defines* sports medicine. In spite of the association between athletic injuries and surgical intervention, the quality of treatment differs little with regard to the circumstance of injury. An ankle fracture, for example, is treated the same whether it occurred as the result of a slide tackle in soccer or tripping over the family cat. But the intensity and duration of treatment are quite different for the soccer player chafing to return to the sport and the sedentary person content with the ability to walk from the car

1

to work without an obvious limp. The second difference is *a need for more complete and comprehensive rehabilitation*—a subject all but ignored in most medical training programs.

The unique aspects of managing athletic injuries fall into a number of categories, among them the injury itself, the rehabilitation program, the influence of coaches and parents, the physician's responsibilities, and prevention. The remainder of this section is a discussion of these areas.

THE INJURY

Although the injuries seen in athletics may not be unique, the circumstances under which they are seen may be. The team physician, standing on the sidelines, may have the opportunity to see (and manage) an injury sooner after its occurrence than under any other circumstance. In some instances this urgency offers treatment options not generally available. For example, reduction of a shoulder dislocated moments before is often easily accomplished without the benefit of analgesics, muscle relaxants, or heroic amounts of traction—a contrast to the usual situation in the emergency room.

The sideline physician may also be called on to provide first aid—another departure from one's usual practice. Although the principle of "splint 'em where they lie" is a good one, theory and practice might be quite different when one is faced with an unconscious football player exhibiting apnea and wearing a helmet and face mask (see Fig. 7–1).

Even in the absence of a physician on site, athletic injuries may be managed in a manner so ideal as to confuse initial diagnostic impressions. The athlete sustaining an ankle sprain in the ideal sports medicine environment—that is, under the direction of a certified athletic trainer—will have the injury evaluated, iced, compressed, elevated, and rested in a matter of moments. Such an ideally treated injury may appear deceptively benign later in the emergency room, where the staff is accustomed to seeing such problems only after 24 hours of attempted weight bearing and warm soaks.

The adult recreational athlete, on the other hand, often sees a physician about an injury only after a variety of sportsman's home remedies have failed and even the activities of daily living are compromised. What started as a mild case of chondromalacia patellae develops into a swollen knee accompanied by hamstring spasm (preventing extension) and calf pain from walking on the partially flexed knee.

TREATMENT

Initial treatment is dictated by the type and severity of the injury rather than the athletic inclination of the patient. The athlete, however, usually requires an earlier appointment for a return visit because of a generally higher level of compliance. Most physicians expect patients to follow instructions in a desultory manner. Thus, although told to ice and elevate the sprained ankle, the usual patient elevates it only during TV watching at night and finds removing the wrap and icing the ankle too much bother. Because the appearance of an ankle so treated will not change much in 48 hours, the return visit is scheduled for 1 week. In contrast, the athlete may apply ice as many as eight times a day and be equally scrupulous in elevating the limb. The athlete's ankle will be ready for the next, more active phase of treatment in

48 hours. Additionally, because impatience is a group characteristic of athletes, if athletes are not seen soon enough they will take further treatment into their own hands, substituting zeal for appropriate advice.

Under ideal circumstances, treatment of the athletic injury can require a minimum of time and effort on the part of the physician. Such circumstances surround virtually every athlete with ready access to a certified athletic trainer. Once apprised of a definitive diagnosis, the trainer is, in the majority of instances, able to carry out the complete treatment and rehabilitation program with a minimum of guidance on the part of the physician. Unfortunately, such circumstances rarely exist outside major team sports such as football or basketball.

It is usually erroneous—and unwise—to assume that coaches will play a major role in the supervision of the treatment/rehabilitation program. Coaches usually find time to function as trainers only after their coaching duties have been discharged. Additionally, coaches may be no better informed than athletes, thus requiring written instruction no less complete than if the athletes were going to oversee their own program. If left to their own devices, coaches often treat athletes the way they have treated their own ankle sprain, which may have occurred 25 years earlier. These comments should in no way be construed as being critical of coaches; rather they reflect the fact that an individual who wanted to spend a lifetime treating athletic injuries would have become a medical professional and not a coach.

In the absence of an athletic trainer, the physician should be prepared to spend an inordinate amount of time precisely describing—teaching—the treatment and rehabilitation program. Athletes must be told exactly what they can and cannot do. Exercises must be described in detail and be demonstrated correctly by the patients. The frequency with which the exercises are to be done and the number of repetitions should be provided in writing.

"Occasional athletes" present yet another problem, that is, wanting to be treated in a "sports medicine" manner but to be relieved of any personal involvement. These patients view treatment as consisting of an hour spent every day in the physical therapist's office. When asked what they are doing for their injuries, occasional athletes reply, "Going to physical therapy." Athletic injuries cannot be treated passively—they require the active involvement of the athletes. Thus, in addition to the daily physical therapy, athletes must be taught their own personal rehabilitation program.

COACHES

The physician must realize that the coach enjoys the ultimate in credibility with the athlete—even concerning medical issues. Physicians, unaccustomed to having their advice or judgment questioned, often react badly when athletes justify their participation in a (medically) forbidden activity because the coach thought they should do it. Questioning (or worse, criticizing) the (medical) veracity of the coach's advice serves no purpose other than to increase the athletes' reluctance to provide honest answers. Accept the fact that, in the athletic world, the coach is king—just as the physician might be in the medical world.

We have dealt with athletes and coaches for an aggregate of more than 50 years. In our experience, it is rare when coaches are not genuinely concerned about the well-being of their athletes. When a coach gives medically questionable advice, it is the result not of malice toward the physician but rather of operating in a medical vacuum. Physicians cannot expect coaches to provide valid medical information if the medical world ignores them.

Communication with coaches is essential if good sports medicine care is to be provided. Providing a diagnosis (in layperson's terms, if necessary), an outline of the treatment program, and an estimate of the length of disability is all most coaches ask of physicians. If available, an athletic trainer provides the most effective bridge of the gap between the physician and the coach: The trainer resides comfortably in both camps. In the absence of a trainer the physician must bear this responsibility.

Communicating with coaches may be difficult—not because they do not want to communicate, but because they are more difficult to contact than physicians. Teaching responsibilities and the unavailability of a telephone at athletic facilities make telephone contact a virtual impossibility.

The most effective means of communication seems to be written injury (status) reports. The athlete sent to a physician should not be allowed to return to participation in the sport without the written authorization of the physician. Interim reports during treatment are also valuable as they allow the coach to organize practices and create team rosters that take into account the presence or absence of the athlete.

Finally, written communications protect the physician, the coach, and the athlete. It is unwise to assume that verbal advice and instructions will be accurately conveyed through the athlete to the coach. If the physician expects the coach to oversee running drills, "half-speed" practices, and other rehabilitative tasks, the instructions must be precise.

PARENTS

Parents, like coaches, generally want what is best for their children athletes. Unfortunately, sometimes what the parent thinks is best for the child is at odds with the thoughts of the physician, the coach, or even the child. The physician should bear in mind that the child is the patient, and it is thus the physician's responsibility to serve as the child's advocate.

Most people are familiar with the "baseball father" or the "tennis mother"—those parents driven to promote their children's athletic careers with pathological zeal. Although a joint parent-child effort is a relationship to be encouraged in any activity, it becomes unhealthy when the parent's zeal is directed toward an apathetic child. In this situation the physician may be called on to resolve "severity disputes," in which the child says that he or she cannot participate because of the injury and the parent contends that the child can.

Because the treatment of most athletic injuries is symptom dependent, the physician must accept the child's appraisal of the complaints. If a boy reports that his Osgood-Schlatter disease is too painful to allow him to play football, then he should not play football, regardless of what his father says.

The committed child athlete often has problems of a different sort. Such a child may approach a sport with a level of zeal beyond the comprehension of the parents. In this circumstance, the parent may be looking for an excuse to attenuate the child's athletic activities. This is particularly true when the child has suffered a succession of sport-related injuries and the parent is genuinely concerned about the child's health. Unless continued participation is truly contraindicated medically, the physician's responsibilities are to the patient, and the physician must avoid thinking or acting like a parent. In general, greatly involved child athletes are good patients, excellent students, and committed to something, even though their parents may not understand them.

Other aspects of caring for the child athlete are not so simple. From a medicolegal standpoint, one can care for the child athlete only with the parents' consent. This becomes a problem when the adolescent is sent to the physician by the coach, sometimes without the parents' knowledge. Aside from the fact that the parents may disavow responsibility for any costs incurred, the physician cannot legally treat the child without the parents' permission.

In addition to obtaining consent for treatment, the physician has a responsibility to convey to the parent some information regarding the diagnosis and treatment of the injury. As with the coach, this can be accomplished by a written note—with a copy kept in the patient's record. Admittedly there is some uncertainty whether the note will ever be delivered to the parents, but short of mailing a report to the family there seems no realistic alternative.

THE MEDIA

The media play a role in the treatment of athletic injuries in two ways: their appetite for information concerning injuries to newsworthy athletes and their promulgation of information concerning the treatment of newsworthy athletes' injuries.

Just because a physician does not care for a professional football or basketball team does not mean the physician is not going to have to answer media queries. The fate of the injured high school quarterback the week before the "big game" or the figure skater before a regional competition is locally newsworthy. Unfortunately, the newsworthy aspect of those injuries is privileged medical information, information that the athlete may not want shared with either the community or, more importantly, the opposing coach or judges in the competition. Thus medical knowledge should be shared only with the athlete's (or parents', in the case of minors) explicit permission.

Equally problematic are patients'/athletes' questions concerning their treatment compared with news accounts of a famous athlete's encounter with a similar problem. Patients cannot understand why their shoulder complaints do not merit magnetic resonance imaging (MRI) when virtually every professional athlete with a sore shoulder has one performed on the day of injury. Aside from the fact that the economic impact of an MRI for a professional athlete is negligible (to the team), in the majority of instances such tests are performed primarily for confirmatory reasons, as the diagnoses have usually been accurately made before the performance of the test.

The nature and acuity of treatment are also often different for the high-level athlete than for the recreational participant. Few recreational or high school athletes have the time, availability, funding, or inclination to spend 6 hours a day rehabilitating a sports injury—de rigueur for the professional. Likewise, few recreational athletes manifest the level of training and conditioning seen among most high-level athletes *before their injuries*. Such prowess is usually associated with shorter treatment and healing times.

MANAGED CARE

High-level, comprehensive sports rehabilitation—the essence of sports medicine—is increasingly difficult to obtain under cost-conscious, managed care programs. Physical therapy, if approved at all, is often limited to only a few treatments—woefully inadequate to return a gymnast to competitive viability or a marathon runner to acceptable times. Without indications for surgical intervention, approval of orthopedic consultations is frequently delayed, discouraged, or even withheld.

Thus primary care physicians, gatekeepers for athletes as well as the general population, often find themselves in the uncomfortable position of caring for problems beyond the scope of their training and experience. Hallway or telephone consultations with orthopedists and physical therapists and continuing education efforts in sports medicine are helpful but do not adequately address the issue of decreasing patient access to specialty care—a problem bound to worsen before it improves.

SPORTS EDUCATION

If one accepts that the goal of the sports physician is to return the patient safely to athletic participation, it follows that the physician must know just what athletic participation entails. It is impossible to make valid decisions regarding a return to sports activities unless one is more than superficially acquainted with the demands of the sport.

Frequently patients are allowed to return prematurely to their sports simply because the physician or physical therapist had no idea of what that particular activity entailed. For example, teenaged gymnasts are told they can work out but not compete, without the realization that gymnastic practices are much more rigorous than competition and account for 95% of the injuries. Likewise, tennis players with resolving tennis elbow are told they can start hitting balls against a practice wall, without the realization that the average player has much more difficulty avoiding awkward shots against a backboard than when using a ball machine.

Being a spectator at athletic events is usually not sufficient background for a physician, because games and matches fail to typify the activities that often produce sports injuries. With the possible exception of collision sports, the majority of athletic injuries occur during practices. Thus, making an effort to observe workouts enhances the physician's ability to make appropriate medical decisions. Aside from the educational value of such visits, they convey to the athletes and coaches the physician's sincere interest.

INJURY PREVENTION

The physician who treats athletes is frequently called on to speak to parents' groups, coaches' clinics, and sports clubs. Inevitably the sponsors want the talk to deal with injury prevention. A perusal of the literature in preparation for such an address reveals little scientific information on which to base the talk. The physician frequently reads in quasi-medical publications that activities such as stretching, weight-training programs, and equipment fitting result in the prevention of injuries, yet the documentation supporting safety enhancement provided by these programs is less than compelling.

There are, however, examples of research that has resulted in substantial improvements in players' safety. Among these studies are those of Torg and associates[1, 2] dealing with football shoes and knee and ankle injuries and the mechanism of injury resulting in cervical spine injuries in football. The use of helmets and face masks in hockey is the product of sports medicine research, as are improved safety bindings in alpine skiing. Yet such universal problems as shin splints, chondromalacia patellae, tennis elbow, and sprains of the anterior cruciate ligament have prompted little attention from the standpoint of prevention.

Acute injuries are much more difficult to prevent than overuse injuries are. The misstep, the awkward block or tackle, and the off-balance lunge are, unfortunately, the "stuff" of which sports participation is made, and unless the games are substantially altered, these mishaps will continue to occur. Some acute problems can be prevented—those that are *re-injuries*. Roughly one quarter of the acute injuries in most sports are recurrences of old problems. Although some of these may truly be re-injuries, a significant proportion of them result from incomplete treatment or rehabilitation of the original problem and thus are theoretically preventable.

Overuse injuries, on the other hand, are amenable to prevention. Epidemiological studies of overuse injuries reveal that the most common "causes" are classified as training errors. Running too far, jumping too often, hitting backhands improperly, and wearing the wrong shoes are all examples of injury-producing circumstances that can be altered by educational programs. Unfortunately, the research necessary to support such educational programs has prompted little interest. It is paradoxical that research is aimed at the prevention of acute (dramatic) injuries, when the prevention of overuse problems appears to offer a much higher potential for success.

REFERENCES

1. Torg J, Quedenfeld T: The shoe-surface interface and its relationship to football knee injuries. Am J Sports Med 2:261, 1974.
2. Torg J et al: The National Football Head and Neck Injury Registry. Report and conclusions 1978. JAMA 241:1477, 1979.

Acute Injuries

A. OVERVIEW

The pathophysiology of acute sports injuries differs little from that seen in musculoskeletal trauma originating from other sources; thus the early management of acute athletic injuries follows the same well-defined orthopedic principles regardless of the cause.[1] The finer points of management are at the same time easier and more difficult in the athletic community: easier because mechanisms of injury might be more obvious, first aid should have been more appropriate, presentation for treatment should have been more immediate, and the patient population is generally more compliant, motivated, and potentially controllable; and more difficult primarily because of the overpowering climate of urgency and the necessity of returning the athlete to a supranormal state.

The psychological aspects of dealing with acute athletic injuries are vastly different from those surrounding trauma from other origins. Both the physician and the athlete are subjected to pressures not usually seen in other circumstances. The physician not only must make immediate appropriate decisions but also must convey the consequences of those decisions in the framework of specific athletic participation. Particularly stressful to many physicians are athletes' demands for prognostications and precise predictions of the duration of disability. Rather than indicating a lack of confidence in the physician's decisions (as they are sometimes perceived), the athlete's incessant and often penetrating questions are more a reflection of the demands being placed by coaches, teammates, and even parents. The athlete knows, for example, that the first question the coach will ask is, "When will you be back?"

INITIAL MANAGEMENT

Except in team sports, medical advice or care is usually not available at the time of injury. The patient's education regarding the basic principles of first aid is an important aspect of the duties of the physician treating athletic injuries. Regardless of how the injury was initially managed—or mismanaged—the patient should be told how it should have been treated, as this information will be valuable in dealing with subsequent problems.

The initial efforts in dealing with an acute injury should be directed toward prevention of bleeding and edema. Most injuries involve rupture of blood vessels; thus, halting hemorrhage is the primary concern. With most injuries the effects of hemorrhage produce far more disability than the loss of a few fibers of muscle, tendon, or ligament. The majority of athletic injuries are of the mild or moderate variety, and thus, by definition, the injured structure generally retains its continuity and ability to function. The accompanying bleeding, however, distorts normal anatomical relationships, resulting in pain and loss of motion.

For example, the disability associated with an inappropriately managed mild ankle sprain is not a reflection of the lost integrity of a few ligament fibers. The bleeding and edema that occur after such an injury result in pain on motion, which is then consciously or unconsciously avoided. Consequently, muscles cease to be used in a normal fashion and become weak. Also, when motion becomes uncomfortable, the muscles responsible for that action become incapable of producing it, and the joint is robbed of the stability afforded by muscular support, thus increasing the likelihood of a recurrent sprain. Had the original hemorrhage been prevented, this entire chain of events could have been avoided.

Compression is the most effective means of stopping hemorrhage, but to be effective, compression must be selective. A cross-section through the ankle at the level of the malleoli reveals that the structures injured in an ankle sprain are actually located in depressions—areas unaffected by a circumferential elastic wrap. Indeed, such a wrap encourages swelling in those areas not in contact with the bandage. Thus, inappropriate compression encourages swelling in the very areas where it will do the most damage.

To be effective, compression must be applied selectively to the injured structures. This is best accomplished by placing padding beneath the wrap at these locations. The padding can consist of six to eight layers of ABD pads or disposable diapers or ½- to ¾-in. felt. At the ankle, a horseshoe effectively applies pressure in front, behind, and beneath the malleolus. Similarly, folded ABD pads can be used to apply focal compression almost anywhere in the body.

We have found elasticized stockinette to be superior to elastic wraps. This material comes in various sizes, provides good, uniform compression, can be applied easily over padding, and is less expensive than elastic wraps. In addition it is less likely to wrinkle and, perhaps most importantly, can be removed and reapplied properly by the athlete. It is our experience that when the athlete attempts to reapply an elastic wrap, more often than not it is too tight or too loose to be maximally effective. It is, however, especially important that the athlete be able to reapply the wrap properly when it is necessary to remove it for such activities as contrast baths and showering.

Elasticized stockinette has the added advantage of providing compression with little bulk, thus permitting shoes and clothing to be worn over the wrap.

The *application of cold* to an acute injury is also helpful but not as important as compression. Scientific documentation of the efficacy of ice is difficult to find. However, the ill effects of applying heat to a fresh injury are well recognized. Thus, of the two, ice is far preferable.

Cold should be applied in the form of crushed ice so that it can be contoured much the same as with a compression pad. To avoid skin irritation, a single layer of loosely applied elastic wrap should be interposed between the ice bag and the skin. The ice bag should be held in place firmly so that it provides focal compression as well as cold. Icing should be continued for a minimum of 20 minutes and repeated every 2 to 4 waking hours.

A number of alternatives to frozen water are available. One of these produces an endothermic chemical reaction—"instant ice." Although appealing because of the ease of transportation, these ice packs usually last less than 10 minutes and, in warm ambient temperatures, do not become cold enough for maximal effectiveness. These products are also more expensive than frozen water in a plastic bag.

Another popular product is the frozen gel. This material holds its cold well, is reusable, and, because it is a gel, can be contoured to irregularly shaped body parts. Like ice, it requires transportation in an insulated container. A potential problem lies in the fact that the material achieves the same temperature as the freezer in which it has been kept. Although melting ice produces temperatures of 33° F or above, the ice gels frequently remain at temperatures below freezing for some time. If the gel is applied directly to the skin, frostbite is not an uncommon occurrence.

We have seen the emergence of an entire industry aimed at cooling injured extremities. First used in the immediate postoperative period for surgical patients, these devices and techniques quickly found a home in athletic training rooms, physical therapy treatment centers, and, now, homes. Most consist of a reservoir, pump, tubes, and a sack to envelop the injured part. The cooled fluid (usually ice water) is circulated, under pressure, around the injured part, thus providing both compression and cooling. Such devices can be either leased or purchased by the injured person.

Although such pumping systems are surely more convenient than making repeated trips to the sink and freezer, they have not been shown to be more clinically efficacious than the repeated application of crushed ice. They are, however, much more expensive.

We have found that a bag of frozen corn (both cheap and readily available) contoured about the injured part and held in place with an elastic wrap is the most satisfactory alternative to crushed ice.

Elevation, or at least the avoidance of dependency, is the third element of the initial treatment of an acute injury. Although athletes usually quickly realize that dependency increases discomfort, they should nonetheless be reminded to elevate the injured part.

Finally, painful activities should be avoided. The term *rest* is probably inappropriate in that it is often taken literally, and the athlete ceases all activity. The injured part should be rested only to avoid pain. For example, if the freshly sprained ankle allows comfortable ambulation, then such activity should be allowed.

Compression, ice, and elevation should be employed as long as the swelling threatens or exists—usually for at least the first few days after injury. The athlete should understand that these are means of preventing and reducing swelling; thus they are appropriate as long as swelling is present. As a general rule, athletes are accustomed to taking instructions literally, and if told to use ice for 48 hours, they will stop at the end of 2 days regardless of the appearance of the injured area. Compression, in particular, should be continued until all swelling has disappeared.

Often the athlete is seen a day or two after the injury has occurred, during which time appropriate measures have not been employed. Nonetheless, initial management is the same; it just takes longer to dissipate the swelling than it does to prevent it.

When swelling has been allowed to develop, additional means must be employed to alleviate it. Nonsteroidal anti-inflammatory medication seems helpful, although scientific documentation of this is not impressive. Formal physical therapy, employing high-intensity electrogalvanic stimulation, appears to be an effective adjunct in alleviating swelling. Home programs employing contrast baths also seem empirically to be effective.

The alternate application of heat and cold (contrast baths) is thought to reduce swelling by increasing blood flow to the area being treated. This means of treatment is simple, is inexpensive, and can be realistically carried out by athletes of any age. In our experience, patient compliance is much greater than with other commonly employed methods such as ice water soaks or ice whirlpools.

CONTRAST BATHS. For contrast baths, two watertight containers are used, one filled with warm water (100° F) and the other with cold water and ice. Heat and cold are alternated (e.g., 4 minutes in the warm bath, 1 minute in the cold), beginning with the warm bath and ending with the cold; this procedure is repeated four or five times. During the warm bath, range-of-motion exercises should be employed lest the dependent position result in increased swelling. The "milking" action of the range-of-motion exercises may be the most important part of this treatment.

The entire sequence should ideally be repeated three or four times daily until all swelling has disappeared. From a practical standpoint, most patients are able to use the contrast baths on arising in the morning and just before retiring at night.

All the techniques aimed at the reduction of edema should be started as soon as the initial swelling has stabilized—usually within 36 hours of the time of injury—and continued until the appearance is identical to that of the uninjured extremity.

Range-of-motion exercises should start as soon as the swelling has stabilized. The involved and adjacent joints should be repetitively moved through the painless range of motion. At first, this may involve only 5 to 10 degrees, but with repetitions the painless range gradually increases. This exercise should be carried out for a minimum of 5 minutes, four to five times a day. Using motion "tasks," such as writing the alphabet with the foot, makes the exercise less tedious and ensures that all planes of motion are used. Compliance seems much better when patients are told to write the alphabet 20 times a day with the foot than when they are instructed to dorsiflex and plantarflex and invert and evert the foot 200 times. (Range-of-motion tasks are suggested in the sections dealing with specific injuries.)

Strengthening exercises should be started simultaneously with the range-of-motion program. Working against the resistance afforded by Theraband or surgical tubing can be undertaken even if only a few degrees of comfortable motion are available. Likewise, if pain on motion is minimal or absent, isometric exercises—against the pressure of the other leg, a table, or a partner—should be employed. As a general rule, strength is lost at least twice as fast as it is regained; thus periods of "rest" should be as short as possible.

ISOMETRIC EXERCISES

Isometric or "tightening" exercises employ muscle actions without any motion of the involved joint. The simplest method of accomplishing this is to "contract" the muscle against an equal contraction of its antagonist; thus, isometric exercise of the quadriceps is done against isometric action of the hamstrings. Such an exercise requires no equipment and can be done under almost any circumstance.

Unfortunately, many patients have difficulty accomplishing this seemingly simple task; thus isometric exercises are often done against the resistance of an immovable object. Triceps isometrics, for example, can be done by sitting with the forearms resting on a desk and pushing downward, or by pushing downward on the arms of a chair.

When the patient is doing isometric exercises, the contraction should be held for 5 or 6 seconds, followed by relaxation for an equal period of time. We suggest that the patient do three or four such contractions at least hourly during the day. Using external prompts as reminders to do the exercises is often helpful. For example, students are told to do the exercises at the beginning of each class during the school day. Doing the exercises during each commercial break in a television program is also an effective memory jogger.

Performing a few exercises many times during the day is, in our estimation, much more effective than attempting to do the more commonly suggested 20 or 30 contractions two or three times a day. In addition, patient compliance seems much greater. Observation of patients reveals that after the fourth or fifth repetition the contractions are desultory.

In all likelihood, the quality of the isometric exercises is much more important than the quantity. The patient must be taught exactly how to do the exercise and must demonstrate the ability to muster a significant contraction for the physician or therapist. The best way to accomplish this is for the physician or therapist to point out the location of the muscle being exercised and have the patient palpate it for a firm contraction during the exercise. It is not uncommon to encounter patients who are using the wrong muscle groups because of inadequate instructions.

The disadvantages of isometric exercises are twofold: They are boring, and the strengthening that occurs is limited to the position in which the exercise is practiced. The former is dealt with by explaining to the patient that this is a means of preparing the muscle for the more formidable task of lifting weights, and that if the athlete fails to do the isometric exercises, the onset of weight lifting will be needlessly delayed. The latter, position specificity, is dealt with by having the isometric exercise done in various positions throughout the range of motion.

ISOTONIC EXERCISES

During isotonic exercises, the muscle action is used to move weight through the range of motion. That weight might initially consist of nothing more than the limb itself. Indeed, as illustrated by the five *fungo exercises* (see Fig. 4–40) used for shoulder rehabilitation, external weights are not employed, and progression is accomplished by increasing repetitions rather than weights.

Isotonic exercises are used to increase both strength and muscular endurance—strength by lifting increasing amounts of weight a small number of times (usually fewer than 12 repetitions) and endurance by lifting smaller amounts of weight many times.

As a general rule, isotonic exercises should be undertaken only throughout the comfortable range of motion. If painful, the exercise may result in swelling, muscle spasm, or both, which will limit subsequent activities. All too often the athlete has been taught "no pain, no gain" and attempts to lift in the presence of increasing discomfort. A mild burning sensation in the muscle should be the only discomfort encountered during any of these rehabilitative exercises. Joint pain should be avoided at all costs. Frequently this can be accomplished by decreasing the range of motion through which the exercise is performed. Ideally, however, isotonic exercises, especially those aimed at increasing strength, should be carried out through the full range of motion.

After an injury, it is safest to begin progressive resistance rehabilitation exercises (PREs) with more repetitions and lighter resistance. We advise athletes to select weights with which they can handle three sets of 10 to 20 repetitions per set. If they cannot do at least 10 repetitions on the third set, the weight is too heavy. When three sets of 20 repetitions becomes too easy, they may add weight. Skeletally immature athletes and older athletes are advised always to stay within these guidelines. Some athletes may chafe at this because they have to know what their "max lifts" are. A rule of thumb that should satisfy this need is that their "10-rep max" for a given lift will be about 70% of the "single-rep max."

For "pure" strength training, as opposed to strength/muscular endurance training, a modified Delorme PRE formula may be used.[2] Athletes first determine the maximal amount of weight they can lift through the range of motion, that is, the single repetition maximum (SRM). Using this weight the following scheme is used:

10 repetitions with 50% SRM
10 repetitions with 75% SRM
Up to 10 repetitions with 100% SRM
20 repetitions with 25% SRM

The lifts of 50%, 75%, and 100% SRM are done slowly, with 2 or 3 minutes of rest between sets; the 25% lifts are done more rapidly. When the athlete is able to lift 100% of SRM 10 times, then the SRM is increased (usually by 10%) and the entire process started over. At the outset, when relatively light weights are being used, the exercises may be done daily, or even twice daily. As the weights get heavier, longer rest intervals between workouts may be required. The rule of thumb is that there should be full recovery (no residual muscle soreness, fatigue, or the like) before the next strength workout is attempted.

The ultimate goal of SRM weight varies with different athletic activities. As a general rule, it should be at least the SRM of the opposite (uninjured) extremity.

ISOKINETIC EXERCISES

During the past 2 decades another form of exercise—isokinetic—has become increasingly popular. These exercises employ a variable amount of resistance at a fixed speed. Thus, lifting harder means greater resistance, rather than greater speed, as is the case in isotonic lifting. Because athletes have absolute and moment-to-moment control of the amount of resistance, they are less likely to injure themselves by the overzealous application of inappropriate weights. In addition, the muscle can produce an appropriately resisted maximal muscular action throughout the entire range of motion, an almost impossible task with the devices used for isotonic lifting.

Lifting weights at higher, "athletic," speeds may be desirable, as there appears to be an element of speed specificity in muscle training. Strength gains made as a result of slow resistance training (most weight machines) may be less evident at higher, more functional speeds. Because the speed is controlled and can be varied, isokinetic exercises can be carried out at velocities considerably higher than those attainable with most weight machines. Unfortunately, greater gains in functional performance resulting from isokinetic training have yet to be documented. Indeed, the only resistance exercises that truly approach powerful athletic speeds, and that have been shown to enhance performance the most, are those done with free weights, e.g., "power cleans" and Olympic lifts, and plyometric exercises.

Isokinetic devices measure the force produced by the exercising muscle and present it as a numerical value. Thus, progress can be documented and these values compared with those produced by the uninjured extremity, yielding a rough estimate of the attainment of the rehabilitative goals. Although it is tempting to regard the athlete who has not yet attained the isokinetic measurements of the opposite side as still disabled, there is little scientific documentation that this is universally true. Likewise, attainment of the isokinetic capabilities of the opposite extremity does not mean that the athlete is cured. Despite the appeal of a device that purportedly enhances (and measures) a muscle's return to full, functional capacity, isokinetic training is not a necessity for complete rehabilitation.

KINESTHETIC SENSE

Much of the success in athletic endeavors is due to the individual's ability to know without conscious effort where the various body parts are and what they are doing. This ability is necessary not only to accomplish the complicated musculoskeletal tasks necessary for sport performance but also to avoid injury or re-injury. Perhaps the function of the ankle is the best example of how this latter system operates. Under normal conditions, executing a running left turn places the right ankle in a position of almost abnormal inversion, yet the athlete is unaware of this, lacking any feedback to suggest an impending ankle sprain. A period of immobilization for, say, chronic Achilles tendinitis results in atrophy and weakness of the peroneal muscles—those prime evertors responsible for preventing inversion (lateral) ankle sprains. Attempting to execute that same running left turn under these circumstances results in a sense of apprehension and instability with regard to the ankle and may even result in an ankle sprain. Although much of this perceived instability is due to muscle weakness, strengthening the peroneal muscles will not completely solve the problem. Only the gradual resumption of increasingly sophisticated athletic tasks will dispel the sense of instability, that is, restore the kinesthetic sense of the ankle.

Restoration of the kinesthetic sense requires, first, a return of nearly normal strength and range of motion. Only then can one begin to test the injured part. With lower-extremity injuries, some degree of kinesthetic restoration can be accomplished by balancing. Merely balancing on the toes of the injured extremity is an excellent starting point, and indeed the ability to balance (for as long a time as on the uninjured extremity) is a good test of progress and a reasonable predictor of the ability to begin jogging. Once static balance is possible, more complicated balancing tasks are introduced, such as the use of a tilt or biomedical ankle platform system (BAPS) board (see Chapter 11 and Fig. 11–11). These more complex tasks require not only balance but also the ability to instantly restore disturbed balance, in a sense comparable to abruptly changing direction while running.

An added advantage in using the kinesthetic training devices is the protected environment of the physical therapy facility or training room— important if the patient is not quite ready for the balancing task. Once the athlete becomes accustomed to the exercises, they can be done at home or school. Single-plane tilt boards can be easily fashioned from a piece of ½-in. plywood and a 1- or 2-in. (diameter) dowel. Multiple boards can be made using a croquet ball cut in half and nailed to the underside of a piece of plywood.

The final stages of kinesthetic sense training can be accomplished only by a gradual resumption of athletic activities. Because the majority of athletic injuries involve the lower extremities, running, jumping, and cutting activities must be reintroduced. We have employed a simple, graduated program that is easily taught and requires no special equipment or facilities.

The athlete is first started on a rapid-walking program (almost a race-walking pace) beginning at 5 minutes per day and increasing by 1 or 2 minutes each succeeding day. When 20 minutes of rapid walking is possible without the presence of a limp, swelling, or pain, jogging is exchanged for the walking. After a brief warm-up, the athlete starts by jogging the first 3 to 5 minutes of the 20-minute period, then walking the remainder. The jogging is increased in 2- or 3-minute increments as the walking is decreased by a similar amount. Thus, jog 7 minutes, walk 13; jog 9, walk 11; and so on. The more demanding activity—running—is always done early in the activity period before fatigue sets in. Once the athlete is able to jog for 20 minutes, brief periods of sprinting can be introduced—again, early in the activity period.

When the athlete can satisfactorily jog and sprint, straight-ahead turning maneuvers are introduced. We start with the wide, sweeping turns accomplished by running figure of eights and gradually tighten the turns as outlined in Chapter 11, Ankle Injuries.

Even the successful return of the ability to do these drills will not absolutely ensure an equally successful return to full athletic participation. On the other hand, the inability to do these drills is an excellent predictor of unsuccessful return to athletic participation.

RULES

Although acute injuries differ with regard to severity, the preinjury conditioning state, the demands of the specific sport, the motivation of the athlete, and a host of other variables, a series of truisms seems to exist. We find these invaluable in patient education as a means of explaining or justifying treatment regimens.

It takes longer to get well than it did to get hurt. Any experienced athlete knows that it is far more difficult to get in shape than it is to get out of shape. This same phenomenon occurs at the level of individual muscles. As a general rule, it takes at least twice as long to recover as it does to decay. Thus if the leg is encased in plaster for a month in treatment of an ankle sprain, it requires at least 2 months of demanding and specific exercises to bring the muscles back to their preimmobilization status. Rest may be necessary for healing to occur, but care should be taken to rest only those structures that have been injured. For example, the use of a sling for an elbow injury results in deconditioning of the entire upper extremity.

Misuse is worse than disuse. In the event of a painful injury, the body is remarkably resourceful in doing what it has to in spite of some localized disability. The athlete with the residuals of a painful ankle sprain continues to ambulate, but with the entire lower extremity externally rotated, the hip abducted, the knee extended, and the ankle locked in partial plantar flexion. This new method of ambulation places unaccustomed stresses on a myriad of muscles and joints, often resulting in symptoms much more difficult to deal with than the original ankle sprain. As a rule, if the exercise—walking, running, throwing, jumping, and so on—cannot be done right, it should not be done at all.

Strength and motion are lost and gained in a parallel fashion. After an injury, some degree of splinting usually occurs. In spite of the fact that the splinting is usually the result of muscle contraction or spasm, the muscle is not working properly and progressively weakens because of the lack of normal function. Range-of-motion exercises alone, although seemingly appropriate because the lack of motion is most readily apparent, will not result in full motion of the joint because the weakened muscles are incapable of supporting the joint in a normal fashion. Thus splinting continues, no longer the result of pain, but rather in an attempt to protect the joint. Range-of-motion and strengthening programs should always be carried out concomitantly.

Athletic participation is not a substitute for rehabilitation. Resolving athletic injuries often allows return to a sport before the completion of rehabilitation. Once back in the athletic activity, athletes think they can play their way back into shape. A common example is athletes who have sustained knee injury and have been treated/rehabilitated to the point at which they can run comfortably. When it is pointed out to them that their obvious quadriceps atrophy is probably responsible for their recurrent effusions, their inevitable response is, "But isn't my running making me stronger?" Indeed it is, but neither running nor any other bilateral activity will bring the strength of the deficient quadriceps up to that of the uninjured side. A unilateral strength deficiency will respond only to a unilateral rehabilitation program.

B. SPRAINS

Sprains are injuries to ligaments.[3] The term *strained ligament* is sometimes used to describe the biomechanical circumstance of the injury, but it is really a misnomer. As a diagnostic classification, a strain is an injury to a musculo-tendinous unit.

The scheme presented here for the diagnosis and management of sprains is based on two premises: (1) that, in many joints, ligaments share with muscles the responsibilities of stabilizing those joints and (2) that ligaments prevent only abnormal joint motion.

The fact that ligaments are not the exclusive stabilizers of joints is readily evident. Consider the wide variation of joint stability, or laxity, among individuals. At one end of the spectrum are those loose-jointed individuals whose joints assume seemingly pathological positions when tested, yet they report no history of prior injury and have no complaints referable to the apparent laxity. At the other end are the "tight" individuals whose joints yield little if at all to abnormal forces. Yet, were the normally lax knee of the loose individual found on one side of an otherwise tight person, it would be interpreted as evidence of a significant injury.

Obviously something more than the static stabilizing force of ligaments is operating to allow functional stability despite widely differing degrees of laxity on examination. Carried one step further, it is our premise that the muscles and tendons acting on a joint not only have the capability of stabilizing a physiologically lax joint but are also able, in many instances, to stabilize a joint that is pathologically lax as a result of injury. This fact is abundantly documented in the references in Chapter 11, Ankle Injuries.

By definition, ligaments do not limit physiological motion. Likewise, through the range of physiological motion, ligaments are not damaged. Thus, even if injured, a ligament should not be further compromised by moving the involved joint through a normal range of motion.

Finally, one must bear in mind that the secondary effects of a ligament injury are often more troublesome to treat than the ligament injury itself. The swelling and protective muscle spasm, both of which limit motion and normal usage, lead to disuse of those very structures, primarily muscles, that will later be expected to assume greater responsibility for joint stabilization.

HISTORY

MECHANISM OF INJURY. Sprains occur as a result of a joint's being forced beyond its normal range of motion (a hyperextended knee) or forced in a plane through which little or no motion normally exists (a lateral ankle sprain). Almost by definition, any significant sprain requires some subluxation of the joint, and some sprains are the result of frank dislocations. (Although usually not viewed in this light, the management of dislocations or subluxations is nothing more than treating the ligaments that were sprained in the process.)

The abnormal forces producing the sprain can be applied quickly, as with a clipping injury in football, or slowly, as with a slow twisting fall in skiing. Although ligaments behave differently, depending on how quickly or slowly they are stretched, either mechanism can produce injury.

SYMPTOMS. Pain is the most prevalent symptom associated with a ligament injury. It is sharp in character and often well localized to the area of actual ligament damage. It may be lasting, but in more severe (grade III) sprains, it may disappear in a minute or so. Thus, with complete ligament tears, the pain may be disproportionately less than the severity of the injury. The corollary of this is often true, i.e., less severe injuries may be associated with more pain than might be expected, given the amount of damage to the ligament.

Swelling to some degree is usually present. The amount of swelling depends on the severity of the sprain (e.g., more swelling with more torn ligament fibers) and the initial management. If, for example, a sprain is initially managed with the application of heat, a substantial amount of swelling might occur, making the injury appear much worse than it actually is. Likewise, allowing the injured extremity to remain in a dependent position encourages swelling out of proportion to the severity of the injury.

Limitation of motion is often present as the result of pain and swelling. As a general rule, motion becomes more restricted with the passage of time. It is important to inquire as to the motion possible immediately after the injury, as most athletes test the joint when the initial shock of the injury has subsided. Likewise, if the physician is fortunate enough to be able to examine the joint immediately after the injury, it is important to determine exactly the extent of painless motion.

A sense of instability often accompanies the more severe sprains. The athlete often describes this as looseness, going out, or wobbling. In our experience, athletes describing any sensation that could be construed as laxity are perceiving the situation correctly and should be heeded.

The history of a *pop* or *snap* at the time of injury should also be heeded, as it often signifies a significant ligament injury.

PHYSICAL EXAMINATION

The most important part of the physical examination is determination of whether *abnormal instability* exists. The presence of swelling, tenderness, ecchymosis, or loss of motion is of only peripheral importance compared with the stability of the joint. *If the examiner is unable to competently test the integrity of the ligaments in question, the athlete should be referred for specialty care.* This is not to suggest that the nonorthopedist is incapable of adequately evaluating joint stability, as this is surely not the case. The ability to accurately assess joint stability requires a great deal of practice, and if the examiner is not utterly confident of his or her capabilities, decisions regarding ligament integrity should be left to others with more experience.

Grading of ligament injuries (Table 2–1) is based on the extent to which the integrity of the ligament has been compromised, that is, how much of it has been torn. Ligaments consist of thousands of collagen fibers aligned in a parallel fashion. When the ligament is stretched beyond its elastic limits, individual fibers fail and break, but at different locations within the ligament. Thus the ligament might lengthen because the torn fibers slide over one another, yet allow the ligament as a whole to appear intact. *Grade I* sprains result in no discernible lengthening of the ligament and thus no abnormal laxity on examination. Lengthening or partial tearing of a ligament that retains some degree of integrity distinguishes the *grade II* sprain. *Grade III* sprains are the result of total loss of integrity of the ligament, that is, a complete tear. The distinguishing factor on examination is not so much the amount of abnormal motion present but rather the absence of an *end point*—the sharp cessation of abnormal motion. Sensing the presence of the end point is much the same as pulling tight a shoelace held loosely between the hands.

The other findings on physical examination are, for the most part, a result of the bleeding and edema that occur at the site of injury. Thus, signs such as *pain, swelling, ecchymosis*, and *loss of motion* are partially the result of the extent of the ligament damage, but they are more the result of the initial management

Table 2–1. GRADING OF LIGAMENT INJURIES

Grade	Abnormal Laxity	End Point
I	Absent	Present
II	Present	Present
III	Present	Absent

of the injury. If the injury was initially managed with ice, compression, elevation, and rest, these signs may be almost totally absent even in spite of a completely torn ligament. On the other hand, if the injured part was allowed to hang dependent in a tub of warm water, the picture may be one of a significant injury regardless of its severity.

RADIOGRAPHIC EXAMINATION

Unless the ligament "failed" by avulsing one of its bony attachments, radiographs contribute little in the evaluation of sprains. Avulsion fractures occur only with complete loss of the stabilizing effect of the ligament; thus there seems little purpose in obtaining radiographs in grade I or II sprains.

Stress radiographs are frequently obtained in an attempt to evaluate the severity of sprains. To quantify the degree of instability, both ipsilateral and contralateral joints must be stressed with the same degree of force and radiographed in exactly the same plane, difficult tasks at best and virtually impossible unless undertaken personally by the examining physician. It seems to us that if one is able to "open the joint" to obtain radiographs, then it should be possible to accomplish the same maneuver in clinical testing and make any decisions on the basis of clinical evidence. Given the obvious potential inaccuracies associated with this test, we also think it inappropriate to base major treatment decisions (i.e., whether to operate) on the presence of a few millimeters or degrees of abnormal motion. More importantly, stress radiographs give no indication of the presence or absence of an end point.

In the skeletally immature, an apparent sprain may in fact be a fracture through a growth plate. Stress views, which essentially involve reproducing the injury, that is, displacing the fracture fragments, may indeed confirm the diagnosis, whereas standard views may not. However, unnecessary or repeated manipulation of the fracture may cause additional injury to the growth plate and is generally contraindicated. A decision to obtain stress views, rather than simply to treat the possible growth plate injury as such, is best left to an orthopedist. Stress radiographs may have a place in the measurement of laxity for research or medicolegal purposes.

OTHER DIAGNOSTIC TESTS

Magnetic resonance imaging may be of assistance in confirming the extent of ligamentous injury or disruption, or both, but rarely provides additional information helpful in the design of management regimens. A thorough history and physical examination usually provide all the information necessary to formulate treatment options and avoid the exceedingly high costs associated with imaging studies.

INITIAL TREATMENT

The immediate management of sprains is described in the overview. Immobilization in a splint may be necessary for the control of pain. Motion is allowed, even encouraged, if painless.

It is our current practice to start treating patients immediately with nonsteroidal anti-inflammatory medications and to continue their use through the definitive treatment phase. Grade I sprains are sometimes inordinately painful. If we can be absolutely certain that no instability exists, we sometimes place the patient on a regimen of a 6- or 8-day oral corticosteroid "burst" (e.g., prednisone 15 mg four times a day for 2 days, 10 mg four times a day for 2 days, 10 mg twice a day for 2 days, and 5 mg twice a day for 2 days). We reserve this treatment for patients we feel will follow through with the appropriate range-of-motion and strengthening exercises even in the absence of discomfort.

REFERRAL

Grade III sprains should generally be referred to an orthopedic surgeon. Many of these more severe injuries require surgical intervention—or, at least, surgical decisions, and if such is necessary, it is generally agreed that the best results are obtained if the repair is undertaken within 5 days from the time of injury.

DEFINITIVE TREATMENT

Treatment is aimed at re-establishing normal strength and motion while simultaneously protecting the injured ligament from re-injury. With few exceptions, the sooner the rehabilitative efforts are started, the less time they require. Immobilization of grade I or II sprains for longer than a few days (for the control of discomfort) only further compromises motion and promotes disuse atrophy of the involved muscles. Splinting may be necessary to carry out the activities of daily living, but the splint should be removed many times during the day in order that the appropriate exercises may be carried out.

Range-of-motion exercises should use the entire pain-free range of motion, as should strengthening exercises. Ideally, exercise periods should be followed by 20 minutes of icing. The use of compression wraps should be continued until all swelling has disappeared and the extremity is the mirror image of the contralateral side. After the initial swelling has stabilized, we have found that Tubi-Grip or similar elasticized stockinette provides sufficient compression for most joints.

General descriptions of the exercise programs are found in the overview, and specific exercises are found in the chapters dealing with individual injuries.

Our management of sprains, particularly of the grade I and II varieties, is predicated on three beliefs: (1) that ligaments limit only abnormal motion, (2) that in many joints, stability is significantly supplanted by the action of the muscles crossing those joints, and (3) that ligaments subjected to some controlled motion and tension heal stronger.

Rigid immobilization of sprains, so common in the past, was presumably undertaken to prevent motion of the torn ends of the ligament so that fibroblast proliferation (scar) occurred undisturbed, allowing the ligament to heal "tightly." Rigid immobilization also results in disuse atrophy of the muscles acting on that joint, as well as in capsular tightness and adhesions. Regardless of how tightly the ligament heals, these last two conditions must be dealt with during rehabilitation—often requiring more time than that required by ligament healing.

Any immobilization beyond 24 to 48 hours seems counterproductive, and immobilization from 1 to 3 weeks seems to make even less sense. At 3 weeks a torn ligament has virtually no more strength than it did the moment following injury. After 3 weeks of immobility, the muscles normally acting on the joint have atrophied significantly, robbing that joint of the stabilizing effects of muscle tone and action. The already-weakened joint is thus even more vulnerable to re-injury.

The essentials of treating sprains consist of protecting the ligament from abnormal stresses while maintaining strength and range of motion. Because both strength and motion are quickly lost, even short periods of immobilization necessitate regaining normal function.

Ice, compression, and rest serve an important purpose during the first 24 to 36 hours, after which local hemorrhage usually ceases and swelling stabilizes. In the more minor sprains, in which little or no swelling is evident, immobilization can be dismissed entirely. Movement through the painless range of motion should be encouraged. Unless specifically contraindicated, as with full knee extension after anterior cruciate ligament injuries, additional motion should be sought each succeeding day, so long as the increased joint excursion is not followed by increased pain or swelling.

Isometric (tightening) exercises are begun immediately. There is nearly always some position of the joint that allows painless, isometric muscle "contractions." The contractions should be held for 5 or 6 seconds and released for 2 seconds. Five contractions are repeated at least every waking hour. Once even a short arc of painless motion is present, isotonic exercises (weight lifting or Theraband) are carried out through that range of motion.

Range-of-motion and strengthening exercises should be employed in virtually every sprain, especially those involving major joints. The use of a splint or brace does not preclude the employment of these exercises. The device can easily be removed during the exercise period. The Velcro-fastening braces hold a joint securely, make removal easy, and, in most instances, obviate the need for casts. *Painless motion in the physiological planes will not compromise healing.*

Exercises should be continued until strength and motion are equal to those on the uninjured side. Gains of strength and motion occur faster early in the course of treatment. As normal values are approached, progress is much slower, and athletes should be apprised of this lest they become discouraged.

C. STRAINS

A strain is an injury to a musculotendinous unit.[3] Although this term is frequently applied to other structures, e.g., a strained ligament, such usage is confusing and should be avoided.

A strain can occur anywhere within the musculotendinous unit: in the tendon, at the musculotendinous junction, or at the bony insertion of the tendon. Some fractures might also properly be considered strains. These avulsion-type fractures are the result of a tendon and its bony attachment pulling loose from the surrounding bone. Such fractures vary from a small flake of barely visible bone, as occasionally seen with tennis elbow, to the large avulsions, many centimeters in length, seen when the hamstring origins avulse a portion of the ischial tuberosity. Because the mechanisms of injury are similar to those seen with the more classic musculotendinous injuries, their treatment employs the same general principles used for pure soft tissue problems—thus their consideration under strains.

Strains are usually thought of as the result of overstretching a muscle. Although this is sometimes the case, more often the injury occurs because the tension within the musculotendinous unit is abruptly and actively increased. This increase in tension can occur because the antagonistic muscle abruptly contracts and the injured muscle fails (tears) before it can lengthen. The increase in tension can also occur from within the muscle itself, that is, pulling itself apart because motion at the involved joint is resisted or abruptly interrupted; examples of this occur when one attempts to lift weights that are too heavy.

The concept that strains result from inappropriately managed internal tension is an important, though empirical, one. If strains are viewed as resulting only from overstretching, erroneous diagnoses will result, because in the vast majority of instances the injuries occur well within the normal, not overstretched, range of motion. In addition, if one views strains only as the result of inadequate flexibility, rehabilitative efforts will be improperly directed and inadequate.

Muscles have two active functions—to produce motion (acceleration, concentric action) and to stop motion (deceleration, isometric and eccentric actions). Tension developed in the musculotendinous unit is actually greatest during eccentric action. From a clinical standpoint, the ability to lengthen rapidly in a controlled manner is the highest order of muscle function. It requires the greatest strength and is the condition in which injuries (strains) are most likely to occur.

A second concept is that a weak muscle is a tight muscle. It makes no difference whether the weakness is primary, that is, the muscle is not strong enough to perform the task, or secondary, the result of fatigue. In either case, when the muscle is faced with a task beyond its capabilities, whether involving strength or endurance, it tightens up.

The failure to appreciate the weakness/tightness relationship is readily apparent in the sports world. Most athletes and coaches recognize that a previously injured muscle is tight; thus, rehabilitative efforts are directed toward stretching. In spite of extensive stretching, many strains become chronically recurrent, as often seen with hamstring injuries. Even though the muscle seems to have normal flexibility when tested, once used the weakened muscle fatigues, tightens, and is re-injured.

We attempt to teach these concepts to patients by telling them that strength and flexibility must be re-established together, that without strength, gains in flexibility are only transient. In the vast majority of instances, recurrences of musculotendinous injuries are the result of inadequate strength or endurance. As pointed out in Chapter 3, Overuse Injuries, the local muscle disuse that follows an injury results in rapid and profound strength loss. These losses are not as readily apparent to the athlete as are the losses in flexibility and thus are often not corrected.

Strains are graded in severity as mild, moderate, or severe. Grade I (mild) strains are generally viewed as microscopic disruptions resulting in no defect in the musculotendinous unit on physical examination. Grade II (moderate) strains involve significant but not complete disruptions of the musculotendinous unit. Grade III (severe) strains are complete disruptions (ruptures) of the musculotendinous unit. Like less severe strains, these injuries seem to occur most frequently at the musculotendinous junction in younger athletes and within the tendon itself in older individuals. Avulsion fractures occur most often in the skeletally immature in whom the tendon is attached to a growth center or traction apophysis (for example, the ischial tuberosity or tibial tuberosity).

HISTORY

MECHANISM OF INJURY. Most strains occur during forceful muscle action. An occasional exception to this rule is the strain that results from ballistic (bouncing) stretching exercises or abruptly assuming a fully stretched position such as the splits in cheerleading. The injury might occur with the initiation of an activity, such as coming out of the blocks at the beginning of a race or an abrupt effort at acceleration, or with an interruption of some motion such as momentarily losing one's footing on a slippery surface.

SYMPTOMS. Grade I strains usually occur in a nondramatic fashion. The athlete usually describes a tightening up of the muscle that occurs over three to five successive steps or motions. The onset is rarely particularly painful. The following day the athlete notes pain with stretching the involved muscle.

Grade II strains occur with a single step or motion and may be accompanied by a pop or snap. The athlete is able to tell the exact moment the injury occurred. It is initially painful and usually is quickly followed by muscle spasm (tightening up) and inability to continue the activity.

Grade III strains are dramatic, abrupt injuries that are immediately disabling, often accompanied by an audible snap or pop (frequently heard by others), and usually quite painful. After the initial burst of pain, however, the athlete may be quite comfortable. Thus from the standpoint of discomfort, the more severe injury may be initially less impressive.

Swelling usually parallels the severity of the injury and, with the more severe injuries, can be massive. Ruptures of the rectus femoris or any of the hamstring muscles may increase the girth of the thigh by 2 to 3 inches. *Ecchymosis*, although often present and even spectacular with the more severe injuries, may not appear until days after the injury. *Limitation of motion*, the result of pain, muscle spasm, or both, also usually varies with the severity of the injury.

PHYSICAL EXAMINATION

The earlier the examination is performed, the more reliably the findings reflect the severity of the injury. If the athlete is examined immediately after the injury, the defects resulting from the more severe strains are often readily palpable. Subsequent bleeding and edema often obscure this finding within hours of the injury.

Initially the area of maximal *tenderness* accurately localizes the exact site of injury. Later, bleeding, edema, and muscle spasm result in more diffuse, though no less severe, tenderness. Contracting or stretching the injured muscle generally becomes more painful during the first few hours after the more severe injuries.

The *obvious deformity* associated with ruptures of the long head of the biceps, the hamstrings, or the rectus femoris may not be readily apparent early in the course of the injury. The deformity is the result of an abnormally bulging muscle rather than a defect, and with swelling and an inability to voluntarily contract the muscle, such a misshapen configuration may not be obvious.

RADIOGRAPHIC EXAMINATION

Radiographs should be obtained with strains occurring at or near bony attachments such as those involving the thigh muscles (arising from the pelvis), the insertion of the quadriceps into the tibial tuberosity, and the insertion of the Achilles tendon into the os calcis.

OTHER DIAGNOSTIC TESTS

Magnetic resonance imaging may be of assistance in evaluating treatment options by revealing the extent of grade II strains and the exact location of grade III injuries, although, in our experience, such circumstances are rare. We do not believe that there is any indication for the routine use of imaging techniques in the management of strains.

INITIAL TREATMENT

The initial management of strains is aimed not only at preventing bleeding/ swelling, but in the case of *incomplete tears*—grade I or II strains—toward lessening the longer-term disability associated with muscle spasm. Thus, *relative rest, ice, compression, and elevation (RICE)* should be augmented, when possible, by maintaining the injured muscle in a relatively stretched position. For example, with a strain of the rectus femoris the knee should be held in flexion; with a hamstring strain, in extension.

If there is *any* evidence of complete rupture of the muscle/tendon unit, the limb should be splinted in the position of maximal comfort—usually one allowing the injured muscle to shorten. For example, an Achilles tendon rupture would be splinted with the ankle in plantar flexion.

Compression is best accomplished by placing a pad over the area of injury to provide focal pressure. Simply wrapping the limb with an elastic bandage, although better than nothing, is usually inadequate. The initial compression wrap should remain in place for at least 24 hours.

Often a substantial hematoma forms rapidly at the site of injury and one is tempted to alleviate it by aspiration. In our experience such attempts are usually futile and introduce the possibility of bacterial contamination to an ideal culture medium.

REFERRAL

Referral is indicated for grade III strains.

DEFINITIVE TREATMENT

Long-term management of strains is aimed at the *re-establishment of both strength and flexibility* of the injured muscle, tasks that must be accomplished simultaneously.

Active range-of-motion exercises are begun at 24 to 48 hours. Using the antagonistic muscles for stretching not only aids in the maintenance of their strength but also lessens the likelihood of re-injury. The injured muscle should be actively stretched to the point of discomfort and held for a minimum of 20 seconds, then released for 10 seconds. This should be repeated three to five times—or until no further motion can be obtained—at least every 2 waking hours. Like strengthening exercises, stretching is most effective when done many times during the day.

Strengthening begins with isometric exercises in the position of maximal comfort. As the range of motion increases, isotonic exercises should be instituted, as already discussed. Once sufficient strength and motion are available, functional activities should be added to the rehabilitation program. Walking with short steps or using a Nordic ski training device both require a minimum of hip, knee, and ankle motion and are effective in building the endurance component of strength. Cycling can be accomplished with little or no ankle motion (by placing the pedal back beneath the heel) but requires roughly 110 degrees of knee motion.

Formal strengthening programs, in the gym or physical therapy facility, should be carried out daily or on an alternate-day basis. Stretching should be done both before and after strengthening exercises.

Occasionally, isotonic exercises are simply too uncomfortable to be accomplished in a meaningful manner. In those instances, we have employed isokinetic devices that provide resistance in proportion to the effort applied, thus allowing some strengthening even in the sadly deficient muscle. Once a modicum of strength is present, we switch the athlete to a more traditional isotonic program. We have not been impressed with the sole use of isokinetic training as a means of re-establishing strength, although once strength is attained equal to that of the contralateral side, a few sessions of high-speed (240 degrees per second or above) isokinetic training seem to hasten the return to athletic function.

Rehabilitation of musculotendinous injuries requires patience and attention to detail. An excess of zeal can be as counterproductive as sloth. We frequently see athletes try to maintain or even to increase their conditioning by attempting feats they are unable to accomplish in anything like a near-normal fashion. For example, the athlete who attempts to run while wearing a knee immobilizer or a motion-restricting brace invites additional problems associated with the abnormal gait accompanying such activities. Although such activities are often touted as aggressive rehabilitation, it seems illogical, and even dangerous, to train one's body to do something that is patently abnormal.

D.   INITIAL ASSESSMENT AND MANAGEMENT OF SEVERE MUSCULOSKELETAL INJURIES

Life- and limb-threatening injuries, although uncommon, do occur in sports. The keys to optimal management are being prepared and attending to priorities. Of paramount importance is to have an efficient plan with priorities established for carrying out the initial assessment and management of the injured athlete. (See the overview in Chapter 7 for further discussion.)

As with multiple-system injuries, there are certain *assessment/treatment priorities* with musculoskeletal (extremity) injuries. Of highest priority (greatest urgency) are *control of hemorrhage, prevention of further injury, and restoration of blood flow to the injured limb.* Of next greatest urgency are reduction of joint dislocations, wound care (especially in the case of open fractures or dislocations), and replantation of amputated parts. Of least urgency are such things as definitive treatment of fractures; repair of tendons, ligaments, and peripheral nerves; and treatment of meniscal tears. The aphorism that a fracture is a soft tissue injury complicated by a broken bone helps keep things in proper perspective.

The examiner must beware of certain pitfalls. In the skeletally immature, for example, "just a sprain" may in fact be a physeal injury; more protection is usually required. "Just a bruise" of the arm (biceps, brachialis) or thigh (quadriceps) may lead to myositis ossificans; protection from further injury is essential. "Just a bruise" of the leg may in fact be an acute compartmental syndrome—a condition that must be diagnosed and treated urgently. A wrist sprain probably is not; carpal fracture must be ruled out by physical examination and bone scan. ("Negative x-rays" do not rule out this diagnosis.) An isolated fracture of a paired bone, e.g., radius and ulna, may not be; look for a fracture or dislocation of the other. Do not undertreat an acute shoulder subluxation; it should be treated exactly as a dislocation. Do not mistake peroneal tendon dislocation for a lateral ankle sprain—the former requires surgical treatment, the latter does not. Do not treat (gamekeeper's) thumb sprains lightly; careful examination, protection, and sometimes surgical treatment are required.

To a large extent, preventing further injury means properly *padding and splinting the injured limb before moving the patient.* The general rule, "splint 'em as they lie," applies particularly to fractures involving the spine, shoulder, elbow, wrist, and knee. With angulated long-bone fractures, however, it is usually best to straighten the limb before splinting, especially if there is any neurovascular impairment or extreme tenting of the skin. Satisfactory alignment can usually be accomplished by first applying gentle in-line traction on the limb (with an assistant providing countertraction as necessary) and then gently bringing the distal part back into its normal anatomical position. While traction is maintained, the neurovascular status of the limb is reassessed (and documented), and then the appropriate splint is applied and secured. (Injury-specific splinting techniques are summarized in Table 2–2.)

Virtually anything that provides some stability can be used as a splint. This includes adjacent body parts, rolled- or folded-up blankets, clothing, and pillows, as well as specifically designed splinting devices. The most appropriate splint depends on the specific injury and circumstances.

Air splints are ubiquitous and in the multiple-trauma situation are certainly expedient. They are used mainly for distal-extremity fractures. They do provide some compression for control of swelling and bleeding, but the pressure can vary considerably with changes in altitude and temperature, and excessive pressure can cause neurovascular impairment. In transport, they can be quite hot and uncomfortable, and they certainly do not immobilize as well as rigid splints. These drawbacks ought to preclude their use except when expediency is the paramount concern.

Military antishock trousers (MAST) are a special type of air splint. They are used to splint pelvic fractures and other lower-limb injuries and to tamponade abdominal, pelvic, and lower-limb bleeding. Any of the problems associated with air splints can occur with the use of MAST, although most

Table 2–2. IMMOBILIZATION OF SPECIFIC INJURIES

Site	Injury	Suggested Immobilization
SC joint	Dislocation or sprain	Figure-of-eight clavicle strap and sling
Clavicle	Fracture	
	Proximal and middle thirds	Sling and swath or figure-of-eight strap and sling
	Distal third	Sling and swath
AC joint	"Separation" or sprain	Sling and swath
Shoulder	Dislocation	
	Anterior	Unreduced, splint as is; postreduction, sling and swath or shoulder immobilizer
	Posterior	Sling and swath as is
Humerus	Fracture	
	Shaft	Rigid splint, sling and swath
	Supracondylar	Splint as is (or as required to restore distal blood flow)
Elbow	Fracture or dislocation	Splint as is, sling
Forearm	Fracture	Rigid splint, air splint, or pillow splint and sling
Wrist	Fracture or dislocation	Splint as is, sling
Hand	Any severe injury	Bandage and splint in intrinsic plus position (MCPs flexed, IPs extended)
Finger	Volar plate injury	Splint PIPJ in 30° of flexion
	All other	Splint in intrinsic plus position
Thumb	UCL sprain	Abduction-limiting splint or thumb spica cast
Pelvis	Fracture	MAST, spine board
Hip	Fracture	Traction splint, rigid splint, or splint to uninjured limb, and spine board
	Dislocation	Spine board and support injured limb and pillows
Femur	Fracture (shaft)	Traction splint and/or MAST
Knee	Any severe injury	Splint as is (or as required to restore distal blood flow); use knee immobilizer, Jones compression splint, or traction type splint without traction
Tibia-fibula	Fractures	Rigid splint, Jones' compression splint, traction splint with some traction, or air splint
Tendo Achillis	Grade III strain	Splint in full plantar flexion with Jones compression splint
Ankle and foot	Any severe injury	Posterior splint, Jones compression splint, air splint, or pillow splint
Toe	Fracture or dislocation	Tape to adjacent toe

Adapted from Caroline NL: Emergency Care in the Streets, 2nd ed. Boston, Little, Brown, 1983.
SC, scapuloclavicular; AC, acromioclavicular; UCL, ulnocarpal ligament; MCP, metacarpophalangeal; IP, interphalangeal; PIPJ, proximal interphalangeal joint; MAST, military antishock trousers.

versions now feature pop-off valves that limit excessive pressure build-up. Congestive heart failure/pulmonary edema can be made worse by MAST and is thus a contraindication to their use. The major problem with MAST, however, is the hypovolemic shock that can follow their abrupt removal. *No one—the physician, emergency medical technician–basic, or chief of surgery—is permitted to deflate the MAST until all the lines are in and either the vital signs have been stabilized or the patient is in the operating room.* When MAST are deflated outside the operating room, first the abdominal part, then one limb, and then the other are gradually deflated while the vital signs are continually monitored.

Rigid or semirigid splints generally provide the best immobilization of a limb. The principal caveat is that they be adequately padded. Of the several types, our personal preference is the Jones compression splint or cotton cast (see Fig. 11–6). Although not usually applicable at the scene of the accident, it is especially useful for long interfacility transports, such as from ski resort emergency room to urban hospital. It provides good comfort, uniform compression with little risk of neurovascular or cutaneous compromise, and excellent immobilization.

Traction splints are special types of rigid splints. They are particularly useful for femur fractures, which are usually associated with considerable muscle spasm. Traction is provided via an ankle hitch, and countertraction by pressure against the ischial tuberosity. Thus, ankle or pelvic injuries may limit their usefulness. However, these ubiquitous devices make fairly good splints for most lower-limb injuries, whether or not traction is required. They can be used, for example, with much, a little, or no traction for the splinting of femur, tibia-fibula, and knee fractures, respectively.

The initial treatment of most acute musculoskeletal injuries includes *rest, ice, compression, and elevation,* as discussed in the overview.

A final important aspect of initial assessment and management is the disposition. As a general rule, an orthopedic surgeon should be involved in the management of all musculoskeletal injuries for which the diagnosis or preferred treatment is uncertain, as well as in those for which surgery is clearly required.

Referral on an *emergent* basis is indicated for fractures or dislocations complicated by neurovascular impairment. It is generally indicated for unreduced dislocations, penetrating joint wounds, open or structurally significant fractures, grade III strains, and mechanical disruption of normal joint function (e.g., locked meniscal tears). With the possible exception of lateral ankle sprains, referral is also indicated whenever severe ligamentous injuries (grade III sprains) are suspected and cannot be ruled out.

REFERENCES

1. Caroline NL: Emergency Care in the Streets, 2nd ed. Boston, Little, Brown, 1983.
2. Delorme TL, Watkins AL: Progressive Resistance Exercise: Technique and Application. New York, Appleton-Century-Crofts, 1951.
3. O'Donoghue DH: Treatment of Injuries to Athletes, 4th ed. Philadelphia, WB Saunders, 1984.

3

Overuse Injuries

A. OVERVIEW

The management of overuse injuries is the most pervasive problem in sports medicine. With the possible exception of injuries from the collision sports such as hockey, wrestling, and football, overuse injuries outnumber acute, instantaneous injuries in almost every athletic activity. Overuse injuries are not instantly disabling and therefore attract less (medical) attention than those that cause an acute and obvious loss of function. As a result, the frequency with which these problems occur is almost always underestimated in surveys of athletic injuries.

The treatment of overuse injuries is made more difficult by a number of factors. Because of their insidious onset, overuse injuries are likely to be initially ignored. Thus when athletes do present themselves for treatment with these problems, the injuries are well established and more difficult to manage. Additionally, overuse injuries rarely seem serious to athletes, making it more difficult to convince them of the necessity for involved management.

Physicians' attitudes toward the athlete with an overuse problem are often inappropriate and frequently result in the athlete's being driven to seek aid at the hands of irregular practitioners. All too often the patient/athlete is told, "If you'll just stop running (or dancing or playing tennis), your knee will be OK." Athletes already know that! They sought medical care not because of the injury, but rather because they are unable to continue athletic participation. Thus, enabling a return to the athletic activity is fully as much a part of the treatment as is alleviation of the symptoms.

ETIOLOGY

Overuse injuries are almost always the result of *change*. These changes can occur in any of three general areas: the athlete, the environment, or the activities. Identification of these changes requires patience, precision in history taking, and a reasonably complete understanding of the demands associated with specific sporting activities. Delineation of these changes is made even more difficult by the fact that the changes become increasingly subtle with heightened athletic expertise.

CHANGES IN THE ATHLETE

The most common cause of overuse injuries arising from changes in the athlete is continued athletic participation despite the presence of symptoms associated with another injury. An example of this is the baseball pitcher who continues to throw even though he has symptoms of tendinitis at the elbow. Because the normal throwing motion is painful, that motion is altered and the shoulder is used in a slightly different manner. The pitcher may then seek help for the shoulder pain, as the elbow symptoms have disappeared. Success in managing the shoulder problem will be short-lived because once the previous (accustomed) method of throwing is resumed, the elbow symptoms will recur and the cycle will be repeated.

Continued participation with an existing injury also occurs as the result of inadequate rehabilitation. In this instance, the athlete has recognized the existence of the original injury and undergone treatment—albeit insufficient. All too often, because the physician is not familiar with the demands of the sport, the athlete is prematurely pronounced cured and allowed to return to full activity. Subtle alterations in muscle function may cause new and inappropriate stresses, with the result being a new injury. A common example is the loss of dorsiflexion that often accompanies an incompletely rehabilitated ankle sprain. This loss of flexibility prohibits a normal heel-to-toe running gait, resulting in the athlete's becoming a "toe runner" with subsequent additional demands and stress placed on the calf musculature. Frequently the result is Achilles tendinitis.

Not all overuse problems originating within the athlete are the result of previous injuries. Some problems arise as the result of normal physiological changes such as growth. During rapid growth spurts, musculotendinous flexibility often decreases. Continued athletic activities, especially those of a ballistic nature such as running and jumping, in spite of muscles that are temporarily too short, can produce tendinitis just as though the muscle were inflexible secondary to an unrehabilitated injury. Osgood-Schlatter disease, in reality a form of tendinitis in the growing child, is a common example of this type of overuse problem.

With the increasing popularity of "fitness activities" it is important to remember that neither athletic participation nor overuse injuries are restricted to the young and the healthy. Increasingly, seniors, including seniors with a surfeit of musculoskeletal abnormalities, are participating in a myriad of sports and fitness activities. Thus a frequent *change* in these athletes is the presence of degenerative joint disease, both idiopathic and post-traumatic. However, the presence of abnormal x-ray films does not necessarily preclude the successful management of overuse injuries.

CHANGES IN THE ENVIRONMENT

Environmental alterations can occur at two levels: the athlete's personal environment and the more global environment of the sport itself. The personal environment includes items of equipment and clothing used by the athlete. The most familiar example is footwear. Achilles tendinitis is often seen in soccer players early in the season even if the athletes have been involved in off-season running and conditioning programs. The problem arises from the fact that the soccer shoe has a flat (nonelevated) heel, as opposed to the running shoe with ½ in. of heel elevation. (This is true of almost every cleated athletic shoe.) Thus, running in the soccer shoe produces the effect of ballistically stretching the Achilles mechanism with every step, as the heel must descend ½ in. farther than it would in a running shoe, with tendinitis being the result.

Some changes in the personal environment result in more direct and obvious problems. A new, stiff figure skating boot often produces pressure over the malleoli that can result in the formation of subcutaneous bursae. Likewise, in an older, broken-in boot, the tongue often migrates laterally, lessening the protection over the medial malleolus, also resulting in bursa formation.

A common day-to-day change that occurs in the personal environment is the tension with which the shoes are laced. Lacing too tightly, for only a single day, can result in unaccustomed pressure over the dorsum of the foot and extensor tendinitis.

Examples of changes in the sport environment are much more familiar to both practitioners and athletes. The symptoms associated with patellofemoral dysfunction (chondromalacia patellae) frequently follow the introduction of running hills into a training regimen previously conducted exclusively on flat ground. Similar complaints may be the result of running the stadium steps as a conditioning drill in preseason football practice or a switch from level to hilly golf courses.

For the high-level athlete, very subtle changes in playing surfaces can result in problems. Tennis players going from clay courts to the less forgiving and more adhesive synthetic surfaces often develop patellar tendinitis. Football players have similar overuse problems when going from natural grass to synthetic fields.

CHANGES IN ATHLETIC ACTIVITIES

Activity changes can be either qualitative or quantitative. Advancing to a higher level of athletic proficiency usually involves changes in both the quality and the quantity of workouts. The gymnast advancing from level II to level I not only spends more time in workouts but also has those workouts filled with practicing increasingly difficult maneuvers, either of which can result in overuse problems. Furthermore, alterations within the workout itself can produce problems, as seen with the gymnast who develops shin splints only when spending an inordinate amount of time on vaulting. Likewise the golfer increasingly frustrated with a chronic slice may develop shoulder problems secondarily to hours spent on the driving range. (It is often helpful to point out that during 30 minutes on the driving range one can hit more drives than during 2 or more weeks of playing 18 holes daily.)

Merely increasing workout time in an abrupt manner can result in overuse injuries. The ballet dancer entering the apprentice year may not have difficulty with the new steps or maneuvers, but the addition of 2 hours of rehearsals to the usual 3 or 4 hours of dance classes can result in fibular or metatarsal stress fractures.

A relative increase in workout time is often seen in athletes attempting to perfect a single, isolated skill. Tennis players accustomed to playing 2 hours a day may develop lateral epicondylitis (tennis elbow) after spending only 30 minutes hitting backhand with a ball machine, not realizing that during that period they will hit more backhand shots than during a week of their usual playing activities.

The learning of new skills should always be viewed with suspicion when one is evaluating overuse injuries. New and more difficult, midair rotational maneuvers being learned by gymnasts often result in landing short, that is, landing in a deep squatting position because the maneuver was incomplete upon hitting the mat. This repetitive dorsiflexion is often the cause of the anterior ankle impingement seen commonly in gymnasts.

A common, yet often unappreciated change, is going on vacation. Most vacations involve some kind of heightened physical activities from simply 10 hours of walking at a theme park to "sports camps" with 4 to 6 hours of daily intensive athletic activities (for example, tennis, golf, football, or soccer camps). Rarely does anyone physically prepare for the rigors of vacations.

At this point it should be obvious that discovering the *changes* that cause overuse problems requires a level of precision in history taking rarely necessary in the diagnosis and management of acute injuries. Moreover, especially when one is dealing with high-level athletes, a thorough knowledge of the nuances associated with specific athletic activities becomes increasingly necessary lest one not know which questions to ask. Fortunately, most athletes are patient if they sense the physician is truly interested in seeking the cause of their overuse injury. The physician's role becomes one of forcing the athlete to remember and identify these changes.

PATHOPHYSIOLOGY

It is important to have an empirical understanding of the pathophysiology of overuse injuries if for no other reason than to be able to explain the mechanisms in terms the athlete can understand. Although athletes seek medical aid for the alleviation of symptoms, they must be made to understand that in the case of overuse injuries they, and not the physician, control their destiny. If they do not understand how the injury occurred in the first place, they will be unable to prevent it from happening again. *The prevention of recurrences is the most important aspect of managing overuse injuries.*

In general, overuse injuries involve bone, ligaments, or portions of musculotendinous units. Stress fractures are the result of bony overuse and are discussed in detail in the section on stress fractures. Overuse injuries involving ligaments are usually the result of nonphysiological loading of joints, as exemplified by the painful medial collateral ligament of the knee resulting from repetitive valgus stresses associated with the breast stroke in swimming. Such injuries might be viewed as multiple minisprains. Although these injuries may occur as chronic problems, they are in reality repetitive subclinical acute injuries.

The vast majority of overuse injuries involve musculotendinous units. Most athletes know what happens to a muscle that has been injured: It becomes tight and painful. The same thing occurs with unaccustomed use or overuse, but at a much more subtle level. Muscle fatigue can occur because of a relative lack of either strength or endurance. Once fatigued, the muscle tightens and, if the activity is continued, probably undergoes actual structural damage, perhaps in the form of hemorrhage or merely localized edema. These changes can occur anywhere within the musculotendinous unit, that is, at bony attachments, within the tendon, at the musculotendinous junction, or within the muscle belly. Although the location within these structures dictates how (and where) the injury occurs, the mechanism is the same, as are the methods of treatment.

The injured musculotendinous unit next fails to respond to the demands placed on it. Now injured—albeit minimally—the muscle appears to react by going into spasm and shortening. Unable to function normally, the muscle becomes weak. When the muscle is next called on to perform, its capabilities are diminished and re-injury occurs with less provocation than was required originally. The *overuse–tightness–pain–disuse–weakness–easier overuse cycle* repeats itself until broken by active intervention.

Unfortunately the athlete usually intervenes by dealing with the only obvious component of the cycle—the pain. The athlete simply stops doing the pain-producing activity and rests the muscle, adding further to the disuse and weakness. Recurrences become more easily provoked, last longer, and ultimately result in the athlete's seeking medical assistance.

B. ASSESSMENT AND MANAGEMENT

HISTORY

MECHANISM OF INJURY. The change causing the overuse problem must be found (see previous discussion). Unlike acute disorders in which one diagnoses and treats the injury, overuse injuries require that one diagnose and treat the cause.

SYMPTOMS. The major symptom in overuse injuries is *pain*. Although swelling, crepitation, loss of strength, and loss of motion may all be noted, most athletes successfully ignore these secondary symptoms so long as there is no pain.

Eliciting an admission of the presence of pain is often difficult in athletes with overuse injuries. They much prefer to describe painful sensations as tightness, aching, discomfort, cramping, or soreness. (It is as though the athlete would like to reserve the term *pain* for those easily understood, acute injuries after which it is acceptable to complain of pain.)

Establishing the *stimulus* for, and the *location* of, the pain is particularly important, as it allows one to concentrate on the involvement of specific anatomical structures. It is not enough for the athlete to say that the pain occurs while running. Rather, it must be known if it occurs with the first few steps of the run (muscle tightness), with just running uphill (specific muscle tightness), after the first 3 miles (lack of muscle endurance), or 2 hours after completing the run (muscle tightness secondary to lack of endurance, postactivity swelling, or pain associated with an early stress fracture). If the pain is initially present only to disappear after 10 or 15 minutes of the activity, it might indicate ligament or capsular swelling that disappears with motion, or muscle tightness that abates with warming up and stretching.

Pain of *increasing intensity* usually indicates injury to some portion of a musculotendinous unit that becomes tight in response to activities beyond its capabilities. Pain that is *sudden and sharp* might suggest an overuse syndrome of the impingement variety such as the anterior ankle problem seen in gymnasts.

PHYSICAL EXAMINATION

The primary purpose of the physical examination is *to define precisely the anatomical structure or structures* involved in the overuse injury. If the examiner is not intimately familiar with the anatomy of the region in question, the physical examination will be less than productive. For example, we frequently see ballet dancers who are referred for management of chronic peroneal tendinitis that has failed to respond to the usual treatments. Although the dancer does indeed complain of pain inferior and posterior to the lateral malleolus (the course of the peroneal tendons) that is worsened by plantar flexion and eversion (the action of the peroneal muscles), palpation reveals that the point of maximal tenderness is actually slightly medial to the tendons. Tenderness at this point is indicative of posterior ankle impingement secondary to an enlarged posterior process of the talus, a condition treated in a manner wholly different from that of peroneal tendinitis.

With musculotendinous injuries, the easiest way to localize the maximally painful area as well as the point of maximal tenderness is to ask the athlete to assume the position that produces the most discomfort and then to point to the painful area. This is usually a position that stretches the involved muscle, which is helpful in devising a therapeutic stretching program.

Stress fractures are usually accompanied by well-localized bony tenderness. As a rule, the tender area is less than 4 cm in diameter. This sign is easily elicited when the involved bone is subcutaneous, as with the anterior tibia, the distal fibula, or the metatarsals. Localized tenderness may not be evident in stress fractures when the involved bone is deeply embedded in muscles, as with the femur or midfibula.

Swelling, increased local temperature, and redness are usually seen only in cases of tendinitis in which the involved tendons are immediately subcutaneous, as with the tendons on the dorsum of the wrist or foot, the origin of the flexor or extensor tendons at the elbow, or the patellar tendon insertion into the tibial tuberosity.

RADIOGRAPHIC EXAMINATION

With the exception of stress fractures, radiographs are rarely of value in establishing the diagnosis of overuse injuries. Exceptions to this rule are listed in the specific anatomical chapters and include such conditions as ankle impingement in dancers and gymnasts or the underlying changes associated with degenerative joint disease.

OTHER DIAGNOSTIC TESTS

Except for radionuclide scanning (for stress fractures), other tests are usually not indicated, although a perusal of the literature concerning magnetic resonance imaging would suggest otherwise. In general we consider the performance of magnetic resonance imaging only if some potential finding *will substantially alter the treatment of the problem.* Documenting the presence of edema within an inflamed tendon or the presence of synovitis in an irritated joint, although fascinating, rarely results in a change in treatment plans. Although one cannot condemn imaging specialists for searching for fertile ground in which to implant new technologies, in all but recalcitrant cases these procedures rarely provide worthwhile information not available from a careful history and precise physical examination.

INITIAL TREATMENT

The first priority in the immediate management of overuse injuries is alleviation of the symptoms. This is accomplished by relative rest (that is, resting the injured structure and not necessarily the entire body), the use of modalities such as ice application, ultrasonography, and high-intensity galvanic stimulation, and nonsteroidal anti-inflammatory medications. The most important of these is the *avoidance of pain-producing activities*. At this point the athlete usually comes up with an (endless) list of "Can I . . . ?" questions (for example, "Can I swim?" "Can I bounce on the trampoline?" "Can I skate figures?"). The response to all of these questions is, *"If it hurts, don't do it."*

REFERRAL

Referral is usually necessary only for specific stress fractures (of the spine, femur, talus, or anterior tibia) or for recalcitrant problems that have failed to resolve with rest and a comprehensive rehabilitation program. In practice, athletes with chronic overuse problems often demand referral to an orthopedic surgeon because they are unwilling to accept the fact that there is no shortcut solution to their problems.

DEFINITIVE TREATMENT

Virtually all overuse injuries can be treated by rest followed by gradual, pain-free resumption of athletic activities. The resumption of activities will be possible only if normal strength (and flexibility if appropriate) is first regained. Formulation of the rehabilitation program thus requires that the injured structure be precisely identified. Stretching and strengthening programs are similar to those described in the individual anatomical chapters and in Chapter 2, Acute Injuries.

Treatment of overuse injuries is not complete until the cause of the original injury has been identified in order that it can be avoided in the future.

C.   STRESS FRACTURES

Stress fractures have been reported in nearly every bone in the body and are exceedingly common in both the sports and the industrial environments.[1, 2, 6–8, 12, 14, 16, 17, 20, 21, 24–27, 29–31, 34–40] Like other overuse injuries, stress fractures possess a high degree of sport specificity. The problems associated with stress fractures are twofold: making the initial diagnosis and preventing recurrence.

As altered demands are placed on bone, its structure changes to accommodate those demands. At one end of the spectrum is the astronaut who, after spending time in the weightlessness of space, returns to earth with a decrease in bone density. At the other end of the spectrum is the highly trained athlete, for example, a ballerina who performs en pointe (on her toes) and develops an obviously thickened and dense second metatarsal.

Because bone is relatively more inert than muscle, these adaptive changes require more time than the sporting activity or the athlete is willing to allow. If bone merely became stronger with increased demands, stress fractures would probably occur far less commonly than they do. What appears to happen, however, is that the newly stressed bone first weakens in preparation for becoming stronger, and if the new demands continue—or even increase, as is so often the case in sports training—during this weak period, the bone fails and microfractures occur.

Some argue that stress fractures are not fractures at all, but rather an adaptive phenomenon gone temporarily awry. They suggest that the strengthening that occurs in bone is actually the result of the healing of many microfractures—adaptive callus, perhaps—and that the pathological entity we call a stress fracture is merely a visible, localized coalescence of microfractures and callus formation.

Regardless of how one perceives this process, a stress fracture should be viewed as failure of the timely adaptation of bone to the stimulus of increased demands. Treatment consists of modulating the demands or the adaptation, or both.

HISTORY

MECHANISM OF INJURY. The mechanism is virtually always an *activity change*. The change may be obvious, as with a runner whose mileage abruptly increases from 15 to 30 miles per week, or it may be subtle, as with the figure skater attempting to learn a new jump. The change may occur in the athlete rather than in the athlete's activities. For example, a systemic illness such as a weeklong bout of the flu that precludes training may result in enough weakening of bone to produce a stress fracture when the normal training regimen is resumed.

Eliciting the mechanism of injury is very important. If the cause is not found, history will repeat itself, and the injury will recur. The essence of managing stress fractures, like all overuse injuries, is the prevention of recurrences.

SYMPTOMS. *Pain* is usually the only symptom. Early in the course of the injury, the pain is often aching in character. Athletes often describe pain in terms with which many physicians are unfamiliar, thus *a weakness* or *cramping* may actually signify pain.

Initially the pain occurs late in the course of the activity, as in the last mile of an 8-mile run. With time, the symptoms occur earlier and last longer, often continuing beyond the period of athletic activity. If ignored, the symptoms may permeate the activities of daily (nonathletic) living.

Although the symptom is pain, the presentation may be one of dysfunction, such as a limp. Athletes are accustomed to discomfort and may successfully ignore it. Dysfunction, on the other hand, results in obviously compromised performance and is heeded more readily.

Swelling, if present, occurs late in the course of the injury and is evident only if the involved bone is accessible, for example, the distal portion of the fibula, the metatarsals, or the anterior tibia. In each of these the bone is located subcutaneously and is easily palpated.

When present as a symptom, *tenderness*, like swelling, is noted only if the involved bone is readily palpable. Occasionally the athlete has only tenderness, noted, for example, at the anterior tibia when putting on a sock. This complaint should not be ignored, as it has been our observation that tenderness often precedes pain in stress fractures.

In some locations, symptoms are notoriously inaccurate as a means of localizing the site of a stress fracture. This is particularly true in a stress fracture involving the femur. Whether involving the neck or shaft, the injury may be noted as pain in the groin (adductor region), the anterior thigh, the area of the greater trochanter, or even the knee.

PHYSICAL EXAMINATION

Tenderness is often the only finding on examination. Even this is difficult to elicit if the involved bone is deeply buried in muscle, as is the femur. When present, the area of tenderness is *well circumscribed*, usually no more than 1 in. in diameter.

Pain may be elicited by stressing or springing the bone. For example, if one suspects a distal fibular stress fracture, compressing the tibia and fibula together at midshaft level might elicit pain distally at the fracture site. Longitudinal percussion, that is, striking the plantar aspect of the heel with the hand, sometimes produces pain at a tibial or fibular fracture site.

Swelling may be palpable, depending on the accessibility of the fracture site. The swelling might be firm, as when callus is present, or boggy, as with periosteal edema.

RADIOGRAPHIC EXAMINATION

Seeking radiographic evidence of the presence of stress fractures is often a study in futility. If the athlete has been symptomatic for less than 3 weeks, it is highly unlikely that radiographs will confirm the diagnosis. Indeed, regardless of the length of time the symptoms have been present, radiographs read as normal do not rule out the presence of a stress fracture. *The radiographic examination for the presence of a stress fracture is of value only if it is abnormal.*

The first sign of a stress fracture is fuzziness of the bony cortex. This is usually followed by localized thickening and increased density of the cortex. In cancellous bones such as the tarsal navicular, or in cancellous portions of long bones such as the proximal tibia, cortical changes may never be seen. The only evidence of a stress fracture in cancellous bone might be an ill-defined streak of increased density.

A fracture line may never be seen. The radiographic diagnosis of a stress fracture is based on the presence of the healing response of bone, that is, new bone formation. The exceptions to this rule usually involve cancellous bones such as the tarsal navicular. In these instances, tomography may be helpful, although it is technically difficult, since for adequate visualization, the fracture line must lie within the plane of the central beam of radiographs.

Both the neck of the femur and the anterior margin of the middle third of the tibia may exhibit a fracture line without any accompanying evidence of new bone formation. These faint, often sharply defined, black lines should be carefully sought and never ignored. Untreated stress fractures in both of these locations are prone to progress to overt, displaced fractures.

OTHER DIAGNOSTIC TESTS

Radionuclide scanning appears to offer the earliest means of obtaining objective evidence for the presence of a stress fracture.[11, 15, 18–20, 22, 23, 28, 41] Admittedly the bone scan lacks specificity; it merely delineates areas of increased metabolic activity, *healing* in this instance. However, the other conditions producing "positive scans" such as tumors and infections are rare among healthy, participating athletes.

We frequently order a bone scan as the first test after history taking and physical examination. In our experience, it is consistently more sensitive than radiographs even when the latter are obtained in multiple planes. The newer scanning techniques allow good delineation of the bone or area of bone involved, permitting discrimination of as small an area as the base of the second metatarsal.

Both *ultrasonography*[33] and various forms of *thermography* are being heralded as noninvasive means of diagnosing stress fractures. The former uses the common ultrasound treatment device to elicit pain at the site of a stress fracture; the latter uses the heat produced in localized areas of increased metabolic activity. In our experience, ultrasonography produces an unacceptable frequency of both false-negative and false-positive results. Thermography, like ultrasonography, seems of less value in the evaluation of bones well covered by muscle—those very locations that often produce the most significant diagnostic challenges.

INITIAL TREATMENT

With the exception of a few specific stress fractures (of the femur, tarsal navicular, and base of the fifth metatarsal—all discussed under those anatomical regions), initial treatment involves *discontinuation of the pain-producing activity* or activities. If the condition has progressed to the point that mere walking is painful, then non–weight-bearing crutch ambulation is indicated. On the other hand, with an early diagnosed stress fracture, only a specific activity, such as vaulting in gymnastics, may have to be discontinued.

Athletes must be told that it is their responsibility to determine which activities produce pain and then to avoid them. Invariably athletes want a list of do's and don'ts—an impossible task, as one cannot list all of the potential activities in which an athlete might engage.

REFERRAL

Stress fractures of the femoral neck, the tarsal navicular, the anterior aspect of the middle third of the tibia, and the base of the fifth metatarsal should be referred to the orthopedic surgeon (see anatomical chapters).

DEFINITIVE TREATMENT

For most common stress fractures, athletes are told that they must be *absolutely pain free for 10 consecutive days*. They are told that on retiring they must be able to say that they felt no pain that day. If they overdo and the pain recurs, the 10 days must be started again. Once the 10 days have passed, activities are gradually resumed so long as the painless state continues.

With the exceptions noted, resort to *cast immobilization is rarely necessary.* Immobilization results in disuse changes in muscle as well as bone. Reversing these changes unnecessarily prolongs the rehabilitation period. Stress fractures occur because a bone was inadequately prepared for some new demand placed on it. Total rest only increases this inadequacy.

The treatment of stress fractures employs a careful titration of activities, allowing, even encouraging, as much activity as possible so long as it is painless.

Treatment ends when athletes are able to participate fully in their activities with no pain. Completion of treatment is not based on the radiographic appearance of bone (with the exceptions noted) or the presence of a normal bone scan. Abnormalities in both of these tests will be present long after the athlete has returned to full participation in a sport.

Surgical management is usually reserved for the exceptions noted previously, particularly stress fractures involving the neck of the femur and the anterior aspect of the middle third of the tibia.

The use of externally applied, electrical bone-stimulating devices in the treatment of stress fractures has been unsuccessful in our hands but continues to have advocates. Even if an enhancement in healing were documented, in the majority of instances the use of bone stimulators would be prohibitively expensive.

D. RELATIVE REST/ALTERNATIVE TRAINING

Of the several things discussed in Chapter 1 that are different about sports medicine, perhaps the unique one is what constitutes the *end point of treatment.* Performance is the athlete's "bottom line." Anatomical reduction, wound healing, radiographic union, mechanical stability, and even complete restoration of motion and strength mean little if they do not lead to safe and effective return to sports participation.

The rest/exercise dichotomy must be viewed within this context. Although rest may be necessary to allow an injured part to heal and to protect it from further injury, it also results in detraining—taking already injured athletes further from their desired goal of returning to a sport. It follows that *more complete rest than is necessary to protect the injured part is undesirable.* Conversely, too much exercise too soon may result in further injury rather than the desired training effect. Although there may not always be a perfect correlation between pain and injury, it can reasonably be assumed that exercise or activity resulting in pain or swelling, or both, is likely to be injurious and therefore counterproductive.

To be sure, many successful athletes have at some time in their careers been able to train through pain and injury. The injured body part simply mends and gets stronger, and the pain gradually goes away, while the athletes continue to train and compete. Sooner or later, however, every athlete is likely to sustain an injury of sufficient severity that the athlete cannot just train through it. The sports physician as educator must then help the athlete unlearn the lesson of ignoring pain—the most reliable indicator that the injury threshold is being exceeded. "No pain, no gain" might better be restated as "no effort, no gain," with pain representing an upper limit to the training effort. Certainly, any pain or swelling apparent the next day should be taken as evidence that the activities of the previous day were excessive.

Often the amount of training stress required to produce successful adaptation is not much less than that which will produce further injury. As discussed previously, *relative rest* simply means avoidance of any exercise or activity that produces pain (immediate or delayed) or swelling. It is a useful clinical guide to the limitations of the kind and intensity of exercise an athlete is able to tolerate at any given time.

Alternative training is simply the opposite of relative rest. It is incumbent on the sports physician as educator and "coach" to help guide the injured athlete in ways of maintaining fitness for the sport while the injury is mending. This can be quite straightforward, assuming the physician is knowledgeable of the athlete's sport and the athlete is willing to listen to the physician. For example, the freestyler with swimmer's shoulder may be advised within the limits of relative rest to do dry land drills, to practice kicks, to swim breast stroke, and the like; the strength athlete with a painful acromioclavicular joint may be advised to substitute triceps pulldowns and limited-arc flies for bench presses; and so forth.

Most sports involve some form of weight bearing by the lower limbs, that is, standing, crouching, pivoting, walking, running, and jumping. Consequently the greatest need for alternative training is with injuries to the lower limbs that preclude such activities. There are a number of innovative approaches to this problem, e.g., wearing a life vest and running in place in a pool as an alternative for the injured runner. However, by far the most logistically feasible and commonly employed alternative exercise for most injured athletes is cycling. The remainder of this section is a discussion of some of the theoretical and practical aspects of cycling as alternative training.

CYCLING AS ALTERNATIVE TRAINING

It usually comes as quite a surprise to our injured and postoperative patients to find that they can indeed ride a bicycle or an exercycle—and get a good workout—often even before they are able to walk without crutches. For several reasons, cycling is generally much "kinder" to the body than are most other forms of exercise.

One reason for this has to do with weight bearing and impact. Cycling can properly be considered partial-weight–bearing/nonimpact exercise, as opposed to full-weight–bearing/impact exercises such as running or dancing. If some form of weight-bearing lower-limb exercise is desirable, for example, to prevent osteoporosis or to maintain fitness for running sports, the intended training can often be accomplished by cycling without risking impact-associated problems. In contrast, with a non–weight-bearing exercise such as swimming, there may be little risk of injury, but also little cross-training effect.

Individual anatomical variations, such as limb-length discrepancies and foot pronation, which often loom as problems for the weight-bearing athlete, are seldom problems for the cyclist. Shin splints, for example, the runner's ailment most clearly related to excessive foot pronation, are really unheard of in cyclists. Moreover, when anatomical problems do occur, they can almost always be rather easily accommodated by adjusting the bicycle or the rider's position on the bicycle (see later).

Another reason has to do with range of motion. Cycling does not require as much joint motion as does running or even walking. Because the pelvis is stable, little or no hip joint rotation is required. Motion at the hip joints comprises essentially flexion and extension in a comfortable midrange (30 to 80 degrees) arc of motion. Similarly, at the knee the required range of motion varies from about 20 to 30 degrees to about 110 degrees of flexion, and at the ankle, from slightly plantarflexed to very slightly dorsiflexed.[9] So whether athletes are trying to protect an arthritic hip joint, recovering from knee surgery, or rehabilitating a sprained ankle, they may very well be able to cycle pain free, even when everything else hurts.

Another reason has to do with the nature of muscular work in cycling. All of the work on a bicycle goes to producing motion (acceleration, positive work, concentric action of muscles), whereas much of the muscular work in walking, running, dancing, and similar activities goes to stopping motion (deceleration, negative work, eccentric action of muscles).[4, 9] With concentric work, less tension is developed in the muscle/tendon unit, and muscles and tendons are less likely to be injured (see Strains in Chapter 2).

Admittedly, athletes may at first be unable to get as good a workout on the exercycle as at their primary sport. However, once their muscles have adapted to the new exercise, if they work just as hard (i.e., get their heart rate up as much), just as long, and just as frequently on the bike as they did at any other endurance exercise, they will derive the same aerobic training effects. Indeed, nonelite athletes may actually be able to improve their aerobic power while recovering from an injury. Elite running athletes can at least expect to slow the rate of detraining.

Adjustment of the Bicycle

The optimal position of the cyclist on the bicycle has been the subject of much scientific and not-so-scientific discussion. In considering this topic, the first question might well be, "Optimal with respect to what?" A sprinter, for example, may be concerned about the most effective application of muscular force for propulsion of the bicycle (mechanical efficiency). A road racer may be most concerned about how to accomplish a given amount of work with the least expenditure of energy (physiological efficiency). On the other hand, an athlete recovering from an injury may mainly be concerned about not hurting a knee again. A number of studies have shown that certain parameters, such as saddle height, cleat position, crank length, and pedaling cadence, can indeed be optimized with respect to mechanical and physiological efficiency.[5, 9, 13] However, although opinions abound, there is a dearth of hard data, and there are no prospective studies that relate such parameters to injury prevention. The following discussion, therefore, mainly reflects our own clinical observations over a number of years of many injured and uninjured elite and nonelite cyclists.

We believe that the case for "pathomechanics" as the major cause of overuse injuries in cycling has been overstated. Most overuse injuries are multifactorial in origin, and in our practices, in cycling just as in most other sports, the most common causes of overuse injury are training errors and incomplete rehabilitation of prior injuries. Certainly most of the world's cyclists, whether bowlegged, knock-kneed, or flatfooted, have, without benefit of scientific fitting of their bicycles to themselves, somehow managed to avoid disabling overuse injuries.

This is not to say, however, that mechanical incompatibility between cyclist and bicycle is never a problem. Gross incompatibility can produce injury in a single ride, and the body seems to become less forgiving of even minor mechanical incompatibilities as the frequency, duration, or intensity, or all of these, of exercise increases or after an injury has occurred.

Obviously it is much easier to adjust the bicycle to fit the cyclist than for the cyclist to adapt to fit the bicycle. Individual anatomical variations must be accommodated. It should not be necessary to point out, but nevertheless it is sometimes forgotten, that not all cyclists are built the same. A case in point is one of our patients, an elite triathlete, who was told by a friend with whom she trained that she ought to lower her saddle, toe her feet in on the pedals, and keep her knees tucked in close to the frame. This seemed to have worked for her friend, a member of the United States National Cycling Team, but in our patient, the results were severely disabling patellofemoral dysfunction, iliotibial band tendinitis, Achilles tendinitis, and patellar tendinitis, the last of which ultimately required surgical intervention. It must also be remembered that a given individual's right side is not necessarily a mirror image of the left side.

It has been our observation that most of the pathomechanical injuries in cyclists seem to be the result of excessive tension on the injured structures. Thus, for example, toeing the foot in may lead to excessive internal rotation torque at the knee, excessive tension on the iliotibial band while cycling, and subsequently iliotibial band tendinitis. Conversely, toeing the foot out to relieve tension on the iliotibial band may permit the cyclist with tendinitis to continue training. These and similar observations with regard to the quadriceps mechanism, hamstring tendons, Achilles tendon, paraspinous muscles, and the like, form the basis for several of the specific recommendations discussed below and summarized in Table 3–1.

In helping cyclists to set up their bicycles, or in trying to sort out cycling-related overuse injuries, it is best to observe the cyclists either on their own bicycles on a wind trainer or rollers or on the exercycles they will be using. The cyclist is observed while stationary and while pedaling—from the front, in back, and both sides. For clinical purposes, particular attention is paid to the saddle height, fore-and-aft position of the saddle, position of the feet on the pedals, path of motion of the knees, crank length, and bicycle length. If

Table 3–1. ADJUSTING THE BICYCLE TO ACCOMMODATE INJURY: SOME GENERALIZATIONS

a. Accommodate knee problems by adjusting saddle, cleats (no-torque position), and/or cranks.
b. Accommodate quadriceps mechanism and Achilles tendon problems with higher saddle, shorter cranks.
c. Accommodate hamstring problems with lower saddle.
d. Accommodate femoral (thigh) shortening with shorter crank.
e. Accommodate tibial (leg) shortening with built-up shoe.
f. Accommodate back, neck, and shoulder girdle problems by adjusting stem and handlebars.
g. Accommodate foot and ankle problems with footwear/orthotics.

See text for specifics.

need be, adjustments are made sequentially to the saddle height, fore-and-aft position of the saddle, position of the feet on the pedals, and so on, and the effect on symptoms and on motion of the knees is observed.

SADDLE HEIGHT. *Saddle height* refers to the distance from the top of the saddle to the pedal spindle when the crank is down and in line with the seat tube. Thus, saddle height increases or decreases, respectively, as the saddle is raised or lowered or as the crank length is increased or decreased.

One formula to calculate the proper saddle height states that it should be 107% to 109% of the limb length as measured from the greater trochanter to the floor.[9] However, with respect to both efficiency and injury prevention, there is probably a considerable range (±1 to 2 cm) of anatomically correct saddle heights for a given individual.

Maximal knee extension occurs at the crank angle at which the saddle height is measured, i.e., when the crank is in line with the seat tube just before the pedal reaches bottom dead center.[5, 9, 13] Maximal knee flexion occurs at the opposite point, just before the pedal reaches top dead center. The saddle height should be such that the knee remains moderately flexed and the ankle moderately plantarflexed at the point of maximal knee extension. The saddle is clearly too low if the ankle must be dorsiflexed or if the hip must be abducted to clear top dead center, or if the ankle is dorsiflexed at the bottom of the down stroke. It is clearly too high if the pelvis rocks from side to side as the cyclist pedals (Fig. 3–1). Within these limits, the saddle may be raised to relieve tension on the quadriceps mechanism and Achilles tendon or lowered to relieve tension on the hamstrings.

FORE-AND-AFT POSITION OF THE SADDLE. For a given individual, there is also probably a considerable range of anatomically correct fore-and-aft positioning of the saddle. Within that range, relatively more forward positioning seems to facilitate spinning, whereas more aft positioning seems to facilitate pushing. However, the saddle is probably too far forward if a plumb line through the patella of the forward knee falls in front of the pedal spindle when the cranks are horizontal.

A too-low or too-far-forward position of the saddle may cause excessive knee flexion (excessive tension in the quadriceps mechanism) or excessive mediolateral "wobble" of the knee, or both. The former may result in patellar tendinitis; either may result in patellofemoral pain. Excessive dorsiflexion of the ankle may also lead to Achilles tendinitis.

A too-high or too-far-aft position of the saddle is most likely to be manifested as excessive tension in the hamstrings and hamstring tendinitis. It may also lead to patellofemoral pain, presumably on the basis of improper "tracking" of the patella.[32]

FOOT PLACEMENT ON PEDALS. It is commonly accepted that the ball of the foot should be centered over the pedal spindle. Although there is some evidence that this is not critical with regard to power output,[5] most cyclists do not want to deviate much from this norm.

The more critical factor with regard to injury prevention seems to be the amount of toe-in/toe-out motion of the foot on the pedal, which may be constrained by cleats, toe clips, or even the ridges on the soles of noncleated shoes. The extent to which the foot naturally tends to toe in or out depends, when the individual is seated, mainly on tibial torsion and the anatomy of the ankle and subtalar joints. As have other authors,[32] we have found it useful

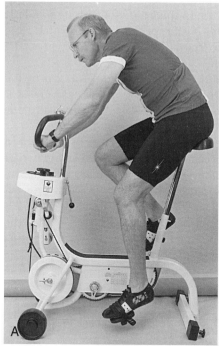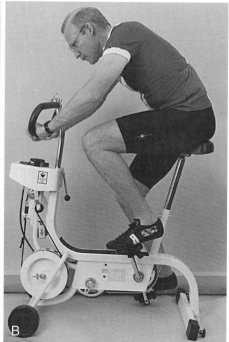

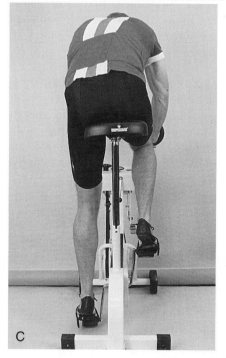

Figure 3–1. *A,* Proper saddle height. There is moderate flexion of the knee and moderate plantar flexion of the ankle at the bottom of the down stroke. *B,* Saddle too low. The ankle dorsiflexes to clear the top dead center or remains dorsiflexed at the bottom of the down stroke. *C,* Saddle too high. The pelvis rocks from side to side.

to have the cyclist sit on an examining table with the knees straight ahead (hips neither abducted nor adducted) and with the legs, feet, and ankles relaxed, and then to observe the amount of toe-in/toe-out motion present (Fig. 3–2*A*). This seems to be the best first approximation of how the feet ought to be placed on the pedals (Fig. 3–2*B*) and the position that minimizes torque at the knee.

Toeing in much more than this (Fig. 3–2*C)* increases tension on lateral structures at the knee and produces an internal rotation torque at the knee. The latter may cause the hip to be adducted and the knee to be held in valgus, and it may be manifested as excessive mediolateral wobble of the knee. Similarly, toeing out much more than this increases tension on medial structures and produces an external rotation torque at the knee. The latter may cause the hip to be abducted and the knee to be held in varus, and it may also be manifested as excessive mediolateral wobble of the knee.

It has been assumed by others and ourselves that it is desirable for the knee not to be held in too much valgus or varus and for it to move smoothly up and down in a parasagittal plane when viewed from the front.[10, 32] Certainly, much side-to-side motion of the knee (mediolateral wobble) as it moves up and down seems to be associated with increased shear forces at the patellofemoral joint and to predispose to patellofemoral dysfunction. It may be that the varus/valgus position of the knee is less critical as long as there is not much wobble. Some cyclists seem to tolerate fairly well riding with their knees tucked in close to the frame, others with their knees pointing outward. These are perhaps cyclists who are at the extremes of femoral anteversion and retroversion, respectively.

We strongly disagree with the author who contends that excessive pronation of the foot is the major cause of overuse injuries in cycling.[10] As the author himself points out, pronation is usually associated with a toe-out position of the foot. We believe that it is the failure to accommodate the toeing out, rather than the pronation per se, that is likely to cause problems. In our experience, orthoses, canted pedals, and the like are very seldom necessary or helpful in managing knee problems in cyclists.

CRANK LENGTH. As discussed previously, crank length is one of the

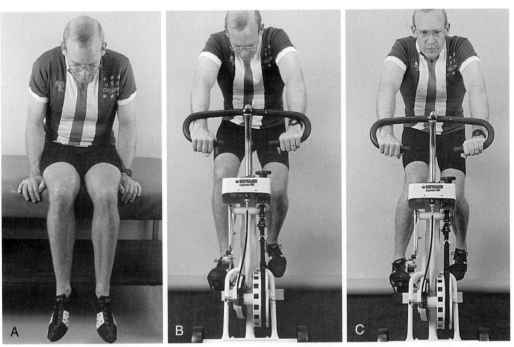

Figure 3–2. *A,* Cyclist seated looking down at relaxed feet and ankles. *B,* Same amount of toe-in/toe-out position is a first approximation of the foot on the pedal. *C,* Excessive toeing-in increases tension on lateral structures at the knee; excessive toeing-out increases tension on medial structures. Either may cause mediolateral wobble, as opposed to smooth up-and-down motion of the knee while cycling.

determinants of the saddle height measurement. For any given saddle height, the amount of both flexion and extension required at the hip, knee, and ankle joints varies directly with the crank length. This is of clinical concern mainly if there is limited joint motion, e.g., after injury or surgery.

Crank length may also be of concern if there is a right/left femoral length discrepancy, such that the range of desirable saddle heights for the right lower limb does not overlap with that of the left. Whereas tibial length discrepancies can be easily accommodated by building up the sole of the shoe, substantial femoral length discrepancies, e.g., after a femoral shaft fracture, are probably best accommodated by adjusting crank lengths.

One formula for calculating the proper crank length, based simply on the observation that average-height males seem to do well with standard 170-mm cranks, states that the crank length should be 0.185 times the limb length as measured in millimeters from the greater trochanter to the floor.[3] The length thus derived should probably be taken as the upper limit of desired crank lengths. From the perspective of injury prevention, it is probably better to have cranks that are too short rather than too long. Certainly if there is marked limitation of joint motion, the crank must not be so long as to force the joint to its limit or limits of motion.

BICYCLE LENGTH. The "length" of the bicycle with respect to the cyclist is a function of the fore-and-aft position of the saddle, the frame size (top tube length), the handlebar stem length, the type of handlebars, and the cyclist's position (upright or horizontal). The bicycle is probably too long if the cyclist's elbows must be fully extended in order to reach the handlebars. It is probably too short if the elbows are flexed more than 90 degrees and the spine is very rounded when the hands are on the bars (Fig. 3–3). In either case, there may be excessive flexion of the lumbar spine and consequently flexion-related low-back problems (see Chapter 7). If the bicycle is too long, there may also be

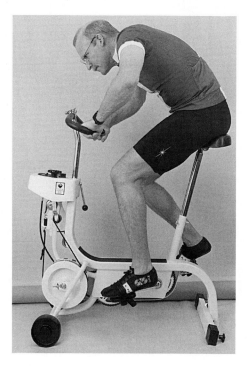

Figure 3–3. Effect of the bicycle fit on the lower back. The fit should be assessed with the cyclist in the usual riding position or positions. If the rider must fully extend the elbows to reach the handlebars, the bicycle is too long. If, as shown, the elbows are flexed more than 90 degrees, and both the thoracic and lumbar spine are quite rounded, the bicycle is too small. Either may be associated with excessive flexion of the lumbar spine and flexion-related low back pain.

excessive protraction of the shoulder girdles, excessive tension on the muscles of the upper back and neck, excessive pressure on the hands, and various related problems (see Chapter 6). Modifications of bicycle length should be made by adjusting the handlebars and stem or, if necessary, selecting another frame, and not by readjusting the fore-and-aft position of the saddle, the proper position for which is determined as described previously.

Equipment

Appropriate equipment can help prevent annoying overuse injuries as well as serious acute injuries. Even the exercyclist is well advised to use proper cycling shoes and shorts. Both cleated racing shoes and noncleated touring shoes are stiff enough to support the foot and transmit power effectively, as opposed to running shoes or sneakers that can deform when the cyclist "pushes." Also, if toe clips are used, relatively wide and bulky sneakers may preclude proper positioning of the foot on the pedal as described previously. Running shorts, sweat clothes, or anything other than clean cycling shorts are likely to cause chafing, saddle sores, and so on.

Once athletes get off the exercycle and out onto the streets or trails, they also become liable to "crash-and-burn" types of injuries, as well as to too-hot, too-cold, too-wet types of problems. A pair of cycling gloves to protect the hands is highly recommended, but clearly the essential piece of equipment is a comfortable (so the athlete will wear it) approved (so it will work) helmet. Our only patient over the past several years who suffered any head injury at all while wearing a helmet is a rider who slid out in a curve into oncoming traffic and had a van come to a stop with its front wheel against his head. In a matter of months he was well recovered and back on his bike. It is no longer true that helmets are too heavy or too hot. Indeed, when radiant heat is a problem, a light-colored, well-ventilated helmet can help keep the cyclist cooler.

Beginning or Resuming Training

It may seem overly negative to approach training for sport from the perspective of avoiding injury. However, it will be readily apparent to most injured athletes that *no lack of training is likely to impair performance more than a nagging injury.*

When starting a training program or when coming back from injury, the athlete is advised to begin with an amount of exercise that may seem ridiculously easy but that can be clearly handled. For some fitness and recreational athletes, this may be no more than 5 to 10 minutes of easy spinning every other day. The athlete gradually builds on this by first increasing the frequency, then the duration, and finally the intensity of exercise as tolerated.

As summarized in Table 3–2, we have defined three levels of training intensity for cycling. The progression is from the least strenuous (and least likely to be injurious) to the most strenuous.

Level I training is basically endurance training or easy spinning. Easy spinning implies pedaling at about 80 to 90 rpm against very little resistance. The athlete is instructed to choose the lowest resistance setting on the exercycle, or to stay in a low gear (small chain ring) and on flat roads on the bicycle. The fitness and recreational athlete is advised to work up to at least

Table 3–2. LEVELS OF TRAINING INTENSITY

Level I Training

a. Endurance training—"aerobic" power.
b. Begin 5–10 min easy spinning (i.e., little or no resistance, 80–90 rpm).
c. Increase cycling time by 5-min increments every 3–4 days, as tolerated.
d. Goal: 30–45 min continuous cycling.
e. Intensity of workouts: Use 6-sec pulse and target heart rate as guide. To work harder, pedal faster rather than against greater resistance.
f. Frequency of workouts: 30 min cycling or equivalent at least $4 \times$/wk.

Level II Training

a. Sprint training—"fast" interval training.
b. After warm-up (5–10 min continuous cycling), pedal 5 sec all-out (stay in same gear, increase rpm) every 2 min.
c. Increase repetitions, decrease rest interval as tolerated.
d. Goal: 5-sec sprint every 30 sec $\times$ 20 min.
e. Finish workout with 5–10 min easy spinning.

Level III Training

a. "Slow" interval training—"anaerobic threshold" training.
b. After warm-up (5–10 min continuous cycling), pedal 30 sec hard (increase resistance, maintain same rpm) every 5 min.
c. Decrease rest interval, increase work interval as tolerated.
d. Goal(s): 30-sec effort every 1 min, 45–60-sec effort every 2 min, etc. $\times$ 20 min.
e. Finish workout with 5–10 min easy spinning.

30 minutes of level I workouts, at least four times a week, before going on to level II workouts. The competitive cyclist is advised to advance to at least 90 minutes of level I workouts five or six times a week before adding level II workouts.

Level II training is sprint training or fast interval training. The interval workout comprises brief (5 to 15 seconds) work intervals of rapid spinning and relatively long (30 seconds to 2 minutes) rest intervals of easy spinning. Athletes should be well warmed up before starting the interval workout and should be fully recovered from one work interval to the next. During the work interval, they simply accelerate the pedaling rate without changing the resistance (i.e., without shifting gears). In a given week, athletes doing five or six cycling workouts may do two or three level II workouts and three or four level I workouts. As training progresses, they increase the repetitions and decrease the time of the rest intervals as tolerated. When they can consistently handle 20 minutes or more of 5-second sprints on the half-minute, they can advance to level III workouts.

Level III training is slow interval training. The interval workout comprises relatively long (30 to 60 seconds or more) work intervals and progressively shorter rest intervals. Athletes should be well warmed up before starting the interval workout. During the work interval, they maintain the same cadence but increase the resistance (i.e., shift to a higher gear). They should not be fully recovered from one work interval to the next and should feel rather fatigued at the end of the workout. As training progresses, they increase the repetitions, increase the time of the work intervals, and decrease the time of the rest intervals as tolerated. In a given week, they may do two level III workouts, two level II workouts, and two level I workouts. When they can consistently handle hard level III workouts, they can resume their usual event-specific training.

No matter how well conceived the training program, if the athlete breaks down, as when overuse injury occurs, the training was somehow too much or too soon. Conversely, no matter how ill-conceived, abrupt, or unscientific the training program, if the athlete holds up, who is to say that any mistake was made? Our philosophical view is, "It's a 'training error' only if the athlete doesn't get away with it." Before the fact, however, it would seem prudent to undertake training in such a manner as to minimize the risk of injury. In this respect, we believe the foregoing to be a useful, but not foolproof, guide for training on a bicycle or exercycle.

REFERENCES

1. Brahms MA et al: A typical stress fracture of tibia in professional athlete. Am J Sports Med 8:131–132, 1980.
2. Butler JE et al: Subtrochanteric stress fractures in runners. Am J Sports Med 10:228–232, 1982.
3. Buttars KR: Crank length and gearing. Bicycling 23:26–37, 1982.
4. Cavanagh PR: They stumble that run fast. Presented at American College of Sports Medicine Annual Meeting. Las Vegas, Nev, May 1987.
5. Cavanagh PR, Sanderson DJ: The biomechanics of cycling: Studies of the pedaling mechanics of elite pursuit riders. In Burke ER (ed): The Science of Cycling. Chicago, Human Kinetics, 1986.
6. Daffner RH et al: Stress fractures of the proximal tibia in runners. Radiology 142:63–65, 1982.
7. Delee JC et al: Stress fracture of fifth metatarsal. Am J Sports Med 11:349–353, 1983.
8. Drez D Jr et al: Metatarsal stress fractures. Am J Sports Med 8:123–125, 1980.
9. Faria IE, Cavanagh PR: The Physiology and Biomechanics of Cycling. New York, John Wiley, 1978.
10. Francis PR: Injury prevention for cyclists: A biomechanical approach. In Burke ER (ed): The Science of Cycling. Chicago, Human Kinetics, 1986.
11. Grahame R et al: Use of scintigraphy in the diagnosis and management of traumatic foot lesions in ballet dancers. Rheumatol Rehabil 18:235–238, 1979.
12. Greaney RB et al: Distribution and natural history of stress fractures in US Marine recruits. Radiology 146:339–346, 1983.
13. Gregor RJ, Rugg SG: Effects of saddle height and cadence on power output and efficiency. In Burke ER (ed): The Science of Cycling. Chicago, Human Kinetics, 1986.
14. Hamilton HK: Stress fracture of the diaphysis of the ulna in a body builder. Am J Sports Med 12:405–406, 1984.
15. Holder LE, Michael RH: The specific scintigraphic pattern of "shin splints in the lower leg": Concise communication. J Nucl Med 25:865–869, 1984.
16. Kaltsas D-S: Stress fracture of the femoral neck in young adults: Report of 7 cases. J Bone Joint Surg Br 63:33–37, 1982.
17. Lombardo SJ, Benson DW: Stress fractures of the femur in runners. Am J Sports Med 10:219–227, 1982.
18. Martire JR: The role of nuclear medicine bone scans in evaluating pain in athletic injuries. Clin Sports Med 6:713–737, 1987.
19. Marymont JH Jr et al: Fracture of the lateral cuneiform bone in the absence of severe direct trauma: Diagnosis by radionuclide bone scan. Am J Sports Med 8:135–136, 1980.
20. Meurman KOA: Stress fracture of the pubic arch in military recruits. Br J Radiol 53:521–524, 1980.
21. Meurman KOA: Stress lesions of the talus. Fortschr Geb Roentgenstr Nuklearmed 132:469–471, 1980.
22. Meurman KOA, Elfving S: Stress fracture in soldiers—A multifocal bone disorder: Comparative radiologic and scintigraphic study. Radiology 134:483–487, 1980.
23. Milgrom C et al: Negative bone scans in impending tibial stress fractures: Report of three cases. Am J Sports Med 12:488–491, 1984.
24. Mubarak SJ et al: The medial tibial stress syndrome: A cause of shin splints. Am J Sports Med 10:201–205, 1982.
25. Mutoh Y et al: Stress fractures of the fibula due to so-called rabbit jump. Orthop Trauma Surg 23:332–338, 1980.
26. Mutoh Y et al: Stress fractures of the ulna in athletes. Am J Sports Med 10:365–367, 1982.
27. Noakes TD et al: Pelvic stress fractures in long distance runners. Am J Sports Med 13:120–123, 1985.
28. Norfray JF et al: Early confirmation of stress fracture in joggers. JAMA 243:1647–1649, 1980.
29. Orava S et al: Stress fractures caused by physical exercise. Acta Orthop Scand 49:19–27, 1978.
30. Pavlov H et al: Stress fractures of pubic ramus. Report of 12 cases. J Bone Joint Surg Am 64:1020–1025, 1982.
31. Pavlov H et al: Tarsal navicular stress fractures: Radiographic evaluation. Radiology 148:641–645, 1983.

32. Pruitt AL: The cyclist's knee: Anatomical and biomechanical considerations. *In* Burke ER, Newsom MM (eds): Medical and Scientific Aspects of Cycling. Chicago, Human Kinetics, 1988.
33. Ridgway GL et al: Ultrasonic assessment of stress fractures. BMJ 286:1479–1480, 1983.
34. Roy S et al: Stress changes of distal radial epiphysis in young gymnasts: A report of 21 cases and review of the literature. Am J Sports Med 13:301–308, 1985.
35. Sacchetti AD et al: Rebound rib: Stress-induced first rib fracture. Ann Emerg Med 12:177–179, 1983.
36. Saunders AJS et al: Stress lesions of the lower leg and foot. Clin Radiol 30:649–651, 1979.
37. Skinner HB, Cook SD: Fatigue failure stress of femoral neck: A case report. Am J Sports Med 10:245–247, 1982.
38. Symeonides PP: High stress fractures of the fibula. J Bone Joint Surg Br 62:192–193, 1980.
39. Torg JS et al: Stress fractures of the tarsal navicular: Retrospective review of 21 cases. J Bone Joint Surg Am 64:700–712, 1982.
40. Van Hal ME et al: Stress fractures of the great toe sesamoids. Am J Sports Med 10:122–128, 1982.
41. Vazelle F et al: Athlete's pubic pain syndrome or "pubialgia": Comparison of radiographic and scintigraphic findings. J Radiol 63:423–428, 1982.

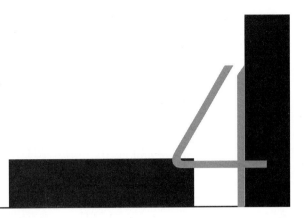

Shoulder Girdle Injuries

Conditions to Be Referred

- Fractures of the acromion, distal clavicle (lateral-to-coracoclavicular ligaments), scapula, or proximal humerus
- Sternoclavicular sprains (and dislocations)
- Grades III to VI acromioclavicular sprains ("shoulder separation")
- Acute, traumatic glenohumeral dislocation, unreduced or complicated by fracture, cuff tear, or nerve injury
- Acute or acute-on-degenerative tears of the rotator cuff
- Acute or acute-on-degenerative tears of the tendon of the long head of the biceps
- Brachioplexitis
- Activity-related pain attributable to primary impingement and unresponsive to activity modification
- Activity-related pain attributable to secondary impingement and unresponsive to rehabilitation
- Activity-related pain of uncertain cause
- Chronic/recurrent frank glenohumeral instability (dislocation, subluxation)

Triage

Indications for Referral

◆ **Acute**

History

Upper-limb neurological symptoms

Abrupt onset of profound weakness

Examination

Deformity (sternoclavicular, clavicular, acromioclavicular, shoulder, arm)

Inability to initiate shoulder abduction

Loss of shoulder rotation

X-ray films

Any fracture but medial and proximal clavicle

◆ **Overuse**

History

Recurrent frank instability

Pain localized to acromioclavicular joint with horizontal flexion activities

Pain localized to lateral arm with overhand activities

X-ray films

Acromioclavicular or glenohumeral arthrosis

"High-riding" humeral head

Indications for X-Ray Films

◆ **Acute**

"Trauma series" indicated for all acute injuries

◆ **Overuse**

"Standard series" indicated for virtually all chronic, recurrent conditions

---

Injuries to the shoulder girdle (sternoclavicular, acromioclavicular, glenohumeral, and scapulothoracic joints and associated structures) account for perhaps no more than 5% to 10% of all sports injuries,[20] but they account for a disproportionately higher percentage of sports injury–related physician visits. That is, these injuries are generally perceived by athletes to be "serious" or disabling, or both, and thus requiring medical attention.

In this chapter, we first discuss an approach to diagnosis and triage based on the typical clinical presentation. We then discuss the specific techniques of sorting out the presenting problem, namely, the problem-oriented history and physical examination, injection techniques, and diagnostic imaging.

A complete discussion of shoulder rehabilitation techniques is beyond the scope of the chapter. For the important, common problems of shoulder dislocation/subluxation and shoulder overuse syndrome, we discuss functional rehabilitation in some detail, including treatment objectives, overall strategy, and specific techniques (parts G and M).

In the usual format we discuss separately sternoclavicular sprains (and dislocations); fractures of the proximal and middle thirds of the clavicle; acromioclavicular sprains; acute, traumatic anterior glenohumeral dislocation; acute, traumatic anterior glenohumeral subluxation; acute, traumatic posterior glenohumeral subluxation; acute or acute-on-degenerative tears of the rotator cuff; acute or acute-on-degenerative tears of the tendon of the long head of the biceps; acromioclavicular degenerative joint disease; the shoulder overuse syndrome (including scapular-stabilizing muscle, glenohumeral capsular, rotator cuff, and impingement problems); osteochondrosis of the proximal humeral epiphysis ("Little Leaguer's shoulder"); and traumatic exostosis of the humerus ("blocker's nodule").

A. PROBLEM-ORIENTED APPROACH TO DIAGNOSIS AND TRIAGE

Shoulder problems in athletes characteristically present in one or more of the following ways:

Acute injury or the immediate sequelae of acute injury
Acute painful episode
Weakness
Loss of motion
Chronic, activity-related pain/disability (overuse injury)
Chronic/recurrent frank instability (dislocation/subluxation)

This section gives an overview of our basic approach to these problems with emphasis on diagnostic and therapeutic pitfalls to avoid and when consultation/referral is appropriate. The discrete diagnostic entities mentioned are discussed in greater detail in subsequent sections.

ACUTE INJURY OR THE IMMEDIATE SEQUELAE OF ACUTE INJURY

"I hurt my shoulder in the game last night." "I hurt my shoulder when I fell 3 weeks ago. The pain has gotten some better, but I still can't . . . ."
Acute shoulder injuries, including contusions, sprains, strains, fractures, and dislocations, are especially common in football, skiing, and wrestling. Some of these injuries, e.g., anterior glenohumeral dislocation, are clinically obvious. Others, e.g., posterior glenohumeral dislocation, are liable to be misdiagnosed even after radiographic examination. Most, at least on the first round, do not require operative treatment, and some aspects of nonoperative treatment are common to all.

Injuries to the clavicle and its articulations may be considered "occupational risks" of participation in those sports in which falls sometimes occur at considerable speeds or from considerable heights onto unyielding surfaces. Bicycling, horseback riding, rock climbing, and skateboarding are notable examples. Clavicular injuries are also relatively common in those sports in which "piling on" sometimes occurs, especially in sandlot football that lacks both referees and shoulder pads. The functional and clinical significance of these injuries is twofold. First, the use of the upper limb in sports is, at least temporarily, impaired. Second, associated injuries to the airway or great vessels, or both, although rare, can be life threatening.

Of primary importance is the establishment of a precise diagnosis. Appropriate initial treatment, indications for referral, definitive treatment, and rehabilitative treatment logically follow. The differential diagnosis of concern includes

Fractures of the acromion, clavicle, scapula, and proximal humerus
Sternoclavicular sprains (and dislocations)
Acromioclavicular sprains ("shoulder separation")
Acute, traumatic glenohumeral dislocation/subluxation
Acute or acute-on-degenerative tears of the rotator cuff
Acute or acute-on-degenerative tears of the tendon of the long head of the biceps

For the most part, given careful clinical assessment and appropriate radiographic examination, diagnosis is straightforward (Fig. 4–1). *The diagnostic pitfalls of greatest consequence are failure to recognize initial acute, traumatic glenohumeral subluxation; extensive rotator cuff tear; and posterior glenohumeral dislocation.*

The first, even the first few, occurrences of glenohumeral subluxation are liable to be dismissed by athletes, their coaches, and often their physicians as inconsequential. Once a pattern of recurrent subluxation has been established, however, the chance of success with nonoperative treatment is considerably diminished. Accordingly, *any shoulder injury in which there is a history of a forced abduction external rotation mechanism of injury, perceived frank instability, or "dead arm" symptoms should be considered as probable acute anterior glenohumeral subluxation and treated accordingly.*

Isolated acute rotator cuff tears with the classic presentation of profound weakness following abrupt forceful loading of the shoulder is unlikely to be missed. However, rotator cuff tear associated with other injuries is liable to be overlooked. For example, weakness following acute anterior glenohumeral dislocation may be the result of pain inhibition of normal muscle function, associated axillary nerve neurapraxia, or associated rotator cuff tear, or all of these. It is most important to maintain a high index of suspicion. The differential diagnosis of profound weakness is discussed later.

Posterior glenohumeral dislocation is liable to be missed because it is rare and because the anteroposterior (AP) radiographic findings are subtle.

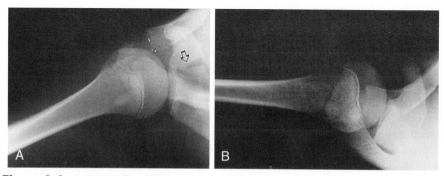

Figure 4–1. Axillary radiographs of a 15-year-old hockey player who sustained a direct blow to the anterior aspect of the right shoulder. The importance of clinical correlation and, in skeletally immature patients, comparison views is well demonstrated. Point tenderness was well localized to the coracoid. The initial "shoulder series" radiographs *(A)* were interpreted by the radiologist as suggestive of acromioclavicular injury, and stress views were recommended. However, correlating precisely with the clinical findings, a fracture of the base of the coracoid (arrow) was demonstrated on the axillary view. That the acromioclavicular "widening" was attributable to incomplete ossification and that the coracoid fracture was not simply an open physis were confirmed by subsequent comparison views of the uninjured left shoulder *(B).*

The hallmark physical finding is that the arm is held adducted and internally rotated, and any attempt to rotate the shoulder externally is painfully resisted. The lateral scapular radiograph is diagnostic (see Fig. 4–20).

A common, but less consequential, diagnostic pitfall is underestimating the severity of the acromioclavicular sprains ("shoulder separations"). The classic "high-riding clavicle" deformity of grade III sprains is typically most obvious subacutely, after any hematoma, soft tissue swelling, and muscle spasm associated with the acute injury have subsided. Because we treat grades I through III acromioclavicular sprains the same, we do not believe precise initial gradation of the injury is critical. However, the physician who has authoritatively reassured the athlete that there is only a low-grade acromioclavicular sprain, only to have the athlete become aware of a pronounced deformity a couple of weeks later, will have (deservedly) suffered some loss of credibility.

The examining physician should also be aware that in the skeletally immature, physeal fractures of the acromion or distal clavicle may be difficult to differentiate from acromioclavicular sprain. However, they can generally be treated similarly.

By far, the therapeutic pitfall of greatest consequence is undertreatment of initial acute, traumatic glenohumeral dislocation and subluxation. Many first-time anterior dislocations and subluxations can be definitively treated by nonoperative means, specifically immobilization (i.e., strict limitation of abduction and external rotation) and subsequent complete shoulder rehabilitation. It is important to appreciate that rigorous nonoperative treatment does not equate with symptomatic treatment. The clinical outcomes of mere symptomatic treatment of acute shoulder dislocation are abysmal, with a recurrence rate of up to 90% in young male athletes. In contrast, with appropriate protective/rehabilitative treatment, the probability of success can be essentially reversed, with a 60% to 70% or better nonrecurrence rate. *The essential therapeutic task is to convince athletes that their only good chance of success with nonoperative treatment is to comply strictly with the treatment protocol.* The primary treating physician is *critically* important in initiating this intervention.

Displaced fractures, intra-articular fractures, unreduced glenohumeral dislocations, suspected extensive tears of the rotator cuff, and musculoskeletal injuries with associated neurovascular injury are relatively common, unambiguous indications for orthopedic referral. The rare grade IV, V, or VI acromioclavicular injuries are also indications for orthopedic referral.

Referral to an appropriate facility on an emergent basis is indicated for fractures or dislocations complicated by vascular impairment. On a less urgent basis, orthopedic consultation/referral is also recommended for dislocations complicated by nerve injury. Although most such injuries appear to be neurapraxias and surgical exploration is generally not indicated, rehabilitation is more complicated, and it is prudent in these cases to defer management to the specialist.

Nondisplaced fractures, grade III acromioclavicular sprains, and tears of the tendon of the long head of the biceps are possible indications for orthopedic referral.

Some primary care physicians may choose to manage some shoulder fractures themselves. Fractures of the proximal humerus with a less than 1-cm displacement of any fragment, a less than 45-degree angulation of any fragment, and a less than 20% impression defect of the articular surface are amenable to nonoperative treatment.[38] Extra-articular scapular fractures are treated nonoperatively, as are minimally or nondisplaced fractures of the distal clavicle. Fractures not meeting these criteria should be referred to an orthopedist.

Fractures of the greater tuberosity of the humerus are frequently associated with anterior dislocations and are usually anatomically reduced when the dislocation is reduced. If they remain more than 1 cm displaced after reduction of the dislocation, orthopedic referral is indicated.[35, 38]

Fractures of the distal clavicle are managed differently from the more common midshaft fractures. The use of a figure-of-eight clavicle strap is relatively contraindicated; it would tend to displace, not to reduce, the fracture. Referral to an orthopedist is generally appropriate.

The management of grade III acromioclavicular sprains is as controversial as any topic in sports medicine. We agree with those authors[23, 28, 40] who recommend nonoperative treatment. Nevertheless we believe that the athlete with acromioclavicular injury should be informed of the possible sequelae of the injury (deformity, degenerative joint disease) and the options regarding primary or delayed surgical treatment. Athletes should be referred if they are unwilling to accept the cosmetic deformity of an overly prominent distal clavicle or if they are unwilling to "allow the shoulder to recover from the acute injury and then see if it still hurts."

As always, for acute injuries in which the precise diagnosis is uncertain after initial evaluation, consultation or referral is indicated.

ACUTE PAINFUL EPISODE

"I woke up in the middle of the night with my shoulder hurting. Since then it's just gotten worse. I can't raise my arm, do my work, sleep . . . ."

Acute, atraumatic shoulder pain is a common presenting symptom in both the general and the athletically active population. In general, intrinsic musculoskeletal causes can be readily differentiated from extrinsic causes (referred pain) on the basis of the shoulder position relatedness and activity relatedness of the pain and confirmatory physical examination findings. The differential diagnosis of usual greatest concern includes

Rotator cuff overuse strain/tendinitis
Calcific subacromial bursitis/rotator cuff tendinitis
Brachioplexitis

In the appropriate clinical settings, inflammatory or septic acromioclavicular or glenohumeral arthritis should also be considered.

"Acute overuse injury" seems to be an oxymoron. Semantics notwithstanding, episodes of acute, quite severe shoulder pain following unaccustomed shoulder-strenuous activity are common. This is especially true for "weekend warriors" and sedentary adults undertaking "honey do" projects. Youth, however, is not immune. Such problems are not uncommon in school-age athletes starting new sports seasons—especially in swimming, baseball, and volleyball.

The common historical finding is an abrupt, marked change in the type, amount, or intensity of shoulder-strenuous work, for instance, an egregious "training error." Symptoms, tenderness, and pain with provocative tests may be moderate to severe. With rest (sling p.r.n.), intermittent icing, and nonsteroidal anti-inflammatory medication, pain usually subsides within a few days.

Narcotics or intra-articular corticosteroids are usually not required. The key to the prevention of recurrence is recognition and avoidance of the training error.

Calcific subacromial bursitis or rotator cuff tendinitis may be idiopathic or associated with "acute overuse" as described previously. The heterotopic precipitation of calcium in soft tissues may be both a cause and an effect of the inflammation. The associated pain is characteristically severe. Patients not uncommonly present in tears, having been unable to sleep or raise the affected arms, and with "touch-me-not" tenderness on examination. Radiographic examination is confirmatory (Fig. 4–2). Nonsteroidal anti-inflammatory medication is usually insufficient for pain relief, and corticosteroid injection is generally indicated. We have found that for most acute cases, injection followed by a series of pulsed ultrasound treatments in physical therapy affords definitive treatment. We have been singularly unimpressed by attempting to aspirate the precipitate, which is of the consistency of Elmer's glue. For recalcitrant cases with persistent pain, we recommend referral for surgical débridement.

Brachioplexitis is a less common cause of severe shoulder pain and profound shoulder weakness. There may or may not be a history of "acute overuse" or of an antecedent acute febrile (viral) illness. Pain is usually the initial presenting symptom. It will not respond well to a trial of rest, intermittent icing, and nonsteroidal anti-inflammatory medication. Typically the pain worsens over time before abating. It can be unrelenting and very severe for many days. Narcotic analgesics are usually indicated, and sometimes even these may not be completely pain relieving. As discussed in the next section (Weakness), consultation/referral is probably indicated.

WEAKNESS

"I can't bench [press] anymore." "I can't even lift my arm up."

Weakness is seldom the only presenting symptom, usually being associated with acute injury or acute or chronic pain conditions. Nonetheless, it is often the symptom that is most disconcerting to the patients, prompting them to seek medical attention, and it is frequently the finding of greatest concern to the examining physician.

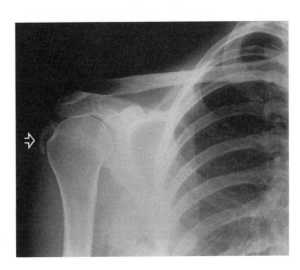

Figure 4–2. Anteroposterior (AP) radiograph of the shoulder demonstrating heterotopic soft tissue calcification (arrow) in the subacromial bursa/rotator cuff tendon.

The differential diagnosis of profound weakness includes

Mechanical musculotendinous disruption
Neuromuscular weakness
Pain inhibition of normal muscle function

To some extent these can be differentiated on physical examination. Smooth giving-way on manual muscle testing, i.e., uniform weakness throughout the range of motion, is characteristic of neuromuscular weakness. In contrast, abrupt or ratchet-like (cogwheel) giving-way is more characteristic of mechanical musculotendinous disruption or pain inhibition.

Differentiation is more reliably accomplished by selective local anesthetization as discussed in Injection/Aspiration in part B. Possible results are as follows. Relief of pain but persistence of profound weakness after intra-articular injection indicates mechanical musculotendinous disruption. Pain relief and improved strength does not rule out intra-articular structural injury, e.g., labral tear, but does effectively rule out an extensive full-thickness rotator cuff tear. Neither pain relief nor improved strength, assuming technically satisfactory injection, indicates an extra-articular problem such as brachioplexitis.

Other causes of weakness include moderate weakness attributable to handedness or muscular disuse atrophy; transient weakness ("dead arm syndrome") associated with brachial plexus traction or compression injuries ("stingers") or acute glenohumeral subluxation; and nonphysiological weakness.

Orthopedic referral is indicated if extensive rotator cuff tear is suspected or cannot be ruled out as the cause of the weakness. Further work-up will likely include magnetic resonance imaging (MRI) arthrography, but a decision to obtain this study is best made in consultation with or is deferred to the orthopedic surgeon.

Specialty (orthopedic or neurological) referral is also recommended for profound weakness, probably attributable to brachioplexitis. Early on, there is severe pain and weakness on the basis of pain inhibition. Subsequently, as the acute, severe pain begins to subside, a profound, neuromuscular weakness becomes evident. Treatment options are actually quite limited. Nonetheless, these conditions are typically very distressing to the patient and even more so to the parents if the patient is a child. Reassurance that "everything possible is being done" is usually appropriate. Further work-up, for both confirmatory diagnostic and prognostic purposes, may include electromyography, usually at about 6 weeks after the onset of symptoms.

LOSS OF MOTION

"I can't reach . . . ." "I can't hook my bra."
Because of compensatory scapulothoracic motion, loss of glenohumeral motion ("frozen shoulder") is generally unnoticed by patients until it gets to the point of limiting customary daily, occupational, or athletic activities. It is virtually always a sequela of constrained active motion—secondary to injury, neuromuscular weakness, pain, inflammation, or prescribed treatment (e.g., immobilization for glenohumeral dislocation). Accordingly, the most important diagnostic and therapeutic challenge is to determine and to address the primary underlying problem or problems.

The mainstays of treating "frozen shoulder" per se are physical therapy (mobilization treatment) and often intra-articular corticosteroid injection (to mute any counterproductive inflammatory response to the mobilization therapy). We do not recommend manipulation of the shoulder under anesthesia, a possible result of which is the creation of a soft tissue Bankart lesion (see the discussions of glenohumeral instability problems).

CHRONIC, ACTIVITY-RELATED PAIN/DISABILITY (OVERUSE INJURY)

"My shoulder's hurt ever since the start of '2-a-days.' " " "It hurts to serve or spike." "I don't even try to bench press or overhead press anymore, because it always hurts afterward." "I can't put anything on the ball now when I throw."

Chronic shoulder pain is a very common clinical problem in both general and athletically active populations. In general, intrinsic, mechanical, musculoskeletal problems (i.e., overuse injuries) can be readily differentiated from other intrinsic and extrinsic causes of shoulder pain on the basis of the history (especially the shoulder position relatedness and activity relatedness of the pain) and confirmatory physical examination findings. Overuse injuries are especially common in baseball, gymnastics, swimming, tennis, volleyball, and weight training, as well as in occupations requiring strenuous or prolonged overhead use of the hand.

As is generally true for overuse injuries, especially early in the course of the problem, activity-related pain is more likely to be noted after rather than during the activity. "Soreness," "stiffness," and difficulty robing and disrobing the day after the provoking activity are common complaints. Also, delayed soreness and overall patterns of pain are more important guidelines for treating and resuming activity than are the odd twinges of pain during activity.

Sometimes, functional impairment, rather than frank pain, is the primary symptom. For example, a coach may notice that a player is "serving funny," or a thrower may notice a loss of accuracy or velocity in throws.

Shoulder overuse injuries represent maladaptations to the repetitive stresses of an activity or activities. Typically there are both structural and functional components of the problem, and also typically more than one structural or functional mechanism is involved. Conversely, simple "isolated" bursitis, tendinitis, or "impingement" problems are uncommon. In all cases, therefore, the examiner should assess each of the following possible components of the problem:

Scapular-stabilizing muscle insufficiency/dysfunction
(Structural) glenohumeral laxity (commonly, anterior laxity/posterior contracture)
Rotator cuff overuse strain, tendinitis, tendinosis, degenerative tear, insufficiency (functional glenohumeral laxity)
Long head of biceps overuse strain, tendinitis, tendinosis, degenerative tear, tendon subluxation, insufficiency
Acromioclavicular degenerative joint disease/distal clavicular osteolysis
Primary impingement (acromial, acromioclavicular, coracoclavicular, coracoid)

Secondary impingement (anterior, posterior, and lateral; secondary to glenohumeral laxity/contracture or rotator cuff insufficiency)
Glenohumeral degenerative joint disease/"cuff arthropathy"

Less severe, shorter-duration problems may respond to basic intervention
comprising relative rest, anti-inflammatory measures, "home program" rehabilitation exercises, and gradual resumption of activity avoiding training
errors. However, unless the patient has the luxury of avoiding the pain-
provoking activity altogether, anti-inflammatory treatment alone, e.g., the
ubiquitous "cortisone shot," will likely prove insufficient. As is true for all
overuse injuries that do not resolve promptly and completely with basic
intervention, *the essential therapeutic task is to identify and to reverse as many of
the causative factors as possible.*

In most cases, patients do not present promptly after the onset of symptoms, but rather after symptoms and function have worsened over time.
During this time, secondary problems (failed compensatory mechanisms) are
likely to have developed. In virtually all such cases, intensive hands-on
physical therapy is necessary for successful resolution of the problem and
return to shoulder-strenuous activity.

Structural injury does not necessarily imply a need for surgical intervention. Depending on the severity of the structural injury and the demands to
be placed on the shoulder, many structural problems (e.g., partial-thickness
and small full-thickness rotator cuff tears) can be well compensated if appropriate functional rehabilitation is carried out.

Physician follow-up is essential and should be scheduled every 3 weeks
or so. Sports medicine/orthopedics consultation/referral is indicated for problems not demonstrably improving over time. Some structural problems, e.g.,
acromioclavicular arthrosis, primary impingement, rotator cuff tear, labral
tears, glenohumeral laxity, glenohumeral arthrosis, and intra-articular osteochondral loose bodies may require surgical intervention. Special diagnostic
imaging, e.g., MRI arthrography, may be required but may be deferred at the
consultant's discretion. Complex problems, e.g., rotator cuff tear associated
with glenohumeral instability, are probably best managed by orthopedic surgeons subspecializing in shoulder problems.

CHRONIC/RECURRENT FRANK INSTABILITY
(DISLOCATION/SUBLUXATION)

*"My shoulder went out again." "Sometimes it seems to go out of place, and I can't
use the arm. Then I shake it or something, and it seems OK again."*

Recurrent shoulder dislocations and subluxations may be attributable to
congenital or acquired joint laxity or simply to being again in the wrong place
at the wrong time. Of these, acquired laxity, i.e., failure of treatment of the
initial injury, is the most common and preventable cause.

The probability of success (nonrecurrence) with nonoperative treatment
is not as good with recurrent as with initial instability episodes. A true pattern
of chronic instability is established if there are multiple recurrences, if the
recurrences occur with increasing ease, i.e., if less force is required to produce
the dislocations/subluxations, if reductions are achieved with increasing ease,
and if associated symptoms become less severe. In such cases, the prognosis
without surgical treatment is indeed poor.

If the recurrent dislocation or subluxation appears to be a truly recurrent acute, traumatic injury, then a trial of protective/rehabilitative treatment is recommended (see part G). Otherwise, especially for athletes intending to return to shoulder-strenuous activities, referral for surgical treatment is recommended.

B.   CLINICAL ASSESSMENT OF SHOULDER PROBLEMS

HISTORY

A careful history is the examiner's most important diagnostic tool. It provides data critical to establishing an accurate diagnosis, determining the cause of the problem, and assessing the clinical significance of the diagnosed anatomic problem in the individual patient athlete. Physical examination and diagnostic imaging are essentially confirmatory or disconfirmatory of hypotheses generated on the basis of the history.

A sample self-administered shoulder injury history questionnaire is given in Table 4–1. Some questions are asked of all patients. Some are specific to acute or overuse problems. All patients are first asked about their age, handedness, occupational history, and sports history. These data are useful in determining the cause of overuse injury and assessing the clinical significance of acute or overuse injury in the individual patient.

Acute Injury

Athletes are asked about the mechanism of the injury, their perception of the severity of the injury, the extent of their disability, any associated symptoms, their postinjury course, and the past history of any shoulder injuries or problems. The mechanism of the injury provides important diagnostic clues. Direct trauma, for example, a direct blow to the acromion such as may occur in a fall or in being struck by an opponent's helmet, may produce a contusion ("shoulder pointer"), an acromioclavicular sprain ("shoulder separation"), or a fracture of the acromion or distal clavicle. Less commonly, direct trauma to the anterior or posterior shoulder may produce glenohumeral dislocation. Indirect trauma, for example, forced abduction and external rotation of the arm such as may occur in arm tackling, is the usual mechanism of anterior glenohumeral subluxation or dislocation and may result in injury to any of the static or dynamic anterior stabilizers of the shoulder. A fall onto the adducted, internally rotated arm or a direct blow to the forearm or elbow with resultant force along the long axis of the humerus may produce a posterior glenohumeral subluxation or injury to the bony or cartilaginous glenoid. Sudden loading of the partially abducted arm is a common cause of rotator cuff strain in the middle-aged.

A tearing sensation at the time of injury is diagnostically nonspecific but is characteristic of more severe soft tissue injury. The athlete's perception of the shoulder's having "come out of place" is probably accurate. Inability to move the arm or to lift the arm immediately after the injury is characteristic

Table 4-1. SHOULDER INJURY HISTORY

Name:
Age:
Handedness (right or left):
   for writing and fine motor skills:
   for throwing:
   for batting:
   for shooting:
   for other:
Present school and/or occupation(s) and past occupation(s):
Present sport(s) and position(s) played:
Past sport(s) and position(s) played:
Number of years pitching or catching:
What are your long-term sport career goals/aspirations?
What other career goals do you have?
What are your immediate goals for this season?
How long do you intend/hope to compete?
How long do you intend/hope to remain regularly active in any competitive, fitness, or
   recreational sport or exercise?

If your present shoulder problem is the result of a recent acute injury (e.g., falling, tackling, being hit or thrown, etc.), please answer questions 1–9 below, then skip to question 13.

1. Which shoulder was hurt?
2. Date of injury:
3. Did injury occur:
   during practice?
   during game?
   other?
4. Did injury involve contact or collision with another player?
5. How did injury occur?
6. At time of injury, did you perceive a tearing sensation, pop, snap, crack, or other noise?
7. Did you perceive anything come out of place/go back into place?
8. Did you have immediate pain? If so, where?
9. Immediately after the injury, were you able to:
   move your arm?
   lift your arm?
   continue to play?

If your present shoulder problem is *not* the result of a recent acute injury (e.g., falling, tackling, being hit or thrown, etc.), please answer questions 10–12 below, and continue with question 13.

10. Which shoulder(s) presently bother(s) you?
11. When did the shoulder(s) begin to bother you?
12. Prior to onset of your present symptoms, had you:
   taken up a new sport, exercise, or other physical activity?
   resumed an activity after a lay-off?
   increased the frequency of your exercise, e.g., working out every day as opposed to every
     other day?
   increased the duration of exercise, e.g., swimming more laps?
   increased the intensity of exercise, e.g., lifting heavier weights, swimming faster?
   changed technique/attempted a new skill, e.g., throwing a new pitch?
   changed equipment, e.g., using a new racquet?
13. How has the problem been treated?
14. Is the shoulder presently painful? If so, where?
15. Do you have any problem or pain:
   with throwing?
   with serving or overhead shots in volleyball or racquet sports?
   with batting?
   with swimming?
   which stroke(s)?
   with weight training?
   which lift(s)?
   with other activity?
   at rest?
   at night?
16. Along with your shoulder pain, do you also have any neck pain or pain down the arm?
17. Do you ever have any numbness or tingling in the arm?
18. Have you lost any shoulder motion?
19. Have you lost any shoulder or arm strength?
20. Does the shoulder seem stiff?
21. Does the shoulder seem too loose or even come out of place?
22. Does the shoulder ever make noise when you move it?

Table 4–1. SHOULDER INJURY HISTORY *Continued*

Please answer yes or no to each of the following questions. If yes, please give details such as right or left, dates of surgeries, etc.

Prior to your present shoulder problem, have you ever had:

23. An acute injury to either shoulder:
    shoulder dislocation?
    shoulder (AC joint) separation?
    rotator cuff tear?
    other?
24. Any shoulder problem or pain:
    with activity?
    at rest?
    at night?
    which limited your ability to throw?
    for which you saw a doctor?
    because of which you missed more than a week of practice, competition, or work?
25. Any neck injury or pain, pain down the arm, numbness or tingling in the arm, a "burner"
    or "stinger," a sensation of the arm's "going dead"?
26. Any shoulder or neck x-rays, arthrogram, MRI, or other diagnostic test?
27. Any shoulder or neck surgery?

---

of rotator cuff tears, dislocations, and subluxations. Holding the arm a bit away from the side and externally rotated and unwillingness to have the arm internally rotated across the torso are characteristic of unreduced anterior dislocation. Similarly, holding the arm internally rotated across the torso and unwillingness to have it externally rotated are characteristic of posterior dislocation. A transiently "dead arm" with perceived loss of sensation and inability to use the arm with quick recovery are characteristic of both acute glenohumeral subluxations and "stinger" nerve injuries.

Overuse Injury

As is true for overuse injury in general, with shoulder overuse injury, successful treatment and prevention of recurrence depends as much on determining the cause of the problem as on establishing a precise diagnosis.

The cause of chronic shoulder problems (activity-related pain, weakness, loss of motion, functional impairment, frank instability, or all of these) is virtually always multifactorial. The two most common causes are (1) physiological—an abrupt increase in the physical demand on the shoulder that, at least in retrospect, would be considered a "training error"—and (2) anatomical—the residuals of undertreated/incompletely rehabilitated prior acute injury. Accordingly, the athlete is asked about changes in the type, frequency, duration, and intensity of exercise and any other circumstances that might have been changing before the onset of symptoms. The athlete is also asked about any antecedent injury and the mechanism of that injury.

More often than not, activity-related pain occurs after rather than during the activity. However, if there is pain during activity, determining the precise circumstances in which pain occurs can provide important diagnostic clues, analogous to determining the mechanism of injury for acute injuries. Pain with overhead use of the hand, for example, with throwing; serving or overhead shots in volleyball or racquet sports; freestyle, butterfly, and back-stroke swimming; and certain weight lifts, is characteristic of what we term the *shoulder overuse syndrome*. Similarly, activities of daily living and occupations involving repetitive use of the elevated arm, for example, painting, plastering, or cello playing, are characteristic of this problem. Pain with daily, athletic, or occupational activities involving horizontal flexion of the shoulder such as occurs with swinging a baseball bat or a golf club is typical of acromioclavicular degenerative joint disease. Also, a painful arc of motion with certain weight lifts, especially overhead press, bench press, bench flies, and dips, is typical of acromioclavicular pain.

Lateral arm pain extending distally to midarm level, about the level of the deltoid insertion, is a very common referral pattern of rotator cuff pain. Pain that extends farther distally, is associated with paresthesias, or is more related to the position or motion of the head and neck or shoulder girdle, as opposed to the shoulder joint, is more typical of nerve impingement. Pain at rest may be attributable either to inflammation produced by a mechanical injury or to any of the nonmechanical intrinsic or extrinsic causes of shoulder pain as discussed previously. A "toothache"-quality pain at night is quite characteristic of rotator cuff pain.

Perception and admission of pain are quite individually variable. Sometimes, functional impairment, rather than frank pain, may be the primary symptom. For example, a coach may say that a player is "serving funny," or a thrower may complain of a loss of accuracy or velocity in the throws.

The athlete is also asked about any previous treatment received. Often treatment has been directed at the relief of pain, swelling, and inflammation, and rehabilitation has been neglected. The athlete may have had some temporary relief of symptoms only to have them recur with resumption of activity.

PHYSICAL EXAMINATION

The principal caveat is to be gentle. Obviously, parts of the examination will cause the patient some discomfort—tenderness on palpation of injured or inflamed structures and provocation of pain or apprehension, or both, with various tests. *The examiner, however, should control the examination in such a way that the information being sought is elicited with minimal discomfort to the patient.* Accordingly, examination of the acutely injured or severely painful shoulder will differ considerably from that for subacute injuries or chronic problems.

To carry out a "complete" examination of the shoulder is an impossible task, since however much one might do, there will always be more tests or different ways of doing tests that someone else might elect. A more realistic objective is to conduct an examination that is "sufficiently thorough" that the possibility of important diagnostic entities is not overlooked. The examiner may or may not be able, on the basis of the physical examination, to confirm or disconfirm all the diagnostic hypotheses but should be able to gauge the index of suspicion for the various entities.

A checklist for our recommended "standard" shoulder examination is presented in Table 4–2. The various components of the examination were chosen because

They are relatively easy to learn and to carry out

They are reliable from examination to examination and from examiner to
　　examiner

They are clinically relevant

Most importantly, they are unlikely to cause the patient undue discomfort
　　or harm

Table 4–2. PHYSICAL EXAMINATION OF THE SHOULDER

(Note right or left.)
Habitus
  Antalgic posture/obvious distress
  Shoulder girdle elevation
  Shoulder girdle protraction
  Thoracic kyphosis
  Scoliosis
  Cervical flexion/atlanto-occipital extension ("sniffing" posture)
  Deformity, e.g., "shoulder separation"
Cervical spine
  Tenderness
  Motion (note abnormal limitation of motion, quality of motion, and pain or "tightness")
  Flexion
  Extension
  Right rotation
  Left rotation
  Right lateral bending
  Left lateral bending
  "Nodding"
  Spurling's test (note neck pain, radicular symptoms)
Scapulovertebral muscle spasm or tenderness/trigger point tenderness
Kibler's test (note for each of Kibler's test positions 1–3 and with forward flexion of shoulder)
  Lateral slide in centimeters
  Winging
  Pain
  Unable to attain or to hold position
"Wall push-up"
Internal rotation reach (note pain, relative limitation of motion)
Combined glenohumeral/scapulothoracic abduction
  Limitation of motion
  Painful arc in neutral rotation
  Painful arc in external rotation
  Early onset of scapulothoracic motion
  Dyssymmetrical pattern of motion
Scar, deformity, soft tissue swelling, ecchymosis
Point tenderness (sternoclavicular, acromioclavicular, coracoid, coracoacromial arch,
  coracoclavicular space, anterior joint line, posterior joint line, lesser tuberosity, bicipital
  groove, greater tuberosity)
Isolated glenohumeral range of motion (standing or seated, scapula, stabilized, note pain and/
  or apprehension)
  Flexion
  Abduction
  Extension
  External rotation in adduction
Impingement test
Acromioclavicular/sternoclavicular compression tests
  Horizontal flexion
  Resisted horizontal extension
  Resisted elevation
Manual muscle testing (note pain, weakness relative to contralateral shoulder)
  Flexion (anterior deltoid)
  Speed's test (long head of biceps)
  "Scaption" (supraspinatus)
  Abduction
  Extension
  External rotation in adduction (infraspinatus)
  External rotation in 90° abduction
  Internal rotation in adduction (subscapularis)
Sulcus and apprehension tests for glenohumeral instability
Glenohumeral range of motion (supine, scapula stabilized, note pain or apprehension)
  External rotation in 90° abduction
  Internal rotation in 90° abduction
Containment (Jobe's relocation) test
Special tests
  Yergason test
  Drawer test
  Iowa shoulder shift test
Upper-limb reflex, sensory, and motor testing

The specific objectives and techniques of the components of the examination are discussed below.

Screening Examination of the Acutely Injured Shoulder

Physical examination begins with simple observation of the athlete and the position of the injured limb.

With acute, traumatic, first-time anterior glenohumeral dislocation, the athlete is in obvious distress. The injured arm is held in an abducted, externally rotated position, supported if possible by the uninjured arm. Any shoulder motion, particularly internal rotation, is painful and resisted by the athlete. The normal rounded contour of the shoulder is lost. The acromion is inordinately prominent, with an indentation beneath it, as shown in Figure 4–3. Examination usually also reveals an anterior fullness caused by the anteriorly displaced humeral head. These findings can usually be appreciated by palpation, e.g., under shoulder pads, as well as by inspection.

The clinical findings with acute posterior glenohumeral dislocation are not as obvious. Pain is likely to be greater than with anterior dislocation.[45] In slender individuals, the coracoid process may be unusually prominent and a posterior fullness may be appreciated. However, these two findings are likely to be obscured in the heavily muscled athlete. The key to making the clinical diagnosis is that the arm is held adducted and internally rotated, and any attempt at abduction or external rotation is blocked and painful.[45]

An acromioclavicular sprain with complete rupture of the coracoclavicular ligaments (grade III or higher sprain) may present with obvious deformity ("high-riding clavicle" or, more correctly, "low-riding scapula"). However, the absence of this sign does not rule out grade III sprain, as muscle spasm can minimize the extent of acromioclavicular separation.

Complete rupture of the tendon of the long head of the biceps is usually

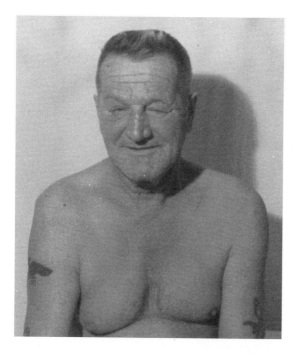

Figure 4–3. Clinical signs of anterior glenohumeral dislocation. The acromion process is quite prominent with an indentation beneath it, giving the shoulder a shortened, squared-off appearance. The arm is held in slight abduction.

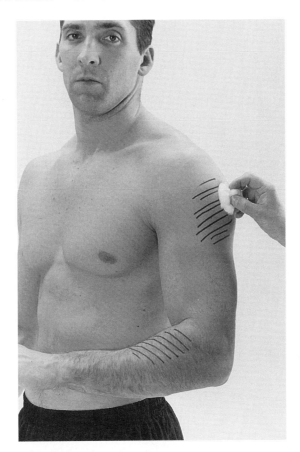

Figure 4–4. Testing for sensation in the distribution of the axillary and musculocutaneous nerves, as described by Rockwood and Wirth.[45]

readily apparent on initial inspection. There may be dependent ecchymosis, and the retracted muscle belly of the biceps is prominent distally.

If none of these injuries are evident, examination continues with systematic inspection and palpation of possibly injured structures (anteriorly: sternoclavicular joint, clavicle, acromion, acromioclavicular joint, coracoid process, coracoclavicular space, lesser tuberosity, bicipital groove; laterally: acromion, subacromial space, greater tuberosity; posteriorly: spine and medial border of scapula, muscle bellies of supraspinatus and infraspinatus). Joint effusion may be detectable as visible or palpable swelling over the anterior joint line, i.e., just lateral to the coracoid process. Inspection can be facilitated by having the patient sit on a low stool.

Assessment of the neurovascular status of the limb is particularly important if any deformity is present. Any of the nerves of the brachial plexus may be injured with anterior dislocation of the shoulder; however, the axillary nerve is particularly at risk. Although sensory testing is usually carried out as shown in Figure 4–4, Blom and Dahlback have shown that this is an unreliable predictor of axillary nerve injury.[13] We have found that the motor function of the nerve can be satisfactorily assessed by gentle isometric testing of the deltoid muscle as shown in Figure 4–5.

Further examination of the injured shoulder is usually deferred until indicated radiographic examination has been carried out. If radiographic examination is negative, gentle muscle testing may be carried out to confirm the diagnosis of musculotendinous injury.

As a quick screening test for active motion, the patients are simply asked

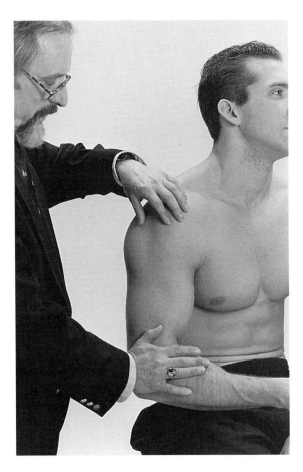

Figure 4–5. Testing for motor function of the axillary nerve. The athlete is asked to press his arm against the examiner's hand. Observation of deltoid action confirms axillary nerve function. Usually, this gently resisted, isometric muscle action is well tolerated by the patient.

to raise their arms forward, raise their arms to the side, put their hands behind their head, and put their hands behind their back, testing flexion, abduction, external rotation, and internal rotation, respectively. Any dyssymmetry or limitation of motion, pain, or apprehension is noted.

Loss of normal synchronization of glenohumeral and scapulothoracic motion with abduction is characteristic of rotator cuff injury (see Fig. 4–10). Normally, with full abduction, the scapula rotates outwardly about 60 degrees. Scapulothoracic motion begins at 30 degrees of abduction, after which abduction comprises 2 degrees of glenohumeral motion for every degree of scapulothoracic motion. With rotator cuff injury, however, scapulothoracic motion begins sooner and abduction comprises relatively more scapulothoracic motion. With acute rotator cuff tears, the patient may be unable to initiate glenohumeral abduction at all but may be able to maintain the position of the arm that has been passively abducted beyond 90 degrees.

As appropriate, additional testing may be carried out as discussed later.

"Standard" Shoulder Examination

SCREENING EXAMINATION OF THE CERVICAL SPINE

In the general population, shoulder pain is a common presenting symptom of intrinsic neck problems. Perhaps even more commonly in the athletic population, neck and scapulovertebral pain are the result of an intrinsic shoulder problem. In either case, screening examination of the cervical and upper thoracic spine is an appropriate part of the standard shoulder examination.

Tenderness to palpation is sought over the vertebral spinous processes and over the paraspinous muscles. Active motion and flexion, extension, left and right rotation, and left and right lateral bending are then observed. The examiner looks for abnormal limitation of motion, the quality of motion, and pain or a sensation of "tightness" with motion. The quality of atlanto-occipital motion is assessed by having the patients nod their head. Commonly, contracture of the short cervical extensors is manifested by stiffness or jerkiness in nodding.

Spurling's test is a screen for radicular irritation/impingement. The patient is guided in extending and then rotating the cervical spine, which narrows the neuroforamina. If the position causes no symptoms, the examiner can then gently place longitudinal compression on the spine by gently pressing down on the patient's head. The examiner notes whether this test provokes any pain or paresthesias and, if so, whether it reproduces the patient's presenting symptoms.

As indicated by the history and the screening tests described, the examiner may proceed with a more detailed examination of the cervical spine and neurological examination or continue with the shoulder examination as described later.

SCAPULAR-STABILIZING MUSCLE FUNCTION

In virtually all handed activities, the shoulder joint functions as one mechanical link between the axial skeleton and the hand. Dysfunction at any link in the kinetic chain, especially adjacent links, can adversely affect the shoulder. Accordingly, assessment of the muscles that position and stabilize the scapula is an important part of the basic shoulder examination.

Kibler's test is a test of scapular-stabilizing muscle function that meets our criteria of simplicity, reliability, and relevance. Kibler's test is a static test of scapular-stabilizing muscle function in which the positions of the scapulae relative to the spine are noted in each of three test positions as shown in Figure 4–6. A lateral slide or winging of the scapula, or both, is the hallmark sign of scapular-stabilizing muscle dysfunction. Scapular dyssymmetry, however, may also result from thoracic scoliosis or frozen shoulder. Pain or an inability to attain test positions 2 or 3 is commonly noted with rotator cuff injury or inflammation.

Additional tests include forward flexion of both shoulders and the "wall push-up"—the classic diagnostic test for the long thoracic nerve and the serratus anterior, with observation for lateral slide or winging of the scapulae (Fig. 4–7).

In most cases, the specific dysfunction is overactivity of the upper trapezius relative to the lower trapezius. This problem, if identified, can be readily and appropriately addressed by physical therapy including McConnell's techniques and biofeedback.

We recommend that Kibler's test be incorporated in the preparticipation examinations of throwing and racquet sport athletes. Addressing the problem of scapular-stabilizing muscle dysfunction in the preseason can obviate clinical problems during the season.

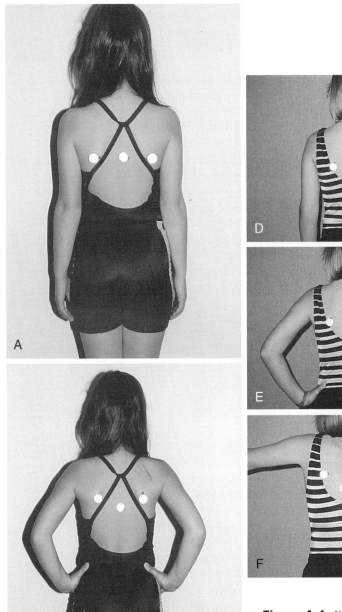

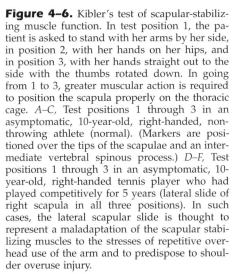

Figure 4–6. Kibler's test of scapular-stabilizing muscle function. In test position 1, the patient is asked to stand with her arms by her side, in position 2, with her hands on her hips, and in position 3, with her hands straight out to the side with the thumbs rotated down. In going from 1 to 3, greater muscular action is required to position the scapula properly on the thoracic cage. *A–C,* Test positions 1 through 3 in an asymptomatic, 10-year-old, right-handed, non-throwing athlete (normal). (Markers are positioned over the tips of the scapulae and an intermediate vertebral spinous process.) *D–F,* Test positions 1 through 3 in an asymptomatic, 10-year-old, right-handed tennis player who had played competitively for 5 years (lateral slide of right scapula in all three positions). In such cases, the lateral scapular slide is thought to represent a maladaptation of the scapular stabilizing muscles to the stresses of repetitive overhead use of the arm and to predispose to shoulder overuse injury.

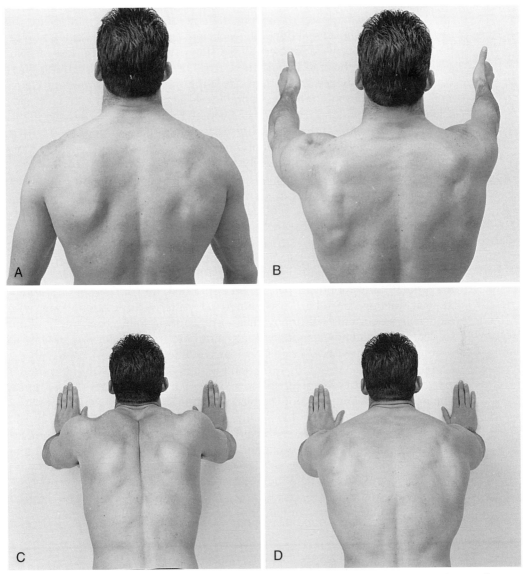

Figure 4–7. Other tests of scapular-stabilizing muscle function. *A* and *B,* Forward flexion of the shoulders. *C* and *D,* "Wall push-up" (actually protraction/retraction of the shoulder girdle without elbow flexion/extension). As in Kibler's test, the examiner observes for lateral scapular slide or winging, or both. (Scapular dyssymmetry in this strength athlete reflects a currently symptomatic left shoulder problem.)

RANGE AND QUALITY OF SHOULDER MOTION

What we consider to be "shoulder motion" is actually a complex of sternoclavicular, acromioclavicular, scapulothoracic, and glenohumeral motion. Depending on the purposes of the examination, it may be appropriate to measure either the total combined motion or the isolated glenohumeral joint motion. For example, for a worker who has to reach overhead shelves, the total range of combined flexion would be useful in assessing the worker's ability to carry out that task. Conversely, in assessing and following the course of a clinical problem such as frozen shoulder, measurement of isolated glenohumeral motion is critical.

Standard orthopedic measurements are of combined motion in the cardinal planes—flexion, abduction, extension, and internal and external rotation with the shoulder adducted to the side. Another common test of combined motion is the internal rotation reach test, measured by the highest vertebral level to which the patient can bring the thumb as shown in Figure 4–8. A difference of up to two vertebral levels less on the dominant hand side relative to the nondominant side is considered normal. These measurements are probably most useful in disability assessments.

Measurement of isolated glenohumeral range of motion is generally more clinically useful. This is most readily accomplished with the patient seated or lying supine with the scapula and shoulder girdle stabilized by the examiner's hand or the examining table as shown in Figure 4–9.

Although arguably less "objective," the quality of motion is probably more significant than the precise range of motion. The first part of the shoulder examination, which is carried out with the patient standing, facing away from the examiner, concludes with observation of combined glenohumeral/scapulothoracic abduction (Fig. 4–10). The examiner looks for abnormal limitation of motion, a painful arc of motion, an early onset of scapulothoracic motion, or other dyssymmetrical patterns of motion. Pain with motion is associated with many diagnostic entities. Pain occurring at about 90 degrees of combined motion or a painful arc from 90 degrees upward is commonly found with acromioclavicular conditions. Increased pain with the shoulder in neutral or internal rotation and less or no pain with the shoulder externally rotated is characteristic of subacromial impingement (of the bursa, rotator cuff, and long head of the biceps tendon). Conversely, greater pain or apprehension, or both, with the shoulder externally rotated and less or no pain with it internally rotated are characteristic of any of the internal derangements associated with anterior glenohumeral instability. An early onset of scapulothoracic motion is seen with scapular-stabilizing muscle dysfunction and with abnormal limitation of glenohumeral motion, such as may be caused by rotator cuff injury or frozen shoulder. Dyssymmetry, especially a "glitch" associated with pain, has similar implications as a painful arc of motion.

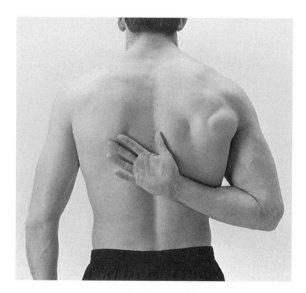

Figure 4–8. Internal rotation reach test. Reach of the dominant hand to within two vertebral levels of the nondominant is considered normal.

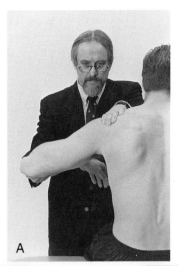

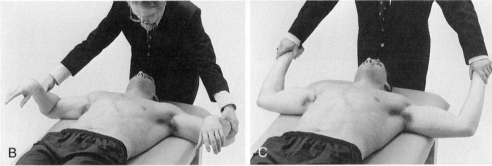

Figure 4–9. Isolated glenohumeral range of motion. *A,* With the patient seated, the examiner stabilizes the shoulder girdle with his hand. True glenohumeral flexion, abduction, and external rotation in adduction are measured. *B* and *C,* With the patient supine, the shoulder girdle is stabilized by the table, and the examiner controls shoulder position and motion. Internal and external glenohumeral rotation in 90-degree abduction are measured.

POINT TENDERNESS

Shoulder examination proceeds with inspection and palpation with the patient seated facing the examiner. Tenderness to palpation is sought over possibly injured or painful structures including the sternoclavicular joint, acromioclavicular joint, coracoid process, coracoacromial arch, coracoclavicular space, anterior glenohumeral joint line, posterior glenohumeral joint line, greater and lesser humeral tuberosities, and bicipital groove. Examination then continues with assessment of the isolated passive glenohumeral range of motion as described previously.

IMPINGEMENT TESTING

Impingement tests are best considered a means of eliciting tenderness of structures not readily accessible to direct palpation. A positive impingement test does not imply a diagnosis of primary impingement. Rather, it implies only that one or more of the structures lying between the humerus and the coracoacromial arch, namely the subacromial bursa, the rotator cuff, and the long head of the biceps tendon, are sensitive to being compressed between

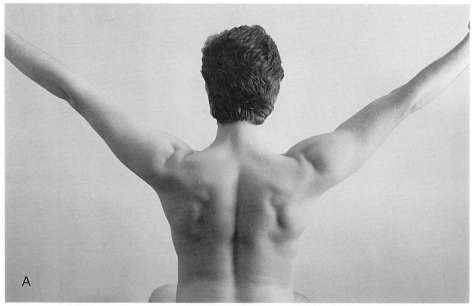

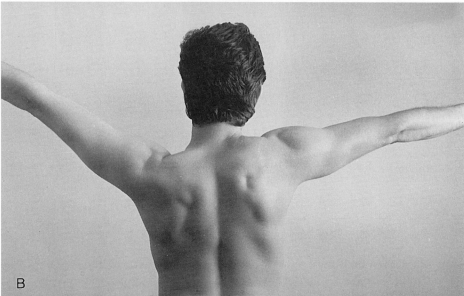

Figure 4–10. *A*, Normal glenohumeral/scapulothoracic pattern of motion. *B*, Altered pattern of motion seen with (right) rotator cuff injury. Scapulothoracic motion begins sooner (the involved shoulder girdle elevates prematurely), and abduction comprises relatively more scapulothoracic motion.

the greater tuberosity of the humerus and the arch. Thus a positive impingement test (impingement sign) can be elicited with any inflammatory condition of or injury to these structures. We commonly employ and recommend the impingement test described by Hawkins and Kennedy,[26] as shown in Figure 4–11.*

---

*Neer differentiates between "impingement sign" and "impingement test" as follows.[39] His impingement sign refers to pain elicited with passive abduction of the glenohumeral joint with the scapula stabilized by the examiner's hand. His impingement test refers to abatement of such pain after subacromial injection of a local anesthetic (see Subacromial Bursa in part B). We believe the more intuitive and more common usage of these terms is as presented in the text.

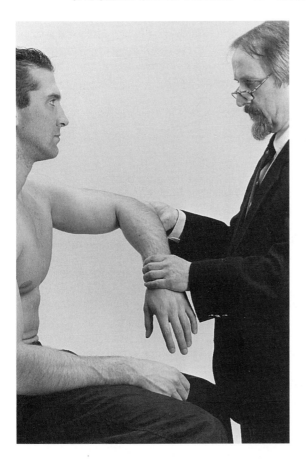

Figure 4–11. Impingement test, as described by Hawkins and Kennedy.[26] With passive flexion and internal rotation of the shoulder, the rotator cuff, the tendon of the long head of the biceps, and the subdeltoid bursa can be impinged between the greater tuberosity and the coracoacromial arch. A positive test, i.e., pain and grimacing, is characteristic of inflammation of the impinged structures.

ACROMIOCLAVICULAR/STERNOCLAVICULAR COMPRESSION TESTS

In addition to a painful arc of motion, pain with compression of the acromioclavicular and sternoclavicular joints is characteristic but not pathognomonic of injury to or inflammation of these joints. Compression of the joints is achieved by passive horizontal flexion of the shoulder, resisted active horizontal extension of the horizontally flexed shoulder, and resisted elevation of the horizontally flexed shoulder as shown in Figure 4–12. Pain localized discretely to the top of the shoulder (acromioclavicular joint) or to the sterno-

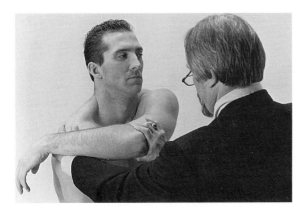

Figure 4–12. Acromioclavicular/sternoclavicular compression tests comprise passive horizontal flexion of the shoulder, resisted active horizontal extension of the horizontally flexed shoulder, and resisted elevation of the horizontally flexed shoulder. These maneuvers also stretch posterior glenohumeral structures.

clavicular joint is highly specific. Diffuse shoulder pain or pain localized to the posterior aspect of the shoulder with these maneuvers is nonspecific and is not uncommonly seen with internal derangement of the shoulder, glenohumeral instability, and muscle injury.

MANUAL MUSCLE TESTING

With manual muscle testing, the examiner looks for pain or weakness relative to the contralateral side, the cause of which then needs to be differentiated as discussed previously. The principal caveat is to do no further harm. The desired information can be safely and reliably elicited by isometric manual muscle testing in positions within the patient's pain-free range of motion. It is important that the examiner control the position of the patient's arm and the amount of muscular force generated by the patient and resisted by the examiner. This is accomplished by the examiner's specific instructions to the patient: "Don't let me push your hands down" or "Don't let me push your hands together," as opposed to "Push up against my hands" or "Push out against my hands." The examiner can then begin with very light pressure and increase it gradually, stopping either at the point when good strength and no pain are clearly demonstrated, or as soon as any pain or weakness is demonstrated. Specific manual resistance tests for anterior, middle, and posterior leaves of the deltoid, supraspinatus, external and internal rotators, and biceps are shown in Figures 4–13 and 4–14.

With testing of the anterior deltoid or supraspinatus, the clavicular part of the pectoralis major may be observed to substitute for them (Fig. 4–15).

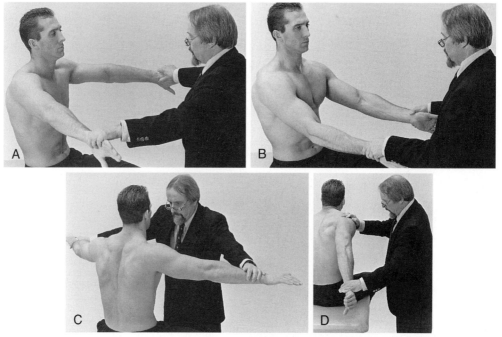

Figure 4–13. *A–D,* Selective testing, respectively, of the supraspinatus and the anterior, middle, and posterior leaves of the deltoid. The patient tries to resist the examiner's downward pressure on his forearms.

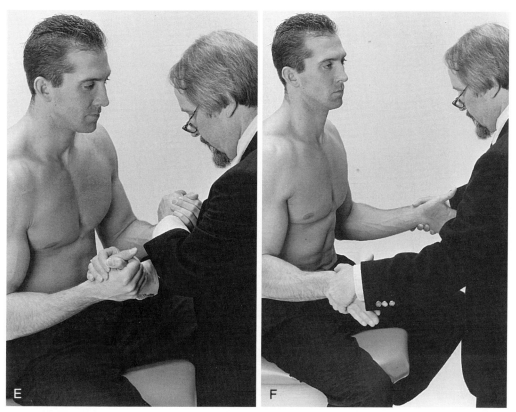

Figure 4–13 *Continued. E* and *F,* Selective testing of the internal and external rotators of the shoulder.

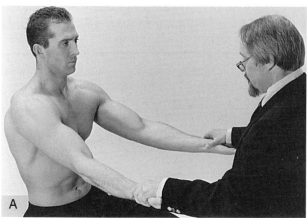

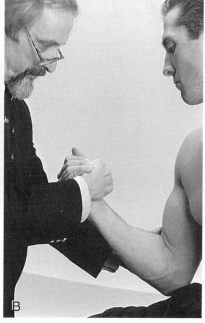

Figure 4–14. Testing of the biceps. *A,* Speed's test. The shoulders are flexed and externally rotated, the elbows extended, and the forearms supinated. The patient tries to resist the examiner's downward pressure on his forearms. *B,* Yergason's test.[59] The elbow is flexed to 90 degrees and the forearm is pronated. The patient attempts to supinate the forearm against the examiner's resistance.

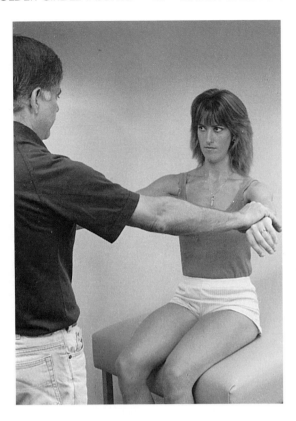

Figure 4–15. Pectoral substitution sign. With specific testing of the (right) supraspinatus, the clavicular part of the pectoralis major is observed to substitute for it.

Protraction of the shoulder girdle and fasciculation of the anterior deltoid may also be noted.

With supraspinatus testing, a "drop arm sign" is elicited when the patient is able to hold the shoulder in 90 degrees of elevation ("scaption," see Fig. 4–13) against gravity, but with slight additional manual pressure the shoulder abruptly gives way and the arm drops. In the authors' experience, this finding may be elicited with any of the conditions causing profound weakness (see previous discussion) and is not pathognomonic of rotator cuff tear.

Smooth giving-way on manual muscle testing, i.e., uniform weakness throughout the range of motion, is characteristic of neuromuscular weakness. In contrast, abrupt or ratchet-like (cogwheel) giving-way is more characteristic of mechanical musculotendinous disruption or pain inhibition.

TESTS OF GLENOHUMERAL INSTABILITY

Various instability tests have been described, many of which strike us as unnecessarily draconian, i.e., they entail an unnecessary risk of causing the patient at least undue pain if not actual injury while not offering the examiner information that can be obtained as readily by other means. We recommend that any such test be used cautiously, if at all, by very experienced examiners and not at all by primary care physicians. The four tests described below meet our criteria for simplicity, reliability, clinical relevance, and, above all, safety.

Sulcus Test

With the patient seated facing the examiner, and with the patient's shoulders adducted with the arms by the sides, the examiner grasps the arms with one hand just above the elbow and gently exerts a downward force. With inferior instability, the examiner and the patient may appreciate the head of the humerus slipping inferiorly relative to the glenoid, and a sulcus between the acromion and head of the humerus may become visible (Fig. 4–16).

In our experience, the sulcus test is as likely to be positive with functional as structural instability of the shoulder. It may be elicited even with rotator cuff insufficiency caused by fatigue, for example, after isokinetic shoulder exercise to exhaustion.

In "normal" shoulders, some inferior subluxation can usually be demonstrated. The extent is probably a measure of how "loose-jointed" the individual is. Dyssymmetry, however, probably represents "abnormal laxity."

Apprehension Test

The seated patient is asked to abduct the shoulders to 90 degrees and then to externally rotate the 90-degree–abducted shoulders. Any symptom of pain or apprehension, or simply an unwillingness to carry out the maneuver, constitutes a positive test. The patient who is able, without symptoms, to rotate the abducted shoulder to 90 degrees of external rotation may then be asked to "flick" the arm backward from that position, thus imparting a mild external rotation impact stress to the shoulder.

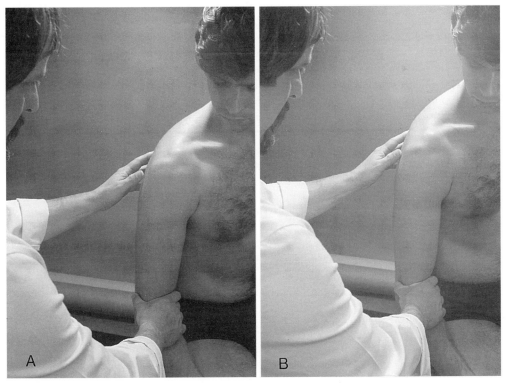

Figure 4–16. Sulcus test. The athlete is seated with his forearm resting comfortably in his lap. The examiner places gentle downward traction on the arm as in *A*. A click may be felt as the shoulder subluxes inferiorly, and a subacromial indentation will be apparent as in *B*. With supraspinatus strain or tendinitis, this motion may produce pain and may be voluntarily or involuntarily resisted.

Containment (Jobe's Relocation) Test

In the containment (Jobe's relocation) test,[34] the patient is asked to lie supine on the examining table with the shoulders 90 degrees abducted as described previously in assessing the range of internal and external rotation in 90 degrees of abduction (Fig. 4–17). If there is pain during or at the limits of external rotation, the examiner, now standing beside the patient and examining just the affected shoulder, uses one hand to control the position and motion of the arm and the other hand to "contain" the head of the humerus reduced in the glenoid socket. This may be accomplished either by direct manual pressure over the head of the humerus or indirectly by pressure over the neck of the humerus. A positive test comprises pain with passive external rotation of the 90 degrees of abducted shoulder, abatement of pain with "containment," and recurrence of pain as the examiner slowly lifts the hand exerting the containing force. The containment test, in our experience, is not pathognomonic of any specific structural injury but is probably the most sensitive test for any functional or structural anterior glenohumeral instability problem.

(Iowa) Shoulder Shift Test

If the containment test is negative or equivocal, and minimally or not pain provoking, a moderately more strenuous instability test may be carried out as follows: Anterior translation of the humeral head relative to the glenoid is effected by gentle anterior force applied by the examiner's hand beneath the humeral head. The patient, with the hand on the examiner's chest, is asked to push the examiner toward the foot of the bench (resisted internal rotation of the shoulder), both when the shoulder is subluxed forward anteriorly and when it is reduced. A positive test constitutes pain or relative weakness, or both, with the effort when the shoulder is subluxed anteriorly.

Admittedly, the "results" of instability testing may depend in large measure on the skill, experience, and enthusiasm of the examiner. As is always the case, if there is clinical suspicion of joint instability, and this possibility cannot be confirmed or disconfirmed by the primary physician, then consultation or referral is recommended. We emphasize that pain and apprehension, as well as frank subluxation, should be considered positive signs of instability.

NEUROVASCULAR EXAMINATION

When the patient presents with symptoms or signs of shoulder weakness or radicular symptoms, neurovascular examination of the upper limb is critical. The screening neurological examination comprises deep tendon reflexes, manual muscle testing, tactile sensation, and two-point discrimination of the palmar surfaces of the digits. The screening examination for thoracic outlet syndrome includes Allen's, Wright's, and Roos' tests, also described elsewhere.

INJECTION/ASPIRATION

In our sports medicine experience, occasions requiring diagnostic arthrocentesis of the shoulder are decidedly rare. The most likely indication is suspected

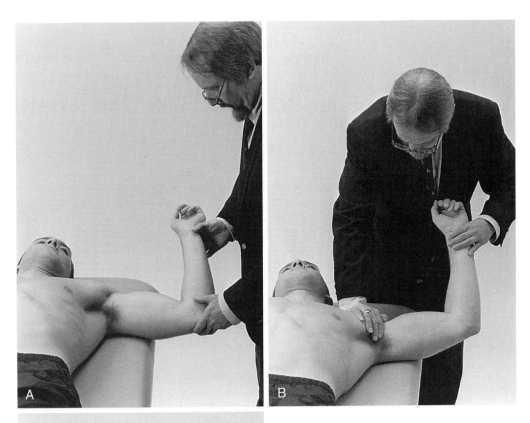

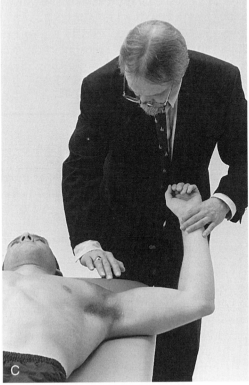

Figure 4–17. Containment test for anterior glenohumeral instability. A positive test comprises pain with passive external rotation of the 90 degrees of abducted shoulder *(A)*, abatement of pain with "containment" of the humeral head in the glenoid by the examiner's manual pressure *(B)*, and recurrence of pain as the examiner slowly lifts the hand exerting the containing force *(C)*.

septic arthritis, e.g., in an immunocompromised individual with atraumatic shoulder pain.

In contrast, local anesthetic injection of sites of tenderness, the acromioclavicular and glenohumeral joints or the subacromial bursa, or both, is frequently useful. As discussed previously, it can help to differentiate weakness secondary to pain inhibition of normal muscle function from other causes of shoulder weakness. It can also help to precisely localize the source or sources of a patient's pain, e.g., in sorting out the relative importance of acromioclavicular degenerative joint disease versus rotator cuff tendinosis in a patient with activity-related shoulder pain. This is particularly important if surgery for pain relief is being considered.

Sometimes combining a corticosteroid with the local anesthetic injection can be both diagnostic and therapeutic. Typically, if the injection is appropriately placed, the patient experiences a prompt offset of pain when the painful structure is anesthetized, a recurrence of pain when the anesthetic has worn off, and then an offset of pain again a day or more later, when the corticosteroid has exerted its full effects. It is important to advise the patient beforehand of this expected course.

The duration of pain relief after corticosteroid injection is quite variable. For the individual fortunate enough to be able to limit or to modify the pain-provoking activity, the pain relief may be indefinite. For the patient who is unable or unwilling to comply with activity and rehabilitation recommendations, pain may recur within a week or two.

All injections are carried out after the skin has been cleansed and prepared (e.g., with povidone-iodine solution or tincture of iodine) and using sterile technique. For diagnostic injections, we use 1% lidocaine with epinephrine. For diagnostic/therapeutic injections, we generally use a 1:1 mixture of betamethasone and 0.25% bupivacaine (1:2 for the shoulder joint).

Provocative tests, e.g., impingement test or manual muscle testing, are carried out before and after injection, and the extent of postinjection pain relief/strength gain is noted. The patients are asked to attend carefully to pain/pain relief they experience, especially during the first few hours after injection. Patients are encouraged to keep a log of activities found to be painful or pain-free for comparison with preinjection symptoms. As a rule, patients are then seen again in 1 week.

Patients are cautioned that after corticosteroid injection they might not have reliable protective pain sensation for 1 to 2 months. Accordingly for the first several weeks after injection, they are asked to limit their activities to the type, frequency, duration, and intensity that were fairly well tolerated before injection.

Acromioclavicular Joint

We prefer a superior approach, as shown in Figure 4–18. This permits, if desired, the injection of the underlying subacromial bursa as well as the acromioclavicular joint with one needle stick. An AP radiograph of the shoulder defines the obliquity of the individual patient's acromioclavicular joint and thereby guides the direction of the needle. In some individuals, marked osteophytosis may preclude easy superior needle entry, in which case an anterior approach may be used. The intact adult acromioclavicular joint accommodates a volume of 3 to 4 mL, after which pressure limits further injection. The needle may then be advanced to inject the bursa. Promptly after

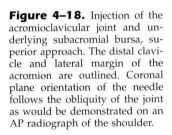
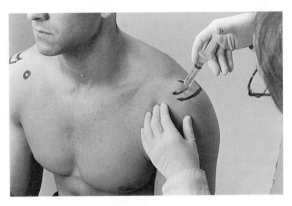

Figure 4–18. Injection of the acromioclavicular joint and underlying subacromial bursa, superior approach. The distal clavicle and lateral margin of the acromion are outlined. Coronal plane orientation of the needle follows the obliquity of the joint as would be demonstrated on an AP radiograph of the shoulder.

injection there should be relief of acromioclavicular pain with compression tests, horizontal flexion of the shoulder, and so forth.

Shoulder (Glenohumeral) Joint

The shoulder joint can reliably be entered anteriorly or posteriorly as shown in Figure 4–19. We generally use an anterior approach with needle entry in the anterior joint line about one fingerbreadth inferior to and one fingerbreadth lateral to the tip of the coracoid. The intact adult shoulder joint accommodates approximately 30 mL, but we generally instill about 10 mL of fluid. We then ask the patient to move the shoulder, e.g., Codman's or "fungo" active motion exercises as described later in this chapter, to help distribute the fluid within the joint. Promptly after injection there should be relief of pain from intra-articular structures with impingement testing, manual muscle testing, and so forth.

Subacromial Bursa

We most often inject the subacromial bursa concomitantly with the acromioclavicular joint as described previously under Acromioclavicular Joint. How-

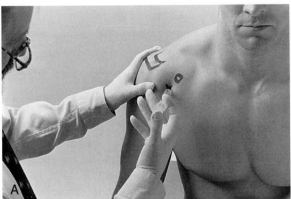
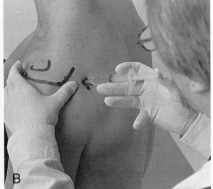

Figure 4–19. Injection of the glenohumeral joint. *A,* Anterior approach. The tip of the coracoid, distal clavicle, and anterolateral margin of the acromion are outlined. Needle entry is a fingerbreadth inferior and medial to the tip of the coracoid. *B,* Posterior approach. The distal clavicle and posterolateral margin of the acromion are outlined. Needle entry is a thumb's breadth inferior and medial to the posterior margin of the acromion. The needle is directed anteriorly toward the tip of the coracoid.

ever, the bursa may be selectively injected using an anterolateral approach with the needle entry beneath the edge of the acromion and above the anterior aspect of the greater tuberosity of the humerus. It accommodates several milliliters of fluid.

C. DIAGNOSTIC IMAGING OF THE SHOULDER

"TRAUMA SERIES" RADIOGRAPHS

With acute shoulder injuries, radiographic examination is generally indicated. A "trauma series," consisting of AP and lateral scapular views, is recommended. (The lateral scapular view is variously referred to as a true lateral view of the shoulder, a trans-scapular lateral view of the shoulder, or a Y view of the shoulder.) *These views can and should be obtained "as is," i.e., without moving the arm or removing it from a sling.* The patient may be standing, sitting, or lying.

The trauma series has some important advantages over "standard" radiographic examination of the shoulder. First, because the views are obtained "as is," discomfort and the risk of further injury to the patient are minimized. Second, these views reveal all the skeletal injuries of concern, i.e., fractures of the distal clavicle, fractures of the proximal humerus, and both anterior and posterior glenohumeral dislocations (Fig. 4–20).

Radiographic examination is not always required before reduction of glenohumeral dislocations. If the clinical diagnosis of anterior dislocation can be made, then gentle reduction may be attempted on the playing field or in the locker room.[35, 48] If there is a possible growth plate injury (elementary or junior high school athlete), or if the injury is a first-time posterior dislocation, then we would recommend radiographic examination before reduction. In all cases, postreduction radiographic examination is indicated.

ACROMIOCLAVICULAR STRESS RADIOGRAPHS

Many orthopedists and radiologists recommend stress views of the acromioclavicular joints whenever the clinical findings are suggestive of grade III or higher acromioclavicular sprains. These AP views of the acromioclavicular joints should be obtained with 5 to 15 lb of weight *suspended* from the patient's wrists. The coracoclavicular distance is measured on the injured and uninjured sides. A difference of 5 mm or more is considered diagnostic of complete disruption of the coracoclavicular ligaments (grade III sprain).

In common practice, the radiographs are obtained with hand-held, as opposed to wrist-suspended, weights, in which case, especially if the shoulder is still painful, protective deltoid muscle action can "reduce" the acromioclavicular separation and result in a false-negative diagnostic test (Fig. 4–21).

In our practice, we generally treat grades I through III acromioclavicular sprains the same and so do not routinely order these films.

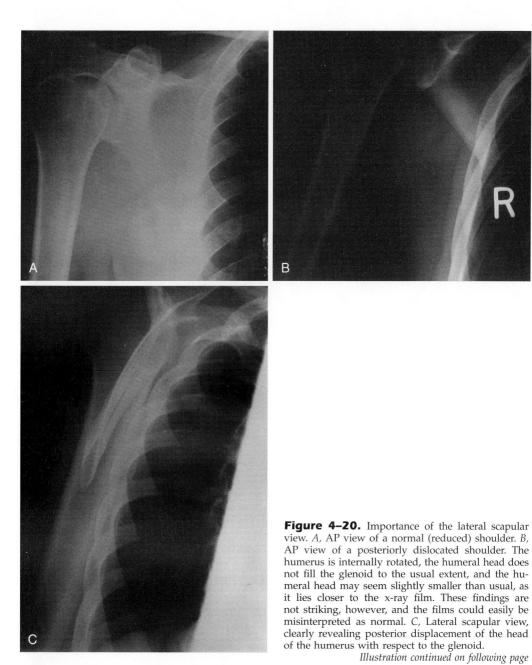

Figure 4–20. Importance of the lateral scapular view. *A,* AP view of a normal (reduced) shoulder. *B,* AP view of a posteriorly dislocated shoulder. The humerus is internally rotated, the humeral head does not fill the glenoid to the usual extent, and the humeral head may seem slightly smaller than usual, as it lies closer to the x-ray film. These findings are not striking, however, and the films could easily be misinterpreted as normal. *C,* Lateral scapular view, clearly revealing posterior displacement of the head of the humerus with respect to the glenoid.

Illustration continued on following page

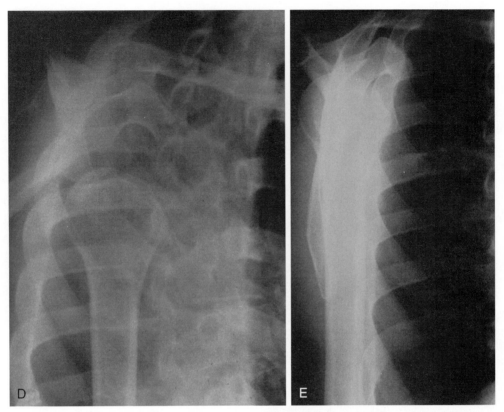

Figure 4–20 *Continued. D* and *E,* Lateral scapular views of anteriorly dislocated and reduced shoulders for comparison. The humeral head is respectively anteriorly displaced and superimposed on the glenoid.

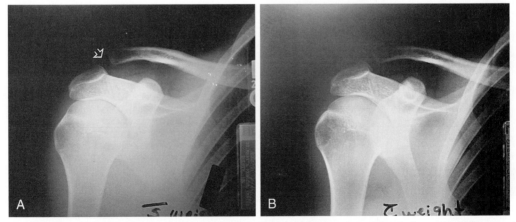

Figure 4–21. Acromioclavicular stress radiographs incorrectly obtained with the weight held, not suspended, from the wrists. The separation (arrow) is greater in *A,* without weights, than in *B,* with weights. Deltoid muscle action/spasm has reduced the grade III sprain.

"SHOULDER SERIES" RADIOGRAPHS

Radiographic examination of the shoulder is generally indicated both for acute injury and for any problem of more than a few weeks' duration. If shoulder joint motion is not contraindicated or very painfully limited, a standard shoulder series, comprising internal and external rotation AP views and an axillary view, may be ordered instead of the trauma series.

Classic signs of anterior glenohumeral instability are the Bankart lesion,[9] a defect of the anteroinferior aspect of the glenoid rim, and the Hill-Sachs lesion,[27] an impression defect of the posterolateral aspect of the humeral head. The Bankart lesion is best evidenced radiographically in a West Point axillary view.[46] The patient is positioned prone with the shoulder abducted 90 degrees. The x-ray beam is directed 25 degrees inferiorly and 25 degrees medially. The Hill-Sachs lesion is best visualized in an AP view with the shoulder internally rotated.

With posterior instability, there may be an impression defect of the anteromedial part of the humeral head. The defect is best visualized in a standard axillary view (Fig. 4–22). It corresponds to the Hill-Sachs lesion with anterior dislocation and is sometimes referred to as a "reverse Hill-Sachs lesion." A more common finding with posterior instability is a defect or irregularity of the posterior glenoid rim, seen best on AP views.

SHOULDER ARTHROGRAPHY

Shoulder arthrography, the former test of choice for diagnosis of full-thickness rotator cuff tears, has now been virtually replaced by MRI, which provides more accurate and more complete information.

RADIONUCLIDE SCINTIGRAPHY

Indications for radionuclide scintigraphy are rare. A bone scan may be useful as a screening test for ruling out uncommon shoulder girdle problems such

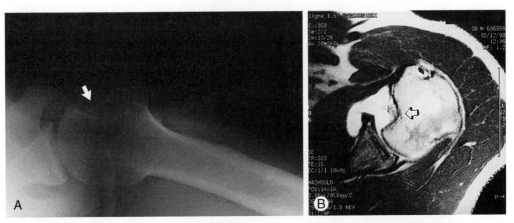

Figure 4–22. Axillary radiograph *(A)* and magnetic resonance imaging (MRI) arthrogram axial section *(B)* demonstrating a reverse Hill-Sachs lesion (arrows), an impression defect of the anteromedial part of the humeral head.

as stress reaction of bone, osteochondrosis (Little Leaguer's shoulder), and bone tumors.

MAGNETIC RESONANCE IMAGING (AND MRI ARTHROGRAPHY)

MRI with gadolinium arthrography is, with certain caveats, the (nonsurgical) diagnostic test of choice for sorting out internal derangements of the shoulder and for assessing structural glenohumeral instability. Partial- and full-thickness rotator cuff tears, rotator cuff tendinitis/tendinosis, glenoid labral tears, SLAP (a mnemonic for detachment of the superior labrum, anterior to posterior) lesions, bony and fibrocartilaginous Bankart lesions, long head of biceps tendon rupture or dislocation, acromioclavicular arthrosis, and various bone lesions can all be well demonstrated (Figs. 4–23 and 4–24).

The reliability and clinical usefulness of MRI is very dependent on the available technology (computer software and shoulder coils) and on the experience of the radiologists and clinicians carrying out and interpreting the studies. A particular pitfall for clinicians is the tendency of radiologists to undercall fibrocartilaginous Bankart lesions as "normal variants." It should be appreciated that

There is not a one-to-one correlation between symptoms and structural abnormality.

A clinical problem results only when physical demands sufficiently stress the abnormal structure or structures.

Accordingly, a physical, radiographic, or MRI finding may be "normal" in the sense of being common in a given population, even in a population of asymptomatic individuals, and nonetheless be "abnormal" in the sense of not being compatible with highly stressful activities such as throwing.

The clinical usefulness of the MRI is not limited to preoperative planning. Information obtained can help with decisions regarding operative versus

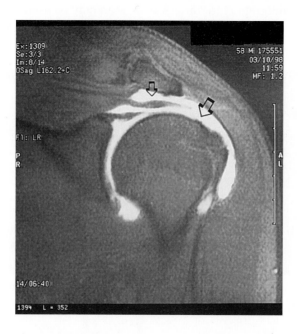

Figure 4–23. MRI arthrogram coronal section demonstrating a full-thickness acute-on-degenerative tear of the supraspinatus (large arrow) in a 57-year-old retired miner and recreational league basketball player. Note that the contrast medium injected into the joint fills the subacromial bursa (small arrow).

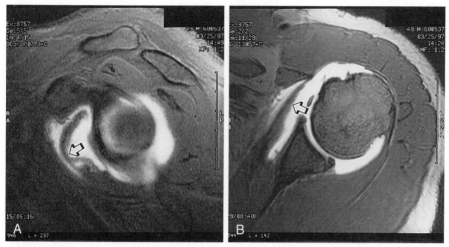

Figure 4–24. MRI arthrogram axial *(A)* and sagittal *(B)* sections demonstrating an acute, traumatic fibrocartilaginous Bankart lesion (arrows), the result of a snowmobiling accident.

nonoperative treatment and the specifics of nonoperative, rehabilitative treatment. The decision to order this test versus some other test or no test is probably best made in consultation with, or deferred to, the sports medicine/orthopedic consultant.

D.   STERNOCLAVICULAR SPRAINS

ANATOMY

The sternoclavicular joint is the only true articulation of the shoulder girdle with the axial skeleton. Some sternoclavicular motion occurs with virtually all motions of the shoulder and shoulder girdle.

The joint has little inherent bony stability. Motion is constrained mainly by the surrounding ligaments, namely, the articular disc ligament, the costoclavicular ligament, the anterior and posterior sternoclavicular ligaments, and the interclavicular ligament. The fact that dislocation is uncommon attests to the strength of these ligaments, most or all of which must be completely disrupted for dislocation to occur.[44]

The brachiocephalic, jugular, and subclavian veins; the brachiocephalic, carotid, and subclavian arteries; the trachea; the esophagus; the lungs and pleurae; and the brachial plexus lie just deep to the sternoclavicular joint and proximal clavicle. Posterior dislocation can cause compression or laceration of any of the underlying structures. Such complications reportedly occur in roughly one-fourth of cases of traumatic posterior dislocation.[44]

HISTORY

MECHANISMS OF INJURY. Sternoclavicular injury may be produced by either *direct or indirect trauma*. The most common mechanism is *lateral compres-*

sion of the shoulder girdle as a result of force applied to the shoulder or upper limb (Fig. 4–25).

Whether direct or indirect, considerable force is required to produce dislocation. This can occur in a number of ways. An equestrian may be kicked or stepped on by a horse. A cyclist may fall at high speed onto the shoulder or outstretched hand. A wrestler or ball carrier may be thrown directly onto the shoulder. An athlete lying on the ground may be jumped on by one or several others.

SYMPTOMS. The hallmark symptom is *pain*, which is well localized and is roughly proportional to the severity of injury. With mild and moderate sprains, the pain is likely to become progressively more limiting during the first 24 hours or so after injury. With dislocation, especially posterior dislocation, the pain is immediate and quite severe.

Other symptoms that may be present with either anterior or posterior dislocation are swelling, pain on motion of the shoulder and shoulder girdle, crepitus on motion, and limitation of motion.

With posterior dislocation, there may be symptoms of associated injury to underlying vital structures. The most ominous symptoms are those of airway obstruction or ventilatory impairment, or both, e.g., dyspnea, dysphonia, stridor, choking, coughing. Compression of the esophagus may cause dysphagia, and compression of the subclavian artery or brachial plexus, or both, may cause upper limb pain and paresthesias.

PHYSICAL EXAMINATION

Attention is first directed to ruling out life- or limb-threatening injury. Are there any obvious signs of respiratory distress, e.g., gasping, choking, stridor, or cyanosis? Can the athlete talk? Is the athlete hoarse? Can the athlete swallow? Are breath sounds decreased? Are the neck veins distended? Is there any marked, rapidly expanding, or pulsatile swelling? Are peripheral pulses or capillary refill, or both, diminished? Are there any motor or sensory neurologic deficits?

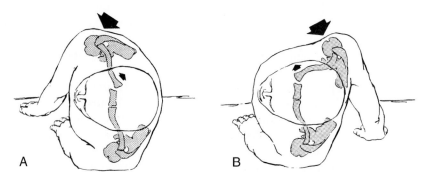

Figure 4–25. Indirect mechanisms of injury to the sternoclavicular joint. *A,* Forcible compression (large arrow) and protraction of the shoulder girdle also tends to displace the proximal clavicle posteriorly (small arrow). *B,* Forcible compression and retraction (large arrow) of the shoulder girdle tends to displace the proximal clavicle anteriorly (small arrow). As anterior dislocation is far more common than posterior, this appears to be the most common mechanism of injury. (From Rockwood CA Jr and Wirth MA: Injuries to the sternoclavicular joint. *In* Rockwood CA Jr, Green DP, Bucholz RW, Heckman JD [eds]: Fractures in Adults, 4th ed, vol 2. Philadelphia, Lippincott-Raven, 1996, pp 1415–1471.)

After vital functions have been stabilized, attention can then be directed to diagnosing the specific musculoskeletal injury. With all sternoclavicular sprains, there is point tenderness over the joint. With anterior dislocation, the clavicle is visibly or palpably, or both, displaced anterior to the manubrium. With posterior dislocation, the usual prominence of the proximal clavicle is lost. Although all these signs can be more or less obscured by obesity or swelling, or both, *careful palpation usually establishes the diagnosis.**

The athlete who has sustained a dislocation usually wants to sit, supporting and guarding the injured limb with the other hand. The athlete's head may be tilted toward the injured side. The shoulder girdle appears shortened and protracted. Any motion of the shoulder or shoulder girdle, especially compression of the shoulder girdle or moving the arm horizontally across the front of the body, is most likely to be painful and resisted. With motion, there is likely to be audible or palpable crepitus, or both, and there may also be palpable subluxation of the joint. These signs are characteristic, but with the exception of joint subluxation, not pathognomonic of sternoclavicular injury. They may also be present with fractures of the sternum or proximal clavicle.

RADIOGRAPHIC EXAMINATION

Radiographic examination of the sternoclavicular joint can be difficult to interpret. However, if the clinical diagnosis is uncertain, fractures of the sternum or proximal clavicle can be ruled out by the appropriate studies.

OTHER DIAGNOSTIC TESTS

Computerized axial tomography or MRI may be useful to confirm the diagnosis of dislocation and to reveal the extent of impingement of underlying structures.[51]

INITIAL TREATMENT

Vital functions are supported as indicated. Definitive treatment on an *emergent* basis is seldom necessary. However, immediate treatment of a complication, e.g., thoracentesis for decompression of a tension pneumothorax, might be required.

Reduction of dislocations, particularly complicated posterior dislocations, is indicated on an *urgent* basis. In nearly all cases, *closed reduction* is the treatment of choice. A possible contraindication might be suspected perforation, as opposed to compression, of a major blood vessel.

Closed reduction of sternoclavicular dislocations can be achieved in several ways, all of which involve direct and/or indirect retraction of the shoulder girdle. Both anterior and posterior dislocations are reduced by this mechanism. Before significant swelling and muscle spasm have occurred, it may be

---

*Before closure of the proximal clavicular growth plate, which occurs at about the age of 25 years, it is practically impossible clinically to differentiate sternoclavicular dislocations from fractures through the growth plate. Indeed, before ossification of the proximal epiphysis, which occurs at about the age of 18 years, it is impossible to do so even radiographically. However, as both injuries are treated the same, the differentiation is not clinically important.

possible to achieve reduction simply by placing a knee between the seated athlete's scapulae and pulling back on the shoulders. In the standard method of closed reduction, the athlete is supine with a sandbag placed between the scapulae. Lateral traction is applied to the abducted and slightly extended upper limb. With anterior dislocation, anterior pressure over the proximal clavicle may also be required. With posterior dislocation, anterolateral traction on the proximal clavicle with the fingers or a sterile towel clip may be required. An alternative method for reducing posterior dislocations is to apply caudal traction to the adducted upper limb while direct anterior pressure is applied to both shoulders. Reportedly, less force is required to effect reduction, and manipulation of the clavicle with a towel clip is usually unnecessary.[15]

If the athlete is seen immediately or soon after injury, it may be possible to achieve reduction without any medication or with just local anesthesia. Usually, however, general anesthesia or intravenous sedation and analgesia is required.

As the joint is reduced, there is usually an audible and palpable snap. Subsequently, palpation confirms restoration of normal anatomical relationships, and the signs and symptoms of associated compression injuries resolve.

After reduction, a figure-of-eight clavicle strap is applied to maintain retraction of the shoulder girdle. As a rule, reductions of posterior dislocations are stable. Closed reductions of anterior dislocations may or may not be stable. Even with the shoulders held back, the joint may sublux anteriorly.

Initial treatment of all sternoclavicular injuries may also include the use of a sling (in addition to the clavicle strap) and intermittent icing until swelling has stabilized.

Posterior dislocations should be considered much the same as penetrating wounds of the neck. Even if stable reduction has been achieved and all signs and symptoms of associated injury have resolved, the athlete should still be admitted to the hospital or closely observed for signs of delayed complications.

REFERRAL

Severe vascular injury may require surgical exploration. If such injury is suspected, referral should be made on an *emergent* basis to a major center with angiographic and cardiovascular/thoracic surgical capabilities.

Orthopedic referral on an *urgent* basis is indicated for all unreduced acute dislocations. Open reduction of acute posterior dislocations is required if stable closed reduction cannot be achieved.

DEFINITIVE TREATMENT

Definitive treatment for mild and moderate sprains is not required. For most dislocations, all that is required for definitive treatment is closed reduction, "immobilization" in a figure-of-eight clavicle strap for 4 to 6 weeks, and complete rehabilitation of the shoulder before resumption of strenuous activity.

The definitive treatment of unstable anterior dislocations is somewhat controversial. Of the reported fatalities associated with sternoclavicular dislocation, most have been the result of complications of surgical treatment, e.g., migration of a Steinmann pin or Kirschner wire into the heart or one of the great vessels. We agree with Rockwood and Wirth that the instability is "less of a problem than the potential problems of operative repair and internal fixation."[44] Recurrent dislocation or subluxation that subsequently proves disabling to the athlete can be definitively treated by resection of the proximal clavicle.

Other possible long-term sequelae of acute sternoclavicular injury are degenerative joint disease and chronic pain. These problems can also be treated definitively by resection of the proximal clavicle, or symptomatically, e.g., by intra-articular corticosteroid injections.

E.   FRACTURES OF THE PROXIMAL AND MIDDLE THIRDS OF THE CLAVICLE

ANATOMY

Lest familiarity with these common and usually uncomplicated fractures create undue complacency, it should be remembered that lying just deep to the clavicle are the pleurae and dome of the lung, the subclavian vessels, and the brachial plexus. Serious and sometimes fatal complications can and do occur as a result of laceration of the underlying structure or structures by a fracture fragment.

HISTORY

MECHANISM OF INJURY. As with sternoclavicular sprains, injury may be produced by either *direct or indirect trauma*. The mechanisms of injury are much the same. With fractures, however, the most common mechanism appears to be *falls onto the outstretched hand*.

SYMPTOMS. Symptoms are for the most part those usually associated with long-bone fractures, i.e., a snapping or cracking sensation at the time of injury, immediate and well-localized *pain*, rapid *swelling, crepitus* on motion, increased pain on motion, limitation of motion, and so forth.

There may also be symptoms of associated injury to underlying vital structures. Pneumothorax may cause dyspnea; brachial plexus injury may cause upper limb pain and paresthesias; and so forth.

PHYSICAL EXAMINATION

Even though the skeletal injury may be strikingly evident, attention must first be directed to ruling out associated life- or limb-threatening injury (see part A).

The most common serious complication is laceration of the subclavian artery, which is evidenced by a large, rapidly expanding, or pulsatile hematoma. The pulsatile nature of the mass can sometimes best be demonstrated by holding a tongue depressor on top of it to amplify the movement.

There may be obvious *deformity*, with anterior and superior angulation.

and possibly penetration of the skin by a fracture fragment. Other physical findings are for the most part those usually associated with long-bone fractures, i.e., *point tenderness* over the fracture site, *false motion*, *crepitus* with motion, pain with motion, and so forth.

RADIOGRAPHIC EXAMINATION

Radiographic treatment is indicated initially to assess position and alignment and in follow-up also to assess the extent of healing.

INITIAL TREATMENT

Immediate treatment of life-threatening complications, e.g., thoracentesis for decompression of a tension pneumothorax, might be required. Such measures are undertaken as the problems are identified.

Open fractures should be débrided of gross contamination, covered with a moist saline dressing, and immobilized "as is." Tetanus prophylaxis should be undertaken according to standard guidelines. Prophylactic antibiotics should be administered only as directed by the consulting orthopedist.

With displaced, angulated, comminuted, or overriding *closed fractures of the proximal and middle thirds* of the clavicle, the position and alignment can usually be improved, though not always completely corrected, by retraction of the shoulder girdles. This should be done with care, particularly if a fracture fragment is tenting the skin, so as not to convert the closed fracture to an open one.

A figure-of-eight clavicle strap is then used to keep the shoulders back. *A clavicle strap is contraindicated for fractures distal to the point at which the strap crosses the clavicle.* It tends to displace, rather than reduce, such fractures.

Initial treatment may also include the use of a sling (in addition to the clavicle strap) and intermittent icing until swelling has stabilized.

REFERRAL

Severe vascular injury may require surgical exploration. If such injury is suspected, referral should be made on an emergent basis to a major center with angiographic and cardiovascular/thoracic surgical capabilities.

Orthopedic referral on an urgent basis is indicated for all open fractures. Otherwise, orthopedic referral is required only for complications, e.g., nonunion.

DEFINITIVE TREATMENT

The standard treatment of proximal- and middle-third clavicle fractures is closed reduction by retraction of the shoulder girdle or girdles, "immobilization" in a figure-of-eight clavicle strap for 6 weeks or so, and complete rehabilitation of the shoulder before resumption of strenuous activity.

When clinical union has occurred *and* some callus has formed, the clavicle strap is discontinued. A sling is used for an additional week or so. The athlete is then allowed to resume noncontact, nonthrowing activities as tolerated.

Complete shoulder rehabilitation is recommended before resumption of throwing and racquet sports, swimming, and so forth. Complete shoulder rehabilitation and radiographic union are recommended before the athlete resumes contact and collision sports, including bicycle racing and horseback riding, as well as football and wrestling.

Both of us are admitted therapeutic nihilists when it comes to these fractures. With standard treatment, complete bony union is the rule, even for severely comminuted fractures. However, most individuals beyond the age of close maternal supervision will not keep a clavicle strap sufficiently tight to maintain end-to-end apposition of the fracture fragments. Accordingly, although nondisplaced fractures remain nondisplaced, displaced fractures almost invariably heal with some overriding or angulation, or both.

Open reduction and internal fixation may seem tempting in the case of the athlete who "must" return to competition as soon as possible, but it is fraught with complications. Nonunion, which is rare with closed treatment, is not uncommon with open treatment. Other possible complications include infection and even death, e.g., as a result of migration of a Steinmann pin or Kirschner wire into the heart or one of the great vessels.

The important fact to remember about clavicle fractures is that *less than anatomical reduction is primarily of cosmetic, rather than functional, significance*. With appropriate rehabilitation, return without impairment to strenuous and demanding use of the upper limb, e.g., baseball pitching or gymnastics, is the rule.

With this in mind, the treatment alternatives can be put in proper perspective. The goal should not be a normal-appearing x-ray film, but rather avoidance of complications, and safe return to sports participation. Clearly, the standard treatment, with some precautions, is the best choice for the athlete. The figure-of-eight clavicle strap should be used to provide comfort, some protection, and an improved, although not necessarily anatomical, position of the fracture fragments. It need not, and should not, be applied so tightly that it causes skin breakdown, edema, paresthesias, pain, or other problems.

Figure-of-eight clavicular braces should not be used for fractures of the distal clavicle, as they would tend to further displace these fractures.

F. ACROMIOCLAVICULAR SPRAINS ("SHOULDER SEPARATIONS")

HISTORY

MECHANISM AND GRADING OF INJURY. The typical mechanism of an acromioclavicular sprain is a *direct blow to the superior aspect of the acromion*, such as may occur in a fall onto the point of the shoulder or in being struck there by an opponent's helmet. The force thus produced tends to drive the scapula inferiorly away from the clavicle. This force is resisted mainly by the coracoclavicular ligaments. Acromioclavicular injury is less commonly produced by direct blows to the clavicle or by indirect forces, such as may occur with falls onto the elbow or outstretched hand.

The extent of acromioclavicular separation depends on the amount of force applied and the corresponding degree of injury to the coracoclavicular ligaments. Allman classified acromioclavicular sprains as grades I, II, and III, representing, respectively, no involvement, partial tearing, and complete disruption of the coracoclavicular ligaments.[4] More recently, Rockwood and colleagues have further classified the more severe injuries as grades III through VI, depending on the direction and amount of acromioclavicular displacement and the extent of associated injury to the deltoid and trapezius muscles (Fig. 4–26).[43]

From a practical point of view, the grading of acromioclavicular injuries is perhaps much ado about nothing. It has been emphasized mainly by those orthopedists who advocate "definitive" treatment of grade III injuries. As discussed later, we believe grades I through III acromioclavicular injuries are best initially treated nonoperatively.

PHYSICAL EXAMINATION

The hallmark physical finding is *point tenderness over the acromioclavicular joint*. Tenderness over the *coracoclavicular space* is characteristic of grade II and III injuries and differentiates these injuries from grade I injuries and contusions ("shoulder pointers").

With complete disruption of the coracoclavicular ligaments (grade III sprains), there may be obvious deformity ("high-riding clavicle" or, more correctly, "low-riding scapula"). However, an absence of this sign does not rule out grade III sprain, as muscle spasm can minimize the extent of acromioclavicular separation.

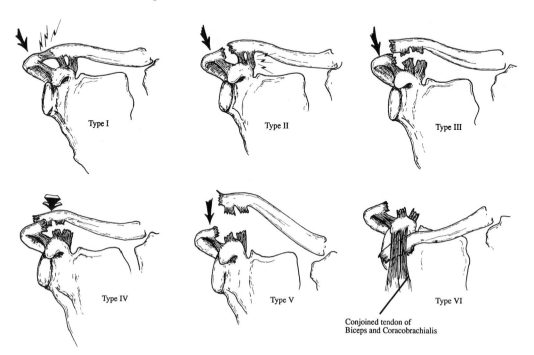

Conjoined tendon of
Biceps and Coracobrachialis

Figure 4–26. Classification of acromioclavicular sprains, as described by Allman[4] and Rockwood and colleagues.[43] Arrow depicts direction of the injuring force.

RADIOGRAPHIC EXAMINATION

Radiographic examination is indicated to differentiate acromioclavicular sprain from distal clavicle fracture. A "trauma series" (see "Trauma Series" Radiographs in part C) suffices for this purpose, although acromioclavicular views are equally appropriate.

Many orthopedists and radiologists recommend stress views of the acromioclavicular joints whenever the clinical findings are suggestive of grade III or higher acromioclavicular sprains. These AP views of the acromioclavicular joints should be obtained with 5 to 15 lb of weight *suspended* from the patient's wrists. The coracoclavicular distance is measured on the injured and uninjured sides. A difference of 5 mm or more is considered diagnostic of complete disruption of the coracoclavicular ligaments (grade III sprain). Because of the likelihood of false-negative radiographs owing to incorrect technique, and because we generally treat all acromioclavicular sprains the same, we do not routinely order these films.

INITIAL TREATMENT

Initial treatment is *symptomatic* and consists of rest (sling or shoulder immobilizer p.r.n.), ice, and analgesics as required. Urgent treatment is required only in the rare event of neurovascular impairment or grade IV through VI sprains.

REFERRAL

Athletes should be informed of the possible sequelae of acromioclavicular injury (deformity, degenerative joint disease) and the options regarding primary or delayed surgical treatment.[37] Athletes should be referred to an orthopedist if they are unwilling to accept the cosmetic deformity of an overly prominent distal clavicle or if they are unwilling to "allow the shoulder to recover from the acute injury and then see if it still hurts."

REHABILITATION

Rehabilitation is carried out as discussed in Rehabilitative Treatment of Shoulder Overuse Injuries in part M. Specific strengthening exercises for the upper trapezius, such as shoulder shrugs with Theraband or weights, are also important.[23]

DEFINITIVE TREATMENT

Our *preferred method* of treating acute acromioclavicular injuries is *initial symptomatic treatment*, as discussed previously, followed by *complete shoulder rehabilitation*, and *operative treatment only if residual symptoms warrant it*.

Definitive treatment is, to say the least, controversial. We tend to agree with Nicol[40] and others[23, 28] that nonoperative treatment cannot achieve the unattainable (restoration of a normal joint), and that primary operative treatment is rarely justified. Acromioclavicular injuries of all grades are associated with some risk of subsequent degenerative joint disease and chronic pain.[11, 43] However, this complication can be satisfactorily treated by resection of the distal clavicle, which need not be done a priori.[37] Furthermore, failure to reconstruct the acromioclavicular joint has not been found to result in impaired strength or functional use of the arm.[23, 28, 57] Indeed, it would appear that the only significant differences in operative and nonoperative treatment of grade III sprains are a longer recovery time with operative treatment, a decreased risk of chronic pain if the distal clavicle is resected, and a trade-off between deformity and surgical scar.

Accordingly, we believe that operative treatment is "definitive" only in the sense that it may prevent or effectively treat chronic pain. When operation is indicated, the procedure of choice involves resection of the distal clavicle as described by Mumford,[37] repair of any trapezius or deltoid tears, reduction of the clavicular displacement, and maintenance of the reduction with a tethering coracoclavicular tape. We have found the results of this operation to be quite satisfactory.

G. ACUTE, TRAUMATIC ANTERIOR GLENOHUMERAL DISLOCATION

HISTORY

MECHANISM OF INJURY. The characteristic mechanism of injury is indirect trauma—*forced abduction and external rotation*, such as may occur in arm tackling in football or in falls onto the abducted, externally rotated arm. Direct trauma to the shoulder is a less common mechanism of injury.

SYMPTOMS. Especially with first-time dislocations, athletes are in obvious distress. They are invariably quite unwilling to continue any athletic activity. They may or may not be aware that the shoulder is "out of place."

PHYSICAL EXAMINATION

The injured arm is *held in an abducted, externally rotated position*, supported if possible by the uninjured arm. Any shoulder motion, particularly *internal rotation, is painful and resisted* by the athlete. The normal rounded contour of the shoulder is lost. The *acromion is inordinately prominent*, with an indentation beneath it, as shown in Figure 4–3. Examination usually also reveals an anterior fullness caused by the anteriorly displaced humeral head. These findings can usually be appreciated by palpation, e.g., under shoulder pads, as well as by inspection.

Assessment of the neurovascular status of the limb is important. Blom and Dahlback reported a 33% incidence of nerve injury with acute anterior dislocations.[13] In patients older than 50 years, the incidence was nearly 50%. Any of the nerves of the brachial plexus can be injured; however, the axillary nerve is particularly at risk. The most reliable clinical test for axillary nerve function is gentle isometric testing of the deltoid muscle (see Fig. 4–5). The significance of nerve injury complicating anterior dislocation would appear to be that rehabilitation is likely to be prolonged. With diligent rehabilitation, eventual full recovery should be expected.

Assessment for possible associated rotator cuff injury is also very important (see part J).

RADIOGRAPHIC EXAMINATION

A "trauma series," consisting of AP and lateral scapular views, should be obtained "as is," i.e., without moving the arm (see "Trauma Series" Radiographs in part C and Fig. 4–20).

Prereduction films are not always required. If the clinical diagnosis of anterior dislocation can be made, and if growth plate injury is unlikely (high school age or older athlete), then gentle reduction may be attempted on the playing field or in the locker room.[35, 48] In all cases, postreduction films are indicated.

OTHER DIAGNOSTIC TESTS

MRI, especially MRI arthrography, is useful for assessing the possibilities of a Bankart lesion (avulsion of the anterior labrum and capsule from the anterior glenoid)[9] or a rotator cuff injury. Acutely, however, MRI is indicated only if an extensive, surgically treatable rotator cuff tear is suspected. More commonly, MRI is carried out for chronic/recurrent instability problems unresponsive to nonoperative treatment. In either case, the decision to order MRI, with or without arthrography, is most appropriately deferred to the surgical consultant.

INITIAL TREATMENT

Acute glenohumeral dislocations should be reduced as quickly, gently, and safely as possible. Early reduction minimizes the amount of muscle spasm that must be overcome to effect reduction and thereby minimizes discomfort and the risk of further injury.

Before any attempted reduction, the physician must be certain that the dislocation is in fact acute. This is not always as obvious in the office or emergency room as it is on the playing field. Chronically dislocated shoulders may present after another acute injury.

Reduction of uncomplicated anterior dislocations can usually be achieved using the techniques of Aronen,[7] Stimson,[53] or Rockwood and Wirth.[45] Each of these techniques is based on the principle of traction and countertraction, and all are safe. We agree with others[18, 45] that leverage techniques, such as the Kocher maneuver,[32] entail an unacceptable risk of further injury to the soft tissues and the articular surface of the humerus. *The use of brute force, levering, or yanking on the arm is contraindicated.* The primary care physician who is unfamiliar with any of the recommended techniques should defer the reduction of the shoulder to an orthopedist.

Of the three recommended techniques, those of Aronen and Stimson are logistically quite simple. They are most useful when reduction is relatively easily achieved, as is usually the case with multiply recurrent dislocations or immediately after injury, before much swelling and muscle spasm have occurred. Both techniques have the advantage of sometimes enabling patients to carry out the reductions by themselves. We make it a practice to teach the Aronen technique to our patients who have sustained shoulder dislocations, as self-reduction may be the only method available to them in certain situations, e.g., solo sailing, backpacking, cross-country skiing, and surfing.

In the technique described by Aronen, the patient is instructed to clasp the hands about the (ipsilateral) knee and then to relax the shoulder muscles, allowing the weight of the lower limb to provide gentle in-line traction on the upper limb as the hip is extended (Fig. 4–27). Countertraction is provided by the patient's own (paraspinous) muscles.

In the Stimson technique, the patient lies prone on a flat surface (examining table, automobile hood, boulder, and so forth) with the injured limb hanging over the side. Traction is applied by weight suspended from the wrist; countertraction is provided by the flat surface. It is important that the weight be tied to the wrist (two half-hitch knots), as opposed to being held by the patient (which would preclude desired relaxation of the muscles of the upper limb). The amount of weight suspended from the wrist depends on the size of the patient. Five pounds is usually sufficient.

With "difficult reductions," e.g., a first-time dislocation in a heavily muscled athlete, the Stimson technique tends to be, at best, rather time-consuming. Standard advice is that the patient be left "undisturbed" for at least 20 minutes. We would caution, however, that the patient *not* be heavily sedated and then left *"unattended."* If reduction is achieved, there will be a dramatic reduction in the level of pain. Without that stimulus, the heavily sedated patient may very well lose consciousness (see later discussion).

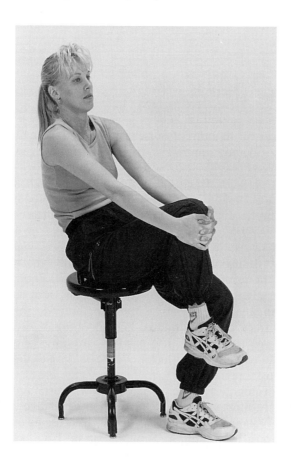

Figure 4–27. The technique of self-reduction of anterior dislocation of the shoulder, as described by Aronen.[7] With her hands clasped about her (ipsilateral) knee, the patient herself applies gentle in-line traction to the dislocated shoulder by extending her hip.

In the Rockwood technique, the patient is supine. A swathe (towel, stockinette, or folded sheet) is placed around the torso and as high up in the (ipsilateral) axilla as possible. An assistant (on the opposite side) holds the free ends. Manual in-line traction on the injured limb is then gently applied and gradually increased against the countertraction provided by the axillary swathe. With adequate analgesia/muscle relaxation, reduction is usually very readily achieved. Sometimes, in addition to this basic maneuver, very slight internal and external rotation or lateral traction may be required.

Although Rockwood's technique does require more "manpower" in most situations—on the playing field, in the locker room, in the office, or in the emergency department—an assistant or two capable of holding a swathe are usually not hard to find. The technique is safe, effective, and expedient. That the patient is not "left alone" is probably an advantage.

Shortly after injury, reduction may be attempted without medication. However, if reduction cannot be readily achieved, or if more than 1 hour has elapsed after the injury, analgesia and sedation are indicated. We recommend starting an intravenous line with Ringer's lactate and administering sufficient intravenous narcotic to obtain good analgesia and sedation. (Usual adult dosages are meperidine 50 mg intravenously [IV] or morphine 5 mg IV.) Intravenous midazolam (Versed) may be administered to attain conscious sedation/muscle relaxation. (The usual adult dosage is 1 to 2.5 mg IV, titrated slowly to the desired effect.) After reduction has been achieved and the pain stimulus is no longer present, the patient may be excessively sedated. Naloxone should be available to reverse the sedative effects of the narcotic analgesic, if necessary.

After reduction, the neurovascular status of the limb is reassessed, the arm is placed in a sling or Velpeau type shoulder immobilizer, and the radiographic examination of the shoulder is repeated. (Shoulder immobilization, i.e., strict limitation of abduction and external rotation, is continued as discussed later.)

Unreduced dislocations should be padded and splinted "as is." Slings are inappropriate for unreduced anterior dislocations, because their application requires internal rotation of the shoulder.

Intermittent icing (i.e., application of crushed ice for 20 minutes at least once every 4 waking hours) is appropriate, whether or not reduction has been achieved. It is continued until any swelling stabilizes.

REFERRAL

Referral to an appropriate facility on an emergent basis is indicated for fractures or dislocations complicated by vascular impairment. Orthopedic referral on an urgent basis is indicated for unreduced glenohumeral dislocations.

Orthopedic referral is also recommended for dislocations complicated by nerve injury. Although most such injuries appear to be neurapraxias, and surgical exploration is generally not indicated, it is prudent to defer their management to the specialist.

Fractures of the greater tuberosity of the humerus are frequently associated with anterior dislocations and are usually anatomically reduced when the dislocation is reduced. If they remain more than 1 cm displaced after reduction of the dislocation, orthopedic referral is indicated.[35, 38]

REHABILITATIVE TREATMENT

Many first-time anterior dislocations can be definitively treated by *immobilization* (i.e., strict limitation of abduction and external rotation) and *complete shoulder rehabilitation*, as discussed later.

The principal overall objective of treatment is to prevent chronic/recurrent instability. Specific, sequential, intermediate objectives are

To keep the avulsed/torn tissues approximated so as to permit healing
To strengthen the muscles, especially the subscapularis, that act as dynamic restraints against hyperabduction/external rotation
To restore normal glenohumeral/scapulothoracic patterns of motion
To strengthen all intrinsic shoulder and scapular-stabilizing muscles

All of these should be accomplished before a return to shoulder-strenuous activity is attempted. (The principal objective of treatment notwithstanding, all patients who have sustained an acute dislocation should be taught the Aronen technique of self-reduction, in case there should be a recurrent injury.)

Based on known principles of wound healing, knowledge gained from arthroscopic treatment of chronic/recurrent shoulder instability, and various outcome studies,[5, 8, 14, 42, 47, 60] we believe that the shoulder should be immobilized for 6 weeks after injury to afford the best chance of healing, and this is in fact what we recommend for our athletic patients younger than 20 years. We hedge a bit for older patients because of the decreasing risk of recurrent instability and increasing risk of "frozen shoulder" with increasing age. For 20- to 30-year-olds, we keep the shoulder immobilized 5 weeks; for 30- to 40-year-olds, 4 weeks; for 40- to 50-year-olds, 3 weeks; and for patients older than 50, we mobilize the shoulder as soon as symptoms permit. During the period of immobilization, the immobilizer may be removed only for prescribed isometric exercises (in which the shoulder is kept adducted and internally rotated) or bathing. It should not be removed for sleeping.

Usually within a few days of the injury, the athlete is no longer in much pain and is reluctant to stay in the immobilizer. *The essential therapeutic task is to convince the athlete that the only good chance of success with nonoperative treatment is to comply strictly with the rehabilitation protocol.* Everyone involved—primary care provider, athletic trainer, team physician, physical therapist, and coach—needs to reinforce this. Compliance is enhanced by reminding the athlete of teammates or acquaintances who either have chronic/recurrent shoulder problems or have had to have surgery for the same.

It has been commonly held that the young athlete who has sustained an anterior dislocation is at very high risk of recurrent dislocation. McLaughlin and MacLellan[36] and Rowe and Sakellarides[49] reported 80% to 95% recurrence rates in patients younger than 20 years.

Recurrence is perhaps related in part to pathoanatomy. It has been reported that recurrent dislocation is more likely with labral detachment types of injury than with capsular tear types.[33] It has also been reported that recurrence is less likely in dislocations associated with fractures of the greater tuberosity.[36]

It appears, however, that the likelihood of recurrence is also importantly related to the specifics of treatment and rehabilitation. In contrast to the studies noted previously are the excellent results reported by Yoneda and coworkers[60] and Aronen and Regan,[8] who have emphasized specific strengthening exercises, as well as the avoidance of abduction (Figs. 4–28 through

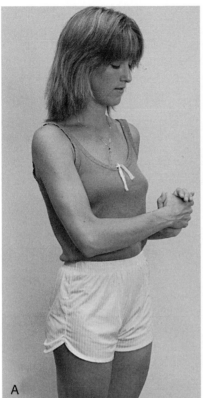

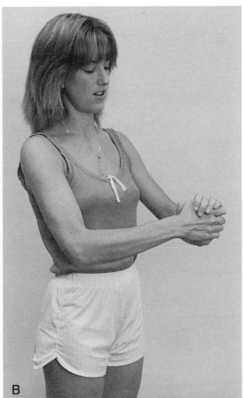

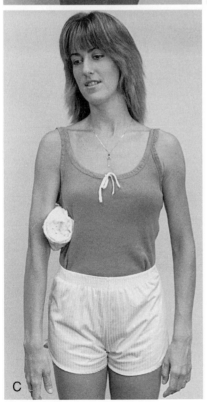

Figure 4–28. *A,* Initial isometric internal rotation exercise as described by Aronen and Regan.[8] The hand of the injured limb is kept close to the body, and the uninjured limb provides the resistance. *B,* As pain-free motion increases, the exercise is performed with the hand farther away from the body. *C,* Isometric adduction exercise. A towel is placed between the torso and the arm.

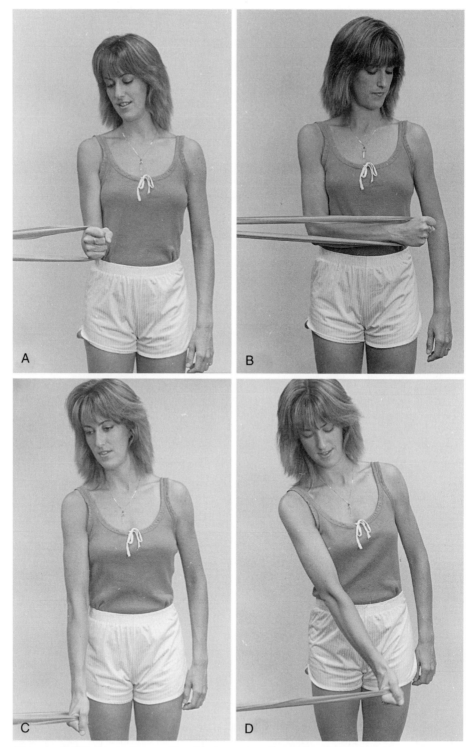

Figure 4–29. Limited-range Theraband exercises for internal rotation and adduction as described by Aronen and Regan.[8] *A*, Start position for internal rotation. *B*, Finish position for internal rotation. *C*, Start position for adduction. *D*, Finish position for adduction.

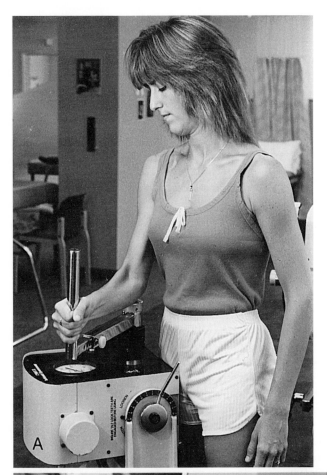

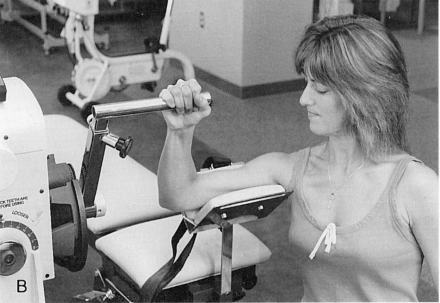

Figure 4–30. Limited isokinetic internal rotation exercises as described by Aronen and Regan.[8] *A,* With the shoulder adducted. *B,* With the shoulder in 90 degrees of flexion. The athlete avoids abduction and external rotation by facing the machine.

4–30). These authors have shown that with appropriate rehabilitation, even the young athlete who intends to return to vigorous athletic activity should have a 75% or better chance of having no subsequent instability.

Ideally, a return to sports participation is simply the final step in the sequence of rehabilitation. There should be full restoration of motion without pain, apprehension, or instability; there should be full restoration of strength as determined by isokinetic testing; and, finally, there should be a gradual resumption of activity as tolerated.

With shoulder injuries, the physician should resist letting athletes return to their sports before full rehabilitation has been carried out. Particularly with dislocations, the risk of reinjury and the consequences of reinjury are too great. At best, athletes only invite overuse injury if they attempt strenuous use of the shoulder before sufficient strength and flexibility have been restored.

With anterior dislocations, abduction- and external rotation–limiting harnesses are sometimes used when, for example, football line play is resumed. These should be used in addition to, rather than in substitution for, adequate rehabilitation.

DEFINITIVE TREATMENT

Recurrent shoulder dislocation is definitively treated by *surgical reconstruction* of the shoulder. Indications are discussed later.

In most handed sports, recurrent shoulder dislocation would be unacceptable. In some, such as rock climbing, it could be life-threatening. The athlete at substantial risk for recurrent dislocation seems to have only two logical choices: limit/modify the athletic activity or undergo surgical treatment.

However, not all authors agree about which athletes are at substantial risk for recurrent dislocation. We do not share the opinion of those who believe that a single dislocation in a young athlete most likely dooms the athlete to recurrent dislocations, and we submit that the extent to which a second dislocation implies substantial risk of recurrence depends on individual circumstances.

A second dislocation is less likely to pose significant risk if more than 1 year has elapsed since the initial dislocation, if there was inadequate rehabilitation after the first dislocation, or if the recurrent dislocation was the result of significant trauma, i.e., force greater than or equal to that which produced the original injury. On the other hand, a true pattern of instability is established if a recurrent dislocation or dislocations occur with increasing ease, i.e., if less force is required to produce the dislocations, if reductions are achieved with increasing ease, and if associated symptoms become less severe. A radiographically or MRI-confirmed Bankart or Hill-Sachs lesion would also imply an increased likelihood of recurrence.

In athletes with recurrent shoulder dislocation, the most common structural abnormality is the fibrocartilaginous Bankart lesion, and the operative procedure of choice in most cases is a Bankart repair. The anterior labrum, capsule, and ligaments are sewed back down to the neck and rim of the bony glenoid, eliminating the potential space into which the humeral head can slip (see Fig. 4–24).

H. ACUTE/RECURRENT ANTERIOR GLENOHUMERAL SUBLUXATION

Subluxation is perhaps best defined as transient displacement of the head of the humerus with respect to the glenoid fossa, associated with momentary disruption of shoulder function.[35] Since first described by Blazina and Satzman,[12] it has been increasingly recognized as an important problem in athletes.[6, 41, 50, 58]

Symptoms and signs of acute shoulder subluxation tend to be underwhelming, and the first, even the first few, occurrences of glenohumeral subluxation are liable to be dismissed by athletes, their coaches, and oftentimes indeed their physicians as inconsequential. For athletes in handed sports, however, recurrent subluxation seems to us to be at least as disabling as recurrent dislocation, and once a pattern of recurrent subluxation has been established, the chance of success with nonoperative treatment is considerably diminished. *Accordingly, any shoulder injury in which there is a history of a forced abduction external rotation mechanism of injury, perceived frank instability, or "dead arm" symptoms should be considered as probable acute anterior glenohumeral subluxation and treated accordingly.*

HISTORY

MECHANISM OF INJURY. The mechanism of injury is the same as previously noted for acute, traumatic anterior dislocation, i.e., *forced abduction and external rotation.*

SYMPTOMS. Pain associated with the acute injury is usually not very severe or prolonged and may be quite transient.

A perception of *frank instability*—"My shoulder went out of place and then popped back in"—is, in our experience, virtually always accurate. (Patients do not always volunteer this information and should be specifically asked about it.) However, an absence of frank instability symptoms does not rule out the possibility of acute subluxation. Some patients are aware only that they somehow hurt their shoulders or arms.

A characteristic, but not pathognomonic, associated symptom is the sensation that "the arm's going dead."[12, 50] This symptom may also occur with cervical spine or brachial plexus injury or with the thoracic outlet syndrome.[50, 54]

Symptoms of recurrent subluxation are positional *pain, apprehension, or frank instability.* Instability is likely to be perceived and described as painful "clicking" or "slipping out of place."

As the shoulder becomes increasingly unstable, the athlete is likely to become increasingly *apprehensive* about those motions that reproduce the symptoms. Symptoms occurring with repetitive abduction, and external rotation motions, such as the cocking phase of throwing or serving, are characteristic of anterior instability.

PHYSICAL EXAMINATION

With acute injury, appreciable swelling and ecchymosis are uncommon, and anterior tenderness is usually not very marked.

The hallmark finding of anterior instability is a *positive containment test* (see Tests of Glenohumeral Instability in part B and Fig. 4–17). With the typical "thrower's shoulder," there is increased external rotation reflecting anterior laxity and decreased internal rotation reflecting posterior contracture (see Fig. 4–37).

There may also be pain, apprehension, or frank instability with combined abduction and external rotation or horizontal extension of the shoulder and a painful arc of combined glenohumeral/scapulothoracic abduction with the shoulder externally rotated more so than with it internally rotated.

RADIOGRAPHIC EXAMINATION

Radiographic examination is indicated. The radiographic findings associated with anterior instability are the Bankart lesion, a defect of the anteroinferior aspect of the glenoid rim, and the Hill-Sachs lesion, an impression defect of the posterolateral aspect of the humeral head.

OTHER DIAGNOSTIC TESTS

The diagnostic imaging test of choice for chronic/recurrent instability is MRI arthrography (see Fig. 4–24). The decision to order MRI, however, is most appropriately deferred to the surgical consultant.

REHABILITATIVE TREATMENT

Rehabilitative treatment follows precisely that discussed previously for shoulder dislocation (see Rehabilitative Treatment in part G and Table 4–3).

Many first-time anterior subluxations can be definitively treated by nonoperative means. *The essential therapeutic task is to convince athletes that their only good chance of success with nonoperative treatment is to comply strictly with the treatment protocol*, a difficult task indeed, given the paucity of symptoms and signs and the general underappreciation of the injury. The primary treating physician is *critically* important in initiating appropriate intervention.

REFERRAL AND DEFINITIVE TREATMENT

If, despite complete rehabilitation, disabling pain, apprehension, or frank instability persists, then orthopedic referral is indicated. Operative treatment is essentially as discussed for recurrent dislocation (see Definitive Treatment in part G). It may include both labral débridement and Bankart repair and is guided by the MRI arthrographic and intraoperative findings.

Table 4–3. MODIFIED ARONEN[8] PROTOCOL FOR SHOULDER DISLOCATION/SUBLUXATION

Level 0 (Immediate Postinjury* or Postoperative†)

Objectives:

Maintain approximation of avulsed/torn tissues

Facilitate healing without abnormal laxity

Protect repair

Rx:

Shoulder immobilizer, continuous except for robing/disrobing, bathing

Instruction re techniques for maintaining adducted, internally rotated position when robing/
   disrobing, bathing

Analgesics, anti-inflammatory medication p.r.n.

Modalities to limit/reduce swelling

Isometric adduction, internal rotation sets as tolerated

Activities permitted:

Virtually no ipsilateral upper limb exercise/handed activities

Lower-limb and contralateral upper-limb exercise as tolerated

Criteria for advancement (generally to level I):

Time as specified by specific protocol, treating physician

Level IA (Immediate Postimmobilization)

Objectives:

Protect from excessive abduction, external rotation, horizontal extension force

Restore endurance and strength of muscles, especially subscapularis, that act as dynamic
   restraints against hyperabduction/external rotation

Restore/maintain scapular-stabilizing muscle endurance, strength, and function

Rx:

Theraband and isokinetic progressive resistance exercises, adduction and internal rotation in
   adduction, as tolerated

Level I AROM exercises (avoid AAROM and PROM/mobilization techniques)

Level I isometric "scap sets"

Activities permitted:

Noncontact sports involving essentially sagittal plane shoulder motion, e.g., running

Criteria for advancement:

Strength and muscle endurance comparable to contralateral side in adduction and internal
   rotation in adduction

Level II

Objectives:

Protect from excessive abduction, external rotation, horizontal extension force

Restore endurance and strength of muscles, especially subscapularis, that act as dynamic
   restraints against hyperabduction/external rotation

Restore/maintain scapular-stabilizing muscle endurance, strength, and function

Restore/maintain intrinsic shoulder muscle endurance

Rx:

Progressive resistance exercise, internal rotation in 90° flexion, as tolerated

Additional progressive resistance exercise for infraspinatus, external rotation in adduction, as
   tolerated

Level I AROM exercises:

   Manual and biofeedback techniques for dynamic scapular-stabilizing muscle function

   Level II Theraband progressive resistance exercises for scapular-stabilizing muscles, as
      tolerated

   Upper limb endurance exercise, e.g., Cybex Upper Body Exercise Machine, rowing, rope
      skipping, as tolerated

Activities permitted:

Same as I

Criteria for advancement:

Strength and muscle endurance comparable to contralateral side in internal rotation in 90°
   flexion

I. ACUTE, TRAUMATIC, POSTERIOR GLENOHUMERAL SUBLUXATION

HISTORY

MECHANISM OF INJURY. In contrast to posterior glenohumeral dislocation, which is rare in sports, posterior subluxation is not uncommon. The principal

Table 4–3. MODIFIED ARONEN[8] PROTOCOL FOR SHOULDER DISLOCATION/SUBLUXATION *Continued*

Level III

Objectives:
  Protection from excessive abduction, external rotation, horizontal extension force
  Strengthen muscles, especially subscapularis, that act as dynamic restraints against
    hyperabduction/external rotation
Rx:
  Progressive resistance exercise, internal rotation in 90° abduction, as tolerated
  Additional progressive resistance exercise for rotator cuff, as tolerated
  Level II AAROM and mobilization techniques
Activities permitted:
  Moderately arm-strenuous daily, occupational, and athletic activities with arm elevation
    limited <90° (e.g., tennis ground stroke practice)
Criteria for advancement:
  Strength and muscle endurance comparable to contralateral side in internal rotation in 90°
    abduction

AROM, active range-of-motion; AAROM, active-assistive range-of-motion; PROM, passive range-of-motion.
  *For example, acute, traumatic glenohumeral dislocation/subluxation.
  †For example, Bankart's reconstruction.

mechanism of injury is axial loading of the arm with the shoulder flexed or horizontally flexed. The force may be applied to the olecranon or ulnar forearm, such as may occur with blocking in football, or it may be applied further distally, such as with a fall onto the outstretched hand.

SYMPTOMS. Pain associated with the acute injury is typically more severe than with acute anterior subluxation, usually sufficient to cause the athlete to seek medical attention.

A perception of *frank instability*—"My shoulder went out of place and then popped back in"—is, in our experience, virtually always accurate. However, an absence of frank instability symptoms does not rule out the possibility of acute subluxation.

Recurrent instability is typically perceived and described as "clicking" or "slipping out of place" with horizontal flexion movements.

PHYSICAL EXAMINATION

A painful click may be appreciated with active or passive motion. There is likely to be pain, localized posteriorly, not superiorly, with "acromioclavicular compression tests" (see Acromioclavicular/Sternoclavicular Compression Tests in part B and Fig. 4–12). Pain, click, and frank subluxation may be found with a posterior drawer test (Fig. 4–31).

RADIOGRAPHIC EXAMINATION

Radiographic examination is indicated. With posterior instability there may be an impression defect of the anteromedial part of the humeral head. The defect is best visualized in a standard axillary view. It corresponds to the Hill-Sachs lesion with anterior dislocation and is sometimes referred to as a "reverse Hill-Sachs lesion." A more common finding with posterior instability is a

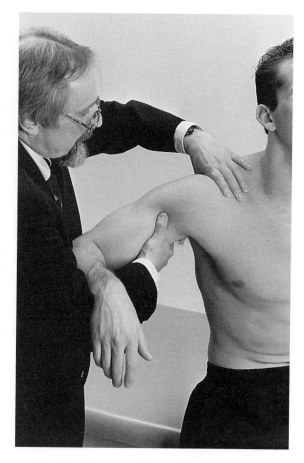

Figure 4–31. Examination of the (right) shoulder for posterior instability, the posterior drawer test.[21] The athlete is seated with his right forearm resting comfortably on the examiner's right forearm. The scapula is stabilized by the examiner's left hand. The shoulder is in 90-degree abduction and neutral rotation. With his right hand, the examiner applies backward pressure on the proximal arm, noting any symptoms or subluxation produced. The pressure is slight, comparable to that used in the Lachman test of the knee.

defect or irregularity of the posterior glenoid rim, the "reverse Bankart lesion," seen best on AP views (Fig. 4–32).

OTHER DIAGNOSTIC TESTS

The diagnostic imaging test of choice for chronic/recurrent instability is MRI arthrography. The decision to order this test, however, is most appropriately deferred to the surgical consultant.

INITIAL AND REHABILITATIVE TREATMENT

The initial and rehabilitative treatment is similar to that previously discussed for anterior shoulder dislocation and subluxation.

With posterior instability the shoulder is unstable with horizontal flexion. However, if it is kept adducted, it is not usually unstable with internal rotation. Accordingly, the acute injury is immobilized in adduction and internal rotation just as for anterior instability.

Postimmobilization rehabilitation follows the rehabilitation protocol presented in Rehabilitative Treatment of Shoulder Overuse Injuries in part M and Table 4–4.

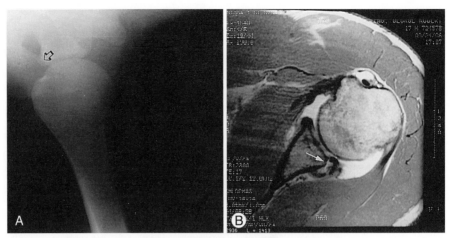

Figure 4–32. AP radiograph *(A)* and MRI arthrogram axial section *(B)* demonstrating an intraarticular fracture of the posterior glenoid (arrows) associated with acute, traumatic posterior shoulder subluxation in an 18-year-old high school football down lineman.

REFERRAL AND DEFINITIVE TREATMENT

If, despite complete rehabilitation, disabling pain, apprehension, or frank instability persists, then orthopedic referral is indicated. Operative treatment is similar to that discussed for recurrent anterior dislocation (see Definitive Treatment in part G). A "reverse Bankart lesion" may be repaired similarly to the anterior fibrocartilaginous Bankart lesion.

J. ACUTE OR ACUTE-ON-DEGENERATIVE TEARS OF THE ROTATOR CUFF

HISTORY

ANATOMY AND MECHANISMS OF INJURY. The rotator cuff comprises four muscles (subscapularis, supraspinatus, infraspinatus, and teres minor) and their tendons. Acting as a force couple with larger muscles that insert farther distally on the humerus (deltoid, pectoralis major, and latissimus dorsi), the rotator cuff and long head of the biceps maintain the axes of shoulder motion centered at the glenohumeral joint.

Tears of the cuff are best described as acute versus degenerative, full-thickness versus partial-thickness, and large or extensive versus small. The term *complete* as applied to cuff tears is ambiguous. Although it has been used synonymously with *full-thickness* to describe tears extending from the articular (deep) surface of the tendon completely through to the bursal (superficial) surface, it also seems to connote extensive tearing that is not always the case.

Large full-thickness tears typically occur with abrupt, forceful, eccentric loading of the cuff. A classic example is that of an individual on a ladder, stairs, rock face, gymnastics apparatus, and so forth who starts to fall and

Table 4–4. REHABILITATION PROTOCOL FOR THE SHOULDER OVERUSE SYNDROME

Level 0 (Acute Painful Episode,* Continuous or Severe Rest Pain, Severe Night Pain)

Objectives:
  Reduce pain, swelling, inflammation
Rx:
  Rest; sling or shoulder immobilizer p.r.n.
  Local anesthetic/corticosteroid injection(s)
    Intra-articular (glenohumeral and acromioclavicular), bursal, peritendinous, trigger point
  Analgesics, anti-inflammatory medication p.r.n.
  Modalities to reduce pain, limit/reduce swelling
  Gentle glenohumeral oscillatory mobilization techniques
  Gentle AAROM (e.g., limited-arc, assisted Codman's) as tolerated
  Static posture correction, isometric "scap sets," as tolerated
Activities permitted:
  Necessary manual activities of daily living and occupation as tolerated
  Active arm elevation limited to <45°
  No prolonged or repetitive arm elevation or shoulder horizontal flexion
  No lifting >10 lb (shoulder adducted)
Criteria for advancement:
  Rest/night pain substantially reduced
  Able to sleep

Level I (Activity-Limiting Pain)

Objectives:
  Reduce pain, swelling, inflammation
  Restore/maintain scapular-stabilizing muscle endurance, strength, and function
  Restore/maintain glenohumeral motion
Rx:
  Relative rest; occasional sling p.r.n. after activity pain, fatigue
  Analgesics, anti-inflammatory medication p.r.n.
  Local anesthetic/corticosteroid injection(s) p.r.n. with precaution re activity
  Modalities to reduce pain, limit/reduce swelling
  McConnell's taping
  Gentle AROM (e.g., Codman's) exercises, as tolerated
  Moderate AAROM exercises (e.g., cane and wall climb exercises), as tolerated
  Isometric "scap sets"
  Osteopathic and "muscle energy" techniques for thoracic dysfunctions
Activities permitted:
  Necessary manual activities of daily living and occupation as tolerated
  Active arm elevation limited to <60°
  No prolonged or repetitive arm elevation or shoulder horizontal flexion
  No lifting >20 lb
  Noncontact sports/exercise involving essentially sagittal plane shoulder motion, e.g.,
    running, as tolerated
Criteria for advancement:
  Activity-related pain substantially reduced
  Rest/night virtually abated

Level II (Activity-Related Pain, Performance Impairment)

Objectives:
  Reduce pain, swelling, inflammation
  Restore/maintain scapular-stabilizing muscle endurance, strength, and function
  Restore/maintain glenohumeral motion
  Restore normal basic patterns of glenohumeral/scapulothoracic motion
  Restore/maintain intrinsic shoulder muscle endurance
Rx:
  Relative test
  Anti-inflammatory medication
  Modalities to reduce pain, limit/reduce swelling
  McConnell's taping
  AROM exercises, as tolerated
  Mobilization techniques (especially posterior capsular stretching), as indicated and tolerated
  Isometric "scap sets"
  Manual and biofeedback techniques for dynamic scapular-stabilizing muscle function
  Theraband and dumbbell progressive resistance exercises for scapular-stabilizing muscles,
    biceps, and triceps as tolerated
  Upper-limb endurance exercise, e.g., UBE, rowing, rope skipping, as tolerated

Table 4–4. REHABILITATION PROTOCOL FOR THE SHOULDER OVERUSE SYNDROME *Continued*

Level II (Activity-Related Pain, Performance Impairment) *Continued*

Activities permitted:
  Active arm elevation limited to <90°
  No prolonged or repetitive arm elevation
  No lifting >50 lb
Criteria for advancement:
  Pain virtually abated
  Negative Kibler's test
  Glenohumeral ROM comparable to contralateral side
  Pain-free, symmetrical arc of combined motion

Level III (Performance Impairment)

Objectives:
  Maintain scapular-stabilizing muscle endurance, strength, and function
  Maintain glenohumeral motion
  Restore normal complex patterns of glenohumeral/scapulothoracic motion
  Restore/maintain intrinsic shoulder muscle endurance and strength
Rx:
  Relative rest
  McConnell's taping
  Stretching as indicated (attention to avoid anterior stretch)
  Isometric "scap sets"
  Manual techniques for dynamic scapular-stabilizing muscle function
  Theraband progressive resistance exercises for scapular-stabilizing muscles, as tolerated
  Upper-limb endurance exercise, e.g., Cybex Upper Body Exercise Machine, rowing, rope
    skipping, as tolerated
  Theraband and dumbbell resistance exercises (flexion, abduction, extension, scaption, 90/90)
    for intrinsic shoulder muscles, as tolerated
  "Fungo" return to throwing, serving program
Activities permitted:
  Tennis ground stroke practice, breast stroke swimming, etc.
  No overhead sports/exercise
Criteria for advancement (to full activity):
  "Fungo" program completed
  Strength on manual muscle testing comparable to contralateral shoulder

AAROM, active-assistive range-of-motion; AROM, active range-of-motion; ROM, range of motion.
*For example, calcific subacromial bursitis/rotator cuff tendinitis.

attempts to arrest the fall by maintaining a handhold. Violent trauma such as this may cause extensive tears in the young or old.

Somewhat less forceful "yanking" on the shoulder, such as may occur with attempting to lift up a heavy suitcase or having a grandchild tug on one's outstretched hand, may be sufficient to cause extensive tearing in an older individual who already has tendinosis (tendon degeneration) or partial-thickness tearing.

Partial-thickness tearing may result from less forceful acute trauma but is typically the result of repetitive trauma (see the section on functional anatomy and mechanisms of injury in Rotator Cuff Overuse Strain, Tendinitis, Tendinosis, Degenerative Tear, Insufficiency in part M).

The previously described mechanisms pertain mainly to the supraspinatus and infraspinatus. Tearing typically occurs just proximal to the insertion, or the cuff may be avulsed from its insertion. Tearing of the subscapularis is typically caused by forced abduction and external rotation. Cuff tear or avulsion or avulsion of the greater tuberosity may be associated with shoulder dislocations.

Injuries to the rotator cuff are not all easily dichotomized as acute or overuse. Attrition from aging, overuse, chronic inflammation, and tendinosis predisposes to acute injury (acute-on-degenerative tear). Conversely, chronic inflammation is often simply a sequela of acute injury that has been neglected, abused, or inadequately rehabilitated, or all of these. Either acute injury or chronic inflammation may lead to the vicious circle of muscular insufficiency, functional instability, and secondary impingement, which in turn may lead to further injury and inflammation (see Primary Impingement [Acromial, Acromioclavicular, Coracoclavicular, Coracoid] in part M).

SYMPTOMS. The characteristic presentation of acute rotator cuff tears is abrupt onset of *pain* and *weakness* (inability to elevate the arm) after forceful loading of the shoulder.

Note that rotator cuff tear associated with other injury is liable to be overlooked. For example, weakness after acute anterior glenohumeral dislocation may be the result of pain inhibition of normal muscle function, associated axillary nerve neurapraxia, or associated rotator cuff tear, or all of these. It is most important to maintain a high index of suspicion. (The differential diagnosis of profound weakness is discussed in Weakness in part A.)

PHYSICAL EXAMINATION

The hallmark findings are provoked *pain* and *weakness* with manual muscle testing (see Manual Muscle Testing in part B and Fig. 4–13). In the acute setting, with large full-thickness tears of the supraspinatus, the patient is typically *unable to initiate shoulder abduction* even against gravity resistance.

A "drop arm sign" is elicited with supraspinatus testing when the patient is able to hold the shoulder in 90 degrees of elevation ("scaption") against gravity, but with slight additional manual pressure, the shoulder abruptly gives way and the arm drops. In our experience, this finding may be elicited with any of the conditions causing profound weakness (see earlier) and is not pathognomonic of rotator cuff tear.

Abrupt or ratchet-like (cogwheel) giving-way on manual muscle testing is more characteristic of either cuff tear or pain inhibition, whereas smooth giving-way, i.e., uniform weakness throughout the range of motion, is more characteristic of neuromuscular weakness.

Point tenderness is typically localized to the greater tuberosity with acute supraspinatus and infraspinatus tears, to the lesser tuberosity with subscapularis tears. Soft tissue swelling and ecchymosis are inconsistent findings. With acute-on-degenerative tears especially, there may be very little bleeding even with extensive tearing.

Subacutely, even with extensive tears, the patient may regain the ability to elevate the arm somewhat, albeit with a grossly abnormal pattern of motion. A characteristic compensatory pattern is to use scapulothoracic motion and lateral bending of the torso to sling the arm upwards. Some patients may be able to attain and hold a position of greater than 90 degrees of combined glenohumeral/scapulothoracic abduction in this manner. However, they are unlikely to be able to attain a full range of active combined abduction.

With subscapularis tears, the patient has pain and weakness with resisted internal rotation of the shoulder. In the acute setting, there is likely to be tenderness, swelling, and ecchymosis localized anteriorly. With isolated infraspinatus tears, the patient has pain and weakness with resisted external rotation of the shoulder.

RADIOGRAPHIC EXAMINATION

Radiographic examination is indicated. Avulsion of the greater tuberosity as opposed to cuff tear may be demonstrated. Also, if the cuff injury is associated with acute shoulder dislocation or subluxation, any of the radiographic findings associated with those injuries may be present. With extensive cuff tears, a "high-riding" humeral head (superior subluxation of the humeral head relative to the glenoid fossa with diminished subacromial space) may be noted (see Fig. 4–39).

OTHER DIAGNOSTIC TESTS

Shoulder weakness can often be differentiated by selective local anesthetization as discussed in Injection/Aspiration in part B. Relief of pain but persistence of profound weakness after intra-articular injection is characteristic of large cuff tears.

The diagnostic imaging test of choice for demonstrating subtle or gross cuff tears is MRI arthrography. Gross tears can also quite reliably be demonstrated with plain arthrography or plain MRI. The decision regarding diagnostic imaging may be deferred to the surgical consultant.

INITIAL TREATMENT

The initial treatment comprises standard symptomatic and protective measures for musculotendinous injury: relative rest (the use of a sling or shoulder immobilizer p.r.n.), intermittent icing, nonsteroidal anti-inflammatory/analgesic medication, and gentle active or active assisted range-of-motion exercises as tolerated (see Rehabilitative Treatment of Shoulder Overuse Injuries in part M, Table 4-4, and Fig. 4–40).

REHABILITATION

Cuff tear does not necessarily imply a need for surgical intervention. Depending on the demands to be placed on the shoulder, many partial-thickness and small full-thickness rotator cuff tears can be very adequately treated with appropriate functional rehabilitation as discussed in Rehabilitative Treatment of Shoulder Overuse Injuries in part M. Nonoperative rehabilitative treatment can also be helpful in reducing pain and maintaining functional motion in patients with large tears who for whatever reason are not candidates for surgery.

REFERRAL AND DEFINITIVE TREATMENT

Very severe injury, e.g., complete cuff avulsion, is a clear indication for surgery in virtually any active patient. Referral on recognition of the problem is appropriate.

Large full-thickness tears with profound weakness are generally best treated surgically. Injury to the dominant side, an intended or desired return to a shoulder-strenuous occupation or sport, and a younger age are factors that favor surgical referral early on. If these factors do not pertain, the patient is averse to surgery, or the patient is a poor surgical risk, a cautious "wait-and-see" approach may be elected. In a month or so, the acute effects of the injury should have subsided; if considerable pain or disability persists, referral is indicated.

A caveat with respect to a wait-and-see approach is that over time, the torn cuff retracts proximally, the gap between the torn ends widens, and repair becomes technically more difficult. As this occurs, some patients develop worsening of their symptoms, further functional impairment, and eventually arthropathy (see Glenohumeral Degenerative Joint Disease/"Cuff Arthropathy" in part M). They (and in some cases their physicians) may belatedly come to the conclusion that surgery would have been appropriate. There is no reliable way to predict which patients will do well and which will not. Certainly, surgical options are greater and outcomes better if surgery is carried out before irreversible changes have occurred. For the primary physician, probably the best way out of this conundrum is to advise patients of the natural history and the uncertain prognosis and to consult early on if surgical treatment might ever seem to be a consideration.

Surgical repair of cuff tears most often entails sewing the proximal edge of the torn cuff down into the humerus, as opposed to sewing the tendon stumps together. Typically, to protect the repair, coracoacromial arch decompression is done at the same time. It is also important to have identified and to address any instability problem, e.g., a fibrocartilaginous Bankart lesion.

Many cases of partial-thickness tears do well with nonoperative treatment. If the patient/athlete is unable to resume a desired level of activity without recurrence of symptoms and is willing to consider surgical treatment, the patient should be referred. Surgery for partial-thickness tears is more likely to comprise cuff débridement, as opposed to cuff repair, with arch decompression and Bankart repair as may be indicated.

K. ACUTE OR ACUTE-ON-DEGENERATIVE TEARS OF THE TENDON OF THE LONG HEAD OF THE BICEPS

HISTORY

MECHANISM OF INJURY. Acute tears of the tendon of the long head of the biceps typically occur with abrupt, forceful, eccentric loading (resisted elbow extension), such as may occur with attempting to catch a heavy object slipping from one's (supinated forearm) grasp. As with rotator cuff tears, acute-on-degenerative tears can occur with lesser external forces.

SYMPTOMS. The acute rupture is commonly associated with a perceptible "pop" or tearing sensation, or both. There may be pain associated with the acute injury, or pain relief with acute tears of an inflamed tendon. Typically, the patient is aware of the characteristic ecchymosis and deformity.

PHYSICAL EXAMINATION

The hallmark physical finding is a *"Popeye" deformity* of the anterior arm (Fig. 4–33). The distal bunching up of the long (lateral) head muscle belly is accentuated with resisted elbow flexion.

Because the tendon is no longer attached at its origin, manual muscle testing is not especially pain provoking, and because of the action of synergistic muscles, there may be little or no weakness with resisted elbow flexion or forearm supination. There is likely to be weakness with Speed's test (see Manual Muscle Testing in part B and Fig. 4–14).

In the acute setting, dependent ecchymosis of the anterior and medial arm is common.

RADIOGRAPHIC EXAMINATION AND OTHER DIAGNOSTIC TESTS

Radiographic examination and other diagnostic tests are not required.

INITIAL TREATMENT

The initial treatment is symptomatic.

REHABILITATION

Specific treatment is not usually required. Any residual disuse shoulder girdle or upper-limb motion or strength deficits can usually be readily and adequately addressed with home program exercises. In the overhand athlete, shoulder overuse symptoms on a return to activity may require physical therapy emphasizing shoulder stabilization (see [Structural] Glenohumeral Laxity/Contracture in part M).

REFERRAL AND DEFINITIVE TREATMENT

Referral and definitive treatment are indicated if the patient is very concerned about cosmesis or if there is residual symptomatic glenohumeral instability

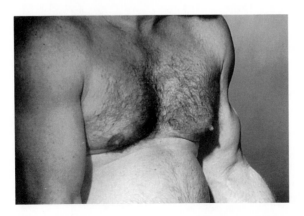

Figure 4–33. Complete rupture of the tendon of the long head of the biceps with prominent retracted muscle belly of the biceps.

unresponsive to rehabilitative treatment (see [Structural] Glenohumeral Laxity/Contracture in part M). Strength deficit is seldom a problem, even in individuals doing heavy manual labor, and is not an indication for surgical intervention. Surgical treatment typically entails tenodesis of the distal stump to the proximal humerus, not reattachment to the superior glenoid.

As discussed in part M, conditions causing degenerative tears of the tendon of the long head of the biceps are also liable to cause degenerative tears of the rotator cuff. The disabling effect of the combined injury has long been appreciated.[18, 22] Thus for the patient who has sustained an acute-on-degenerative tear of the long head of the biceps, referral for assessment of the status of the cuff may be appropriate.

L. ACROMIOCLAVICULAR DEGENERATIVE JOINT DISEASE/DISTAL CLAVICULAR OSTEOLYSIS

HISTORY

MECHANISMS OF INJURY. Acromioclavicular degenerative joint disease is commonly a sequela of acute injury. As discussed in part F, degenerative changes may follow any acute acromioclavicular sprain, regardless of grade.[4, 11, 23, 28, 37, 40, 43, 57]

In weight lifters and male gymnasts, degenerative changes may also occur without definite antecedent injury.[16] With these activities, the joint is subject to repetitive, high combined shear and compression loads.

SYMPTOMS. The hallmark symptom of acromioclavicular arthritis is activity-related, aching *pain* localized to the top of the shoulder. Pain with daily, athletic, or occupational activities, or all of these, involving horizontal flexion of the shoulder, such as occurs with swinging a baseball bat or a golf club, is characteristic. A painful arc of motion with certain weight lifts, especially overhead press, bench press, bench flies, and dips, is also typical but by no means pathognomonic. With any of these activities, the patient may note crepitation as well as pain. Positional night pain with an inability to sleep on the affected side is very common.

In addition, whether or not the joint itself is painful, acromioclavicular swelling and osteophytosis may be a cause of shoulder impingement pain (see Glenohumeral Degenerative Joint Disease/"Cuff Arthropathy" in part M).

PHYSICAL EXAMINATION

The hallmark physical findings are *point tenderness* over the acromioclavicular joint and *pain provocation with acromioclavicular joint compression tests* (see Acromioclavicular/Sternoclavicular Compression Tests in part B and Fig. 4–12). There may also be deformity from antecedent injury, palpable enlargement (effusion or osteophytosis, or both) of the joint, or crepitation with motion, or all of these.

RADIOGRAPHIC EXAMINATION

Radiographic examination is indicated. Degenerative changes of the acromioclavicular joint are usually well demonstrated on standard shoulder views as well as acromioclavicular views. Depending on the stage of the degenerative joint disease, as well as on the effects of antecedent acute injury, the joint may appear abnormally widened or narrowed. A common finding in young strength athletes is concave erosion (osteolysis) of the distal clavicle, as opposed to the osteophytosis and gonarthrosis (joint space narrowing) more typically seen in older athletes.

OTHER DIAGNOSTIC TESTS

The extent to which a given patient's shoulder pain is attributable to acromioclavicular arthritis can be confirmed by selective local anesthetic injection of the joint (see Acromioclavicular Joint in part B). A caveat for the clinician is that although postinjection pain relief is diagnostic, the converse is not true. That is, a lack of pain relief after injection of the acromioclavicular joint does not rule out acromioclavicular degenerative joint disease as a possible cause of shoulder impingement pain.

INITIAL TREATMENT

The mainstay of initial treatment is *relative rest.* This often involves only avoidance or modification of certain offending activities, such as push-ups, bench press, or overhead press. If there is pain with daily and occupational activities, then complete rest, i.e., the use of a sling, is recommended. Other initial treatment measures include nonsteroidal anti-inflammatory medication, ice massage, and physical therapy modalities.

We commonly employ local anesthetic/corticosteroid injection as a diagnostic and possibly therapeutic measure. Since the definitive treatment for chronic acromioclavicular pain is resection of the distal clavicle,[37] there is little cause for concern regarding the use of intra-articular corticosteroids when simpler measures have not afforded satisfactory relief of symptoms.

The duration of pain relief following corticosteroid injection is quite variable. For the individual who is able to limit or to modify the pain-provoking activity, e.g., a strength athlete who has pain only with overhead press at 90 degrees of shoulder abduction, the pain relief may be indefinite. For the patient who is unable or unwilling to comply with activity and rehabilitation recommendations, e.g., an individual whose occupation requires strenuous or prolonged overhead work, pain may recur within a week or two.

REHABILITATION

Associated shoulder motion and (especially deltoid and trapezius) strength deficits are rehabilitated as discussed in Rehabilitative Treatment of Shoulder Overuse Injuries in part M.

REFERRAL

In most cases, symptomatic treatment and activity modification as discussed previously permit the athlete to return to sports participation. The athlete who is unable to resume a desired level of activity without recurrence of symptoms and is willing to consider surgical treatment should be referred to an orthopedist.

DEFINITIVE TREATMENT

Chronic acromioclavicular pain is definitively treated by *resection of the distal clavicle* as described by Mumford.[37] We have found the results of this operation to be generally quite satisfactory. Patients have been able to resume heavy weight wrestling and weight training, football line play, and other very shoulder-strenuous activities without symptoms or functional impairment.

M.   SHOULDER OVERUSE SYNDROME

Shoulder overuse injuries represent maladaptations to the repetitive stresses of an activity or activities. The maladaptations may be structural or functional or both. Any of the bones and joints of the shoulder girdle, the dynamic neuromusculotendinous units acting at these joints, and the static fibrocartilaginous stabilizers of the joints may be involved.

Although "isolated" problems, e.g., rotator cuff tendinitis, do occur, much more commonly several structures/functional mechanisms are involved. The "typical" shoulder overuse injury, therefore, is a composite of several things gone awry, including structural injury or injuries, muscle dysfunctions, and failed compensatory mechanisms, each complicating the other.

Accordingly, we have come to use the term *shoulder overuse syndrome* to describe the clinical problem. Labeling the problem *tendinitis, bursitis, or impingement*, we believe, seems to focus one's attention too narrowly, too quickly, and often incorrectly. We recommend that these terms not be used as synonyms for *shoulder overuse syndrome*.*

The terms *thrower's shoulder, swimmer's shoulder, weight lifter's shoulder,* and so forth do not denote any specific diagnostic entity or entities. These terms simply connote the sports settings in which shoulder overuse injuries commonly occur.

Semantics notwithstanding, the multiple possible components of the clinical problem need to be appreciated (and, as discussed later in Rehabilitative Treatment of Shoulder Overuse Injuries, treated in proper sequence). The examiner should look for each of the following:

---

*Our concept of the pathophysiology and pathomechanics of shoulder overuse injury has evolved over time. Neer's description[39] of clinical stages with progressive deterioration of symptoms, function, and pathologic changes remains valid; however, it now seems clear that not all shoulder pain related to overhand activity is necessarily attributable to impingement of the cuff and long head of the biceps against the coracoacromial arch. Accordingly, we choose not to label overuse strain/tendinitis of the rotator cuff as "stage 1 impingement." Our term, *primary impingement*, corresponds closely to Neer's (stages 2 and 3) *impingement lesions*. Our *secondary impingement* follows the terminology of Jobe.[29]

Scapular-stabilizing muscle insufficiency/dysfunction

(Structural) glenohumeral laxity/contracture (most commonly, anterior laxity/
  posterior contracture)

Rotator cuff overuse strain, tendinitis, tendinosis, degenerative tear, insufficiency (functional glenohumeral laxity)

Long head of biceps overuse strain, tendinitis, tendinosis, degenerative tear,
  tendon subluxation, insufficiency

Acromioclavicular degenerative joint disease/distal clavicular osteolysis

Primary impingement (acromial, acromioclavicular, coracoclavicular, coracoid)

Secondary impingement (anterior, posterior, and lateral; secondary to glenohumeral laxity/contracture or rotator cuff insufficiency, or both)

Glenohumeral degenerative joint disease/"cuff arthropathy"

As is true for overuse injury in general, successful treatment and prevention of recurrence depends as much on determining the cause of the problem
as on establishing a precise diagnosis. The cause of overuse injury is virtually
always multifactorial, and three broad categories of causes are sought:

Physiological—usually an abrupt increase in physical demand on the shoulder, which, at least in retrospect, would be considered a "training error"

Anatomical—frequently the residual of undertreated/incompletely rehabilitated prior acute injury

Mechanical

For most shoulder overuse injuries, and certainly for any injury that does
not resolve promptly and completely with initial basic treatment, *the essential
diagnostic and therapeutic task is to identify and to reverse as many of the causative
factors as possible.*

Structural injury does not necessarily imply a need for surgical intervention. Depending on the severity of the structural injury and the demands to
be placed on the shoulder, many structural problems (e.g., partial-thickness
and small full-thickness rotator cuff tears) can be adequately compensated if
appropriate functional rehabilitation is carried out.

MECHANICS AND PATHOMECHANICS OF THROWING AND CLINICAL CORRELATES

A discussion of the biomechanics of all activities causing shoulder overuse
injuries is clearly beyond the scope of this or perhaps any text. Given the
prevalence of throwing-related overuse injuries, however, an overview of the
mechanics and pathomechanics of throwing as these relate to mechanisms of
injury is appropriate. Although the present discussion focuses on the mechanics of baseball pitching, the mechanics and clinical correlates are quite similar
with serving and overhead shots in tennis; serving and spiking in volleyball;
throwing a javelin; and so forth.

Functionally, the shoulder (glenohumeral) joint is but one biomechanical
link between the axial skeleton and the hand. What we consider to be
"shoulder motion" is actually a complex of sternoclavicular, acromioclavicular, scapulothoracic, and glenohumeral motion.

The "thrower's shoulder syndrome" represents maladaptation to the
repetitive stresses of throwing. Although the presenting symptoms are often

attributable to rotator cuff tendinitis or tear, there is, characteristically, scapular-stabilizing muscle insufficiency or dysfunction and glenohumeral ligament/capsule/labrum changes that seem to predispose to the eventual breakdown of the rotator cuff. These characteristic maladaptations may occur even with "ideal" throwing mechanics. However, certain deviations from the ideal seem to increase the risk of overuse injury.

In pitching, the fundamental biomechanical task is to accelerate the ball. This is accomplished by first accelerating the mass of the body and then transferring momentum to the "cocked" upper limb, accelerating the hand and ball. The pitching motion may be broken down into five phases as follows (Fig. 4–34):[24]

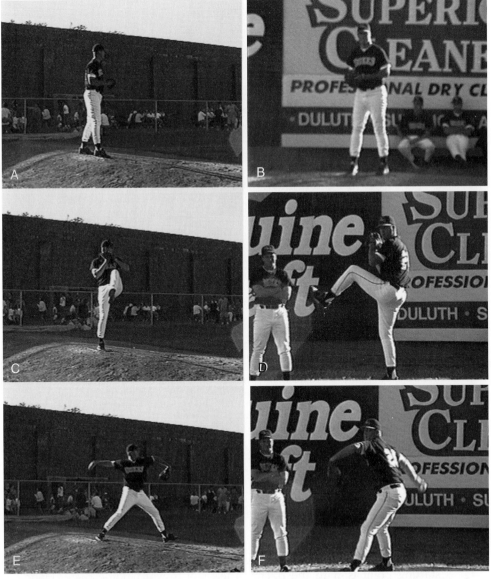

Figure 4–34. Throwing motion. *A* and *B*, Start. *C* and *D*, Windup. Potential energy is stored. *E* and *F*, Early cocking. Potential energy is converted to kinetic energy.

Illustration continued on following page

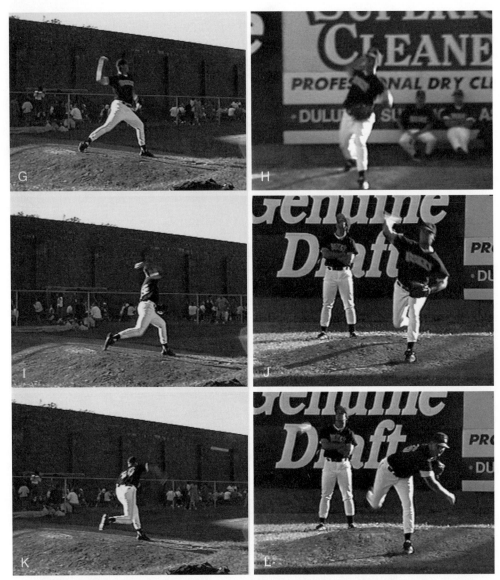

Figure 4–34 *Continued. G* and *H,* Late cocking. Forward momentum is changed to angular momentum. *I* and *J,* Acceleration. Angular momentum is transferred to the cocked throwing arm. *K* and *L,* Deceleration and follow-through. The accelerated throwing arm is brought to a stop. Note the extreme horizontal extension and external rotation of the shoulder in late cocking. Note also that the shoulder remains about 90 degrees abducted throughout late cocking and acceleration. (The main difference between "overhand" and "sidearm" throwing is the degree of elbow flexion/extension, not shoulder abduction.)

Wind-up
Early cocking
Late cocking
Acceleration
Deceleration and follow-through

For simplicity, mechanics are described for a right-handed pitcher. The starting point is with the pitcher's left side toward home plate. Hands are together in front at chest height.

The wind-up phase begins as the pitcher raises the left knee and ends when the knee is at maximal height. Concomitantly, the hands and arms are raised together. Potential energy is stored. The wind-up motion should be smooth and controlled. Kicking out, as opposed to raising the knee, is liable to throw the torso backward off balance. This, in turn, can lead to clinically significant mechanical problems in the next phases of throwing.

Early cocking begins when the left knee has reached its maximal height and ends when the left foot is planted. During this phase, potential energy is converted to kinetic energy. The left shoulder and hip should remain oriented toward home plate throughout, and the torso and left leg should move directly toward home plate. Concomitantly, the hands break, with the left arm moving toward home plate and the right arm moving away from it in symmetrical, smooth, downward-outward-upward, coronal plane motions. Shoulder motion should be essentially combined glenohumeral/scapulothoracic abduction. This motion ends with the right arm cocked at 90 degrees of shoulder abduction.

The most common sin of the early cocking phase is "opening up too soon." Ideally, the left foot should land within 3 in. on either side of a reference line drawn from the right foot on the rubber to home plate. With "open stride offset," the left foot lands more than 3 in. to the left of this line and the hips and torso rotate prematurely toward the plate. This results in increased horizontal extension at the shoulder of the cocked throwing arm and additional stress on the anterior ligaments, capsule, and labrum.

"Kicking and swinging" the left leg, as opposed to "raising and stepping," during the wind-up and early cocking phases are liable to cause open stride offset. "Exploding off the rubber" is also liable to result in stride offset. Early cocking should, in contrast, be characterized by balance and control.

A less common problem of the early cocking phase is not opening up enough. The left foot lands to the right of the reference line. This may limit torso rotation in the acceleration phase, impairing the transfer of momentum to the throwing arm, and may cause additional eccentric loading of the scapular-stabilizing muscles and rotator cuff during the deceleration phase.

Other problems of the early cocking phase are "hooking" and "wrapping." *Hooking* refers to the throwing arm's moving backward out of the coronal plane, with horizontal extension at the shoulder. As with opening up prematurely, hooking places additional stress on the anterior structures of the shoulder. *Wrapping* refers to the throwing arm's being internally rotated at the shoulder during the cocking phase. Ideally, the ball should face down (toward the ground) at the end of the early cocking phase. With wrapping, it faces backward (toward first base). The pitcher who wraps the ball essentially performs an impingement test on himself with each throw.

Late cocking begins with planting of the left foot and ends when the shoulder reaches the maximal horizontal extension and external rotation. Forward momentum is changed to angular momentum as the torso is rotated toward home plate. The "explosive" part of the pitching motion properly begins with late cocking. Tremendous force is placed on the anterior stabilizing structures of the shoulder during this and the acceleration phase.

The acceleration phase begins with maximal horizontal extension and external rotation of the shoulder and ends at the point of ball release. The angular momentum developed in the preceding phases is transferred to the cocked throwing arm. The hand and ball at the end of the kinetic chain are accelerated quite similarly as a whip is cracked. Throughout the late cocking and acceleration phases, the shoulder remains about 90 degrees abducted. During the acceleration phase, it rapidly moves from maximal horizontal extension to neutral extension and from maximal external rotation to less than 90 degrees externally rotated. For a professional baseball pitcher throwing a fast ball, the internal rotation angular velocity at ball release may be as great as 7000 degrees per second. As discussed later, with any anterior laxity or cuff insufficiency, secondary impingement problems are likely.

Deceleration begins with ball release and ends with the cessation of arm motion. The shoulder moves from abduction and external rotation to adduction and internal rotation. In contrast to the preceding phases, during which virtually the entire mass of the body is used to accelerate the ball, only the relatively puny mass of the scapular-stabilizing muscles and rotator cuff are available to decelerate the throwing arm. Not surprisingly, they are liable to breakdown from repetitive tensile overload.

SCAPULAR-STABILIZING MUSCLE INSUFFICIENCY/ DYSFUNCTION

HISTORY

MECHANISM OF INJURY. Overuse injury of the scapular-stabilizing muscles is a problem of throwing athletes, the result of repetitive eccentric overload during the deceleration phase of throwing (or serving in racquet sports and volleyball). Dysfunction, typically overactivity of the upper scapulovertebral muscles relative to the lower trapezius and serratus anterior, may also be the result of habitual compensation for an intrinsic shoulder problem. Much less commonly, dysfunction (paresis) of the serratus anterior is caused by injury to the long thoracic nerve.

Scapular-stabilizing muscle dysfunction is not uncommonly exacerbated by training error. In many athletic activities, especially swimming and weight training, and particularly with inexperienced lifters, there is a tendency to overdevelop the chest muscles and to neglect the upper back muscles. The result is habitual bilateral shoulder girdle protraction (lateral scapular slide).

SYMPTOMS

Most often, scapular-stabilizing muscle dysfunction per se is asymptomatic. It is typically brought to the attention of both patient and examiner in the course of evaluating an associated intrinsic shoulder problem, e.g., rotator cuff tendinitis, or in the course of a preparticipation examination for throwing athletes. Less commonly, a patient may complain of (usually upper) scapulovertebral pain or muscle spasm, or both.

PHYSICAL EXAMINATION

The most reliable sign of unilateral scapular-stabilizing muscle dysfunction is *lateral scapular slide or winging, or both, with Kibler's test* (see Scapular-Stabilizing Muscle Function in part B and Fig. 4–6). Additional tests include forward flexion of both shoulders, observing for lateral slide or winging of the scapulae, and the "wall push-up"—the classic diagnostic test for the long thoracic nerve and serratus anterior. There may also be a habitus of elevation of the ipsilateral shoulder girdle, tightness or frank spasm of the upper scapulovertebral muscles, trigger point tenderness, and a dyssymmetrical pattern of combined glenohumeral/scapulothoracic abduction (see Fig. 4–10).

DIAGNOSTIC IMAGING

Diagnostic imaging is not required.

CLINICAL SIGNIFICANCE

Malpositioning of the scapula (shoulder girdle) constrains glenohumeral joint motion, a fact that can usually be readily demonstrated by having the patient abduct the arms first with the shoulder girdles protracted, then with the scapulae properly "set" (Fig. 4–35). During overhead handed activities, e.g., throwing, serving, and swimming, this probably puts the rotator cuff at a mechanical disadvantage and makes impingement more likely.

SPECIFIC TREATMENT

In most cases, the specific dysfunction is overactivity of the upper scapulovertebral muscles relative to the lower trapezius and serratus anterior. This problem, if identified, can be readily and appropriately addressed by physical

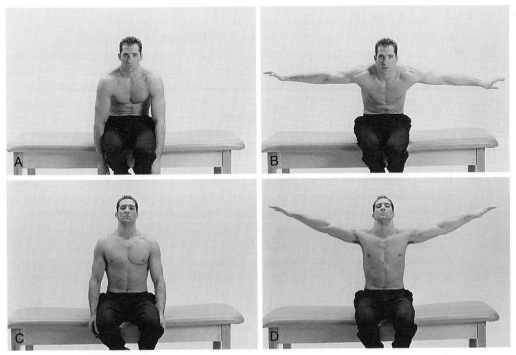

Figure 4–35. Effect of shoulder girdle position on range and freedom of glenohumeral motion. *A* and *B,* Shoulder abduction with the shoulder girdles protracted (slumped posture). *C* and *D,* Shoulder abduction with the scapulae properly "set" ("military" posture). Most individuals note much freer shoulder motion with the scapulae set as in *C* and *D.*

therapy including McConnell's techniques, biofeedback, and progressive resistance exercise (see Rehabilitative Treatment of Shoulder Overuse Injuries later in this chapter).

PREVENTIVE MEASURES

We recommend that Kibler's test be incorporated into the preparticipation examinations of throwing and racquet sport athletes, and that rehabilitation exercise be incorporated into their regular training regimens. Addressing the subclinical problem of scapular-stabilizing muscle dysfunction in the preseason can obviate clinical problems during the season.

(STRUCTURAL) GLENOHUMERAL LAXITY/CONTRACTURE

HISTORY

MECHANISM OF INJURY. As an overuse injury, abnormal glenohumeral laxity occurs when repetitive stresses are applied to the stabilizing structures of the shoulder at a rate that exceeds that of tissue repair.[34] Over time, the capsule and ligaments become attenuated and lax. Degenerative tearing of the glenoid labrum or detachment of the labrum and capsule from the glenoid (Bankart and SLAP lesions*), or both, may occur.

This mechanism of injury pertains mainly to throwing, racquet sports, and swimming. The direction of the resultant instability is anterior. In throwing, the anterior stabilizing structures are subject to repetitive high stress during the late cocking and acceleration phases of the throwing motion; in swimming, during the catch and early pull phases of the strokes.

Laxity of the static (fibrocartilaginous) anterior stabilizing structures has the effect of *permitting* anterior subluxation of the shoulder during overhand activities, if not compensated by action of the dynamic (musculotendinous) stabilizers of the joint. These structures, however, are also liable to overuse injury with the same activities. As compensatory mechanisms fail and subluxation becomes chronic, contracture of the posterior ligaments and capsule can occur. This has the effect of *forcing* the anterior subluxation.

Anterior glenohumeral laxity can be exacerbated by ill-advised strength-training and stretching techniques. Push-ups, bench press (including incline and decline presses), bench flies, and dips place similar stresses on the anterior stabilizing structures as throwing does. The use of the inverted bar for bench pressing or doing deep push-ups between chairs is especially bad in this regard. Classic "pectoralis" stretches, e.g., corner push-ups, wall stretches, door jamb stretches, and buddy stretches, which use the upper limb as a lever arm, actually stretch/stress the anterior shoulder much more than the pectorales (Fig. 4–36).

Abnormal glenohumeral laxity may also be congenital or the result of acute trauma. The clinical significance for the throwing athlete or swimmer is the same as that of laxity resulting from repetitive trauma.

---

*Bony and soft tissue (fibrocartilaginous) Bankart lesions are discussed in "Shoulder Series" Radiographs and in Magnetic Resonance Imaging (and MRI Arthrography) in part C, and in part G.

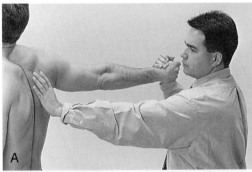
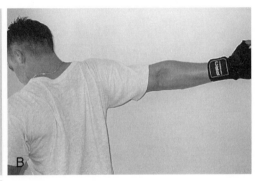
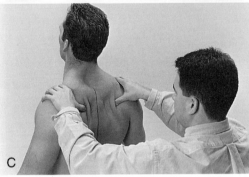

Figure 4–36. *A* and *B*, "Buddy" and "wall" stretches, respectively. Stretches such as these, which use the upper limb as a lever arm, place undue stress on the anterior stabilizing structures of the shoulder. They are generally ill advised, especially for throwing athletes. For individuals with secondary impingement, they are contraindicated. *C*, Appropriate stretching techniques for the anterior chest muscles do not use the upper limb as a lever arm.

SYMPTOMS. Frank instability symptoms—"My shoulder goes out of place"—are uncommon. Pain with overhand activities is most often attributable to rotator cuff overuse strain, tendinitis, or secondary impingement, or both (see Secondary Impingement [Interior, Posterior, and Lateral Secondary to Glenohumeral Laxity/Contracture or Rotator Cuff Insufficiency, or Both] later). Pain associated with labral tear or detachment is characteristically intermittent and positional. For example, in throwing, pain is most likely to be noted at the end of late cocking/start of acceleration, when there is maximal horizontal extension and external rotation of the shoulder. The athlete may also be aware of a click associated with such pain.

PHYSICAL EXAMINATION

The range of internal and external rotation of the 90-degree–abducted shoulder is the best measure of structural glenohumeral laxity. With the typical "thrower's shoulder" there is increased external rotation reflecting anterior laxity and decreased internal rotation reflecting posterior contracture (Fig. 4–37).

In throwing athletes and swimmers, what constitutes "abnormal" anterior laxity versus "physiological" adaptation to the activity is not always clear. Up to 120 degrees of external rotation of the 90-degree–abducted shoulder is probably within normal limits for these athletes. Any limitation of internal rotation or any pain at the limit of external rotation is, however, clearly abnormal.

In the skeletally immature, or in the skeletally mature who began throwing or swimming at an early age, an increased range of external rotation and decreased range of internal rotation may be the result in part of bony torsion, as opposed to capsuloligamentous changes.

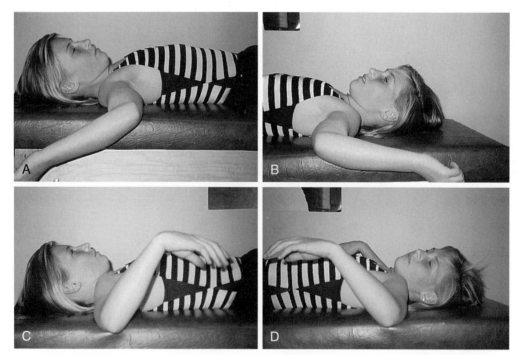

Figure 4–37. Range of external/internal glenohumeral rotation in a 10-year-old right-handed girl who had played competitive tennis since the age of 5 years, demonstrating anterior laxity/posterior contracture of the shoulder of the dominant arm. *A,* External rotation, right shoulder. *B,* External rotation, left shoulder. *C,* Internal rotation, right shoulder. *D,* Internal rotation, left shoulder.

A painful arc of combined glenohumeral/scapulothoracic abduction with the shoulder externally rotated and positive apprehension and containment tests are characteristic, but not pathognomonic, of structural injury such as labral tear or detachment (see Scapular-Stabilizing Muscle Function in part B and Fig. 4–17).

RADIOGRAPHIC EXAMINATION

A shoulder series is indicated if symptoms have been present for more than a few weeks. Bony Bankart's lesions and glenohumeral degenerative changes are sought.

OTHER DIAGNOSTIC TESTS

The diagnostic imaging test of choice is the MRI arthrogram (see Magnetic Resonance Imaging [and MRI Arthrography] in part C and Fig. 4–24).

Isokinetic testing can sometimes corroborate a positive containment test. If the isokinetic device is set up properly so its axis of rotation is centered on the center of the glenohumeral joint, there may be provoked pain and demonstrable weakness on manual muscle testing, but little or no pain and good strength with isokinetic testing. This is indicative of abnormal glenohumeral laxity and secondary impingement.

CLINICAL SIGNIFICANCE

The clinical significance is twofold:

The ligamentous/capsular/labral injury may be painful in and of itself.
More commonly, the abnormal laxity results in secondary impingement problems.

REHABILITATIVE TREATMENT

Structural anterior laxity cannot be changed nonoperatively. However, the ability to compensate for it can be markedly improved by physical therapy (supervised rotator cuff endurance and functional stability training). Posterior capsular contracture can (and should) be readily addressed with an appropriate stretching program.

REFERRAL/DEFINITIVE TREATMENT

Referral/definitive treatment is indicated in the case of failure of nonoperative treatment. Surgical treatment may include both labral débridement and Bankart's repair and is guided by the MRI arthrographic and intraoperative findings.

PREVENTIVE MEASURES

Throwing athletes and swimmers should be instructed to avoid other activities that place undue stress on the anterior stabilizers of the shoulder, e.g., wall stretches and full-arc bench press, as discussed previously. They should be encouraged to maintain flexibility of the posterior capsule and maintain rotator cuff endurance to minimize the clinical consequences of any anterior laxity that may be present.

ROTATOR CUFF OVERUSE STRAIN, TENDINITIS, TENDINOSIS, DEGENERATIVE TEAR, INSUFFICIENCY

HISTORY

FUNCTIONAL ANATOMY AND MECHANISMS OF INJURY. The rotator cuff comprises four muscles (subscapularis, supraspinatus, infraspinatus, and teres minor) and their tendons. Acting as a force couple with larger muscles that insert farther distally on the humerus (deltoid, pectoralis major, and latissimus dorsi), the rotator cuff and long head of the biceps maintain the axes of shoulder motion centered at the glenohumeral joint.

The supraspinatus and infraspinatus are particularly liable to overuse strain and associated muscle soreness and tendinitis with repetitive or prolonged overhand activities. As discussed previously in Mechanics and Pathomechanics of Throwing and Clinical Correlates, the cuff is subject to high tensile loads during the late cocking, the acceleration, and especially the deceleration phases of throwing. When repetitive stresses are applied at a rate that exceeds that of tissue repair, tendinosis (tendon degeneration) occurs. Over time, tendon changes may become irreversible, and degenerative tearing may occur.

In addition, the cuff is liable to abrasion injury with primary and secondary impingement problems (see Primary Impingement [Acromial, Acromioclavicular, Coracoclavicular, Coracoid], and Secondary Impingement [Anterior, Posterior, and Lateral Secondary to Glenohumeral Laxity/Contracture or Rotator Cuff Insufficiency, or Both] later). Over time this also may lead to tendinosis and degenerative tearing.

As a very general rule, cuff failure due to excessive tensile loading is first manifested as fraying of the articular (deep) surface of the tendon or tendons, whereas failure due to anterior and lateral impingement is manifested as fraying of the bursal (superficial) surface. Failure due to posterior impingement involves the posterosuperior aspect of the articular surface.

SYMPTOMS. The hallmark symptom of rotator cuff tendinitis is *a "toothache"-quality pain* related to (i.e., during or after, or both) overhand daily, occupational, and sports activities.

As for other overuse injuries, there is often a progression of symptoms. At first there may be moderate postexercise pain only. Subsequently, there may be increasing pain during athletic activity. By the time the athlete presents for treatment, there may be constant, aching pain, exacerbated even by routine activities of daily living, e.g., lifting a carton of milk.

Characteristically, the pain is not well localized to the shoulder but rather *referred to the lateral arm*, as far distally as the insertion of the deltoid. Pain at night with an inability to sleep on the affected side or with the arm overhead is a common complaint.

PHYSICAL EXAMINATION

The hallmark physical findings of musculotendinous overuse injury are *point tenderness* over the involved muscles and tendons and *pain reproduced with specific muscle testing* (see Manual Muscle Testing in part B and Fig. 4–13). Point tenderness is sought over the muscle bellies of the supraspinatus and the infraspinatus, the greater tuberosity (supraspinatus and infraspinatus insertion), and the lesser tuberosity (subscapularis insertion). Impingement testing is likely to be positive (see Manual Muscle Testing in part B and Fig. 4–11). There is also likely to be a painful arc of combined glenohumeral/scapulothoracic abduction.

RADIOGRAPHIC EXAMINATION

A shoulder series is indicated if symptoms have been present for more than a few weeks or if pain is especially severe. With calcific tendinitis/bursitis, heterotopic calcification may be demonstrated.

OTHER DIAGNOSTIC TESTS

The diagnostic imaging test of choice is the MRI arthrogram (see Magnetic Resonance Imaging [and MRI Arthrography] in part C and Fig. 4–23).

Isokinetic testing provides a quantitative assessment of muscle power and, as discussed previously, may permit muscle testing to be carried out without impingement pain.

INITIAL AND REHABILITATIVE TREATMENT

The mainstay of initial treatment is *relative rest*. If there is pain with daily and occupational activities, then complete rest, i.e., the use of a sling, is recommended. Other initial treatment measures include nonsteroidal anti-inflammatory medication, ice massage, physical therapy modalities, and McConnell's techniques. For calcific tendinitis/bursitis, corticosteroid injection is recommended (see Acute Painful Episode in part A and Injection/Aspiration in part B).

In our experience, treatment consisting solely of symptomatic and anti-inflammatory measures for tendinitis and bursitis is doomed to failure. The pain is bound to recur when the athlete attempts to return to sports. The key to successful treatment is identification and correction of the specific muscle insufficiencies, as discussed later in Rehabilitative Treatment of Shoulder Overuse Injuries. A trial of rehabilitative treatment is generally indicated, even with MRI-confirmed full-thickness cuff tears.

REFERRAL

The athlete who is unable to resume a desired level of activity without recurrence of symptoms should be counseled regarding the risks of continuing the activity, e.g., worsening of the tendinitis/tendinosis, worsening of functional instability, or "wear and tear" on the articular surfaces. The recreational or fitness athlete should be advised of alternative activities that do not place as much stress on the shoulder. A swimmer, for example, may be able to swim breast stroke rather than freestyle. A weight lifter may be able to substitute limited arc lifts for bench press, dips, flies, and so forth. If, despite appropriate rehabilitation and realistic activity modification, disabling symptoms persist, then orthopedic referral is indicated.

DEFINITIVE TREATMENT

A surgical caveat is that unless the associated glenohumeral instability (secondary impingement) and primary impingement problems are appropriately addressed, cuff repair is likely to fail. Preoperative and intraoperative assessment of glenohumeral stability is therefore critical. Therefore, operative treatment may entail, in addition to débridement/repair of the rotator cuff, a Bankart repair and coracoacromial arch decompression.

PREVENTIVE MEASURES

For swimmers and for throwing, racquet sports, and strength athletes, "prehabilitation" rotator cuff progressive resistance exercises, identical to the rehabilitation exercises discussed later in Rehabilitative Treatment of Shoulder Overuse Injuries, should be incorporated into the year-round training regimen.

The frequency, duration, and intensity of exercise should be kept within the limits of relative rest. Athletes should anticipate increased demands, e.g., the start of team practice, allot adequate time for preparation/adaptation, and thereby avoid "training error" problems. Mechanical/technical problems predisposing to injury should be identified and corrected; in this regard, working with a knowledgeable coach is most helpful. Coaches and parents of young athletes should emphasize participation, fun, and motor skill learning over winning—if for no other reason than to lessen the temptation of overusing the shoulders of the most talented young athletes.

LONG HEAD OF BICEPS OVERUSE STRAIN, TENDINITIS, TENDINOSIS, DEGENERATIVE TEAR, TENDON SUBLUXATION, INSUFFICIENCY

HISTORY

MECHANISMS OF INJURY. Similar mechanisms apply as with overuse injury of the rotator cuff. In addition, the long head of the biceps, more so than the rotator cuff, is liable to overuse injury in fast-pitch softball pitching. (The acceleration phase of the underhand pitching motion entails rapid, forceful shoulder flexion from a "cocked" position of extreme shoulder extension.)

SYMPTOMS. The hallmark symptom of tendinitis is activity-related pain, characteristically localized to the anterior shoulder and arm. In addition to pain with overhand activities and softball pitching, there may be pain with activities, especially lifting, that entail forceful shoulder or elbow flexion or forearm supination. Subluxation of the tendon of the long head of the biceps out of the bicipital groove typically presents as painful anterior snapping with shoulder motion.

PHYSICAL EXAMINATION

The hallmark physical findings are *point tenderness* over the bicipital groove and anterior arm and *pain reproduced with specific muscle testing* (Speed's and Yergason's tests; see Manual Muscle Testing in part B and Fig. 4–14). Impingement testing is likely to be positive (see Manual Muscle Testing in part B and Fig. 4–11). Tendon subluxation may be reproduced with a modified Yergason's test in which, concomitantly with supinating the forearm against resistance, the patient also attempts to externally rotate the shoulder against the examiner's resistance.

RADIOGRAPHIC EXAMINATION

If symptoms have been present for more than a few weeks or if pain is especially severe, shoulder series radiographs are indicated as part of the general work-up.

OTHER DIAGNOSTIC TESTS

Other diagnostic tests are not required unless surgical treatment of tendon subluxation or tear is being considered, in which case the clinical diagnosis may be confirmed by MRI.

INITIAL AND REHABILITATIVE TREATMENT

Initial and rehabilitative treatment follow the same general plan as for tendinitis in general and as for rotator cuff overuse injury as discussed previously.

REFERRAL/DEFINITIVE TREATMENT

Referral/definitive treatment is indicated for chronic, painful tendon subluxation or possibly for tendon rupture (see Referral and Definitive Treatment in part K).

ACROMIOCLAVICULAR DEGENERATIVE JOINT DISEASE/ DISTAL CLAVICULAR OSTEOLYSIS

Acromioclavicular degenerative joint disease/distal clavicular osteolysis is discussed as a separate entity in part L. Especially in older athletes, it is more likely to be one component of a shoulder overuse syndrome than to be the sole cause of shoulder symptoms.

The extent to which a given patient's shoulder pain is attributable to acromioclavicular arthritis can be gauged by selective local anesthetic injection (see Acromioclavicular Joint in part B). A caveat for the clinician is that although postinjection pain relief is indicative of an acromioclavicular joint problem, the converse is not true. It must be appreciated that *whether or not the acromioclavicular joint itself is painful,* acromioclavicular swelling and osteophytosis may nonetheless be a cause of shoulder impingement pain. Surgical decompression, e.g., a Mumford procedure, may be required for treatment of the primary impingement.

PRIMARY IMPINGEMENT (ACROMIAL, ACROMIOCLAVICULAR, CORACOCLAVICULAR, CORACOID)

The term *impingement* may properly be used to describe a physical examination finding (see Impingement Testing in part B), a structural abnormality (primary impingement), or a mechanical dysfunction (secondary impingement). Primary impingement implies *bony or ligamentous encroachment* on the subacromial space capable of impinging on the subacromial bursa, the rotator cuff, and the tendon of the long head of the biceps and causing or exacerbating injury, inflammation, or pain, or all of these.

As previously discussed, there is not a one-to-one correlation between activity-related shoulder pain and primary impingement. Rather, the diagnosis of primary impingement is made when characteristic physical, radiographic, and MRI findings, such as osteophytosis, are noted in an appropriate clinical setting, e.g., pain with overhand activities or a positive impingement test (Fig. 4–38).

Primary impingement may be congenital or acquired. The latter is by far the more common, usually the result of degenerative bone and joint changes occurring over years of shoulder-strenuous activity. Encroachment may be from the lateral or anterior aspect of the acromion, the acromioclavicular joint, the coracoacromial ligament, and the coracoid process.

Treatment options are essentially twofold: activity modification/limitation (relative rest) and surgical intervention (coracoacromial arch decompression). A typical operative procedure might include acromioplasty, resection of the distal clavicle (Mumford's procedure), and resection of the coracoacromial ligament.

SECONDARY IMPINGEMENT (ANTERIOR, POSTERIOR, AND LATERAL SECONDARY TO GLENOHUMERAL LAXITY/CONTRACTURE OR ROTATOR CUFF INSUFFICIENCY, OR BOTH)

HISTORY

MECHANISMS OF INJURY. Activity-related shoulder pain may be the result of musculotendinous overuse strain/tendinitis, an internal derangement such as a glenoid labral tear, or impingement of inflamed tendons and bursae between the humeral head and the coracoacromial arch, or all of these. The fact that impingement occurs does *not* necessarily imply that there is insufficient space to accommodate the impinged structures. Especially in the athletically active, impingement pain is commonly *secondary* to structural glenohumeral laxity/contracture (most commonly anterior laxity/posterior

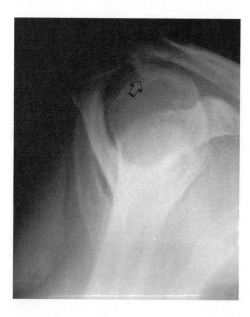

Figure 4–38. Lateral scapular radiograph demonstrating acromial osteophytosis (arrow) causing primary impingement of the underlying rotator cuff in a 69-year-old man with a full-thickness cuff tear.

contracture) or insufficiency of the stabilizing muscles of the shoulder, or both, which results in functional instability of the shoulder (i.e., subluxation during activity).

This mechanism of injury pertains especially to ballistic overhand activities such as throwing. During the acceleration phase of the throwing, anterior laxity permits anterior subluxation of the shoulder. If uncompensated by action of the rotator cuff or if exacerbated by posterior contracture, or both, the axis of humeral rotation moves anterior to the center of the glenohumeral joint. The eccentric rotation in turn may result in impingement of the bursal surface of the cuff anteriorly against the unyielding coracoacromial arch. It may also cause impingement of the articular surface of cuff posteriorly against the sharp posterosuperior edge of the glenoid rim. Abrasion injury of the cuff (mainly to the supraspinatus and the infraspinatus) is a predictable sequela, given the speed of humeral rotation (up to 7000 degrees per second) and the repetitiveness of the activity (often more than 100 pitches per day).

In swimming, glenohumeral subluxation may similarly lead to cuff impingement anteriorly and laterally against the acromion during the recovery phases of the crawl and butterfly strokes.

Specific mechanisms of overuse injury to the anterior stabilizing structures of the shoulder and to the rotator cuff were previously discussed in Mechanics and Pathomechanics of Throwing and Clinical Correlates; the section on mechanism of injury in (Structural) Glenohumeral Laxity/Contracture; and the section on functional anatomy and mechanisms of injury in Rotator Cuff Overuse Strain, Tendinitis, Tendinosis, Degenerative Tear, Insufficiency.

In addition, as with other overuse syndromes, a vicious circle may ensue, whereby pain leads to disuse, which leads to muscle atrophy and dysfunction, which leads to increased vulnerability to injury and recurrence of pain on attempted resumption of activity. Rotator cuff tendinitis/insufficiency is often thus both the effect and the cause of secondary impingement.

In contrast to primary impingement, which is more common in the older athlete, secondary impingement may affect athletes of any age.

SYMPTOMS. The hallmark presenting symptom of secondary impingement is *pain related to overhand activities*—throwing, racquet sports, swimming, weight training, and manual work. Other symptoms of glenohumeral instability or rotator cuff injury, or both may also be present (see the previous sections on symptoms in [Structural] Glenohumeral Laxity/Contracture, and Rotator Cuff Overuse Strain, Tendinitis, Tendinosis, Degenerative Tear, Insufficiency).

Functional instability of the shoulder is often obvious to athletes who have just discontinued the use of a sling or an immobilizer. They may complain that they must "hold the shoulder tight to keep it from slipping out." Or they may complain that if the arm is relaxed they must first "tighten the muscles to get the shoulder back in place" before they can raise it. These symptoms of inferior subluxation usually disappear with re-establishment of some deltoid muscle tone.

Temporary muscle insufficiency and gravity-induced inferior subluxation sometimes also occur after exhausting exercise, such as high-speed isokinetic workouts. If so, the athlete may need to use a sling for up to 12 hours until the muscles have sufficiently recovered from the exercise to prevent the subluxation.

Unfortunately, muscle atrophy and dysfunction, particularly of the rotator cuff, are not always as obvious to the athlete. Attempted return to functional use of the arm before full recovery and rehabilitation can result in recurrence of symptoms.

PHYSICAL EXAMINATION

The hallmark finding of *symptomatic functional anterior instability* is a *positive containment test* (see Tests of Glenohumeral Instability in part B). It is not, however, pathognomonic of any particular structural abnormality. The Iowa shoulder shift test has the same implications. Other findings related to glenohumeral instability or rotator cuff injury, or both, may also be present (see the previous sections on physical examination in [Structural] Glenohumeral Laxity/Contracture, and Rotator Cuff Overuse Strain, Tendinitis, Tendinosis, Degenerative Tear, Insufficiency).

Sorting out the relative contributions of impingement versus tendinitis can help guide both rehabilitative and operative treatment:

A positive impingement test with little or no pain or weakness on manual muscle testing within a pain-free range of motion suggests that the problem is mainly impingement.

A negative impingement test and pain and weakness with manual muscle testing, however, suggest that the problem is mainly rotator cuff strain/tendinitis.

A positive impingement test with acromioclavicular tenderness and positive acromioclavicular compression tests suggests that primary acromioclavicular impingement is likely.

A positive containment test or shoulder shift test indicates that the problem is attributable at least in part to secondary impingement and that injury to anterior stabilizing structures is likely.

DIAGNOSTIC IMAGING

Indications for radiographic examination and MRI arthrography are as discussed for structural glenohumeral laxity, rotator cuff overuse injury, and acromioclavicular degenerative joint disease (see the previous sections on radiographic examination and other diagnostic tests in [Structural] Glenohumeral Laxity/Contracture, and Rotator Cuff Overuse Strain, Tendinitis, Tendinosis, Degenerative Tear, Insufficiency); Radiographic Examination in part L; Magnetic Resonance Imaging [and MRI Arthrography] in part C; and Fig. 4–24).

OTHER DIAGNOSTIC TESTS

Secondary impingement can often be demonstrated in an individual athlete with the use of an isokinetic device. After carefully positioning the patient and the device so that the position of the humeral head is fixed throughout the arc of motion, a previously painful motion can afterward be performed with little or no pain, through a full or nearly full range of motion, and with full or nearly full force. (Corroboration of the containment test in this manner is more of academic than practical clinical interest.)

INITIAL AND REHABILITATIVE TREATMENT

Initial and rehabilitative treatment is as discussed in the later section Rehabilitative Treatment of Shoulder Overuse Injuries. Most cases of secondary impingement not complicated by advanced degenerative changes causing primary impingement or extensive structural injury can be successfully treated by nonoperative means.

REFERRAL/DEFINITIVE TREATMENT

Referral/definitive treatment is indicated mainly for structural glenohumeral laxity that, after an appropriate trial of rehabilitative treatment, remains inadequately compensated (see the section on referral/definitive treatment in [Structural] Glenohumeral Laxity/Contracture).

GLENOHUMERAL DEGENERATIVE JOINT DISEASE/"CUFF ARTHROPATHY"

After extensive full-thickness tear of the rotator cuff, action of the deltoid causes superior subluxation of the glenohumeral joint before initiation of arm elevation. Dynamically, the shoulder joint thus becomes an acromiohumeral joint.

Some individuals seem to tolerate this condition quite well for many years. Once the effects of acute injury have subsided and any residual "frozen shoulder" symptoms have resolved, they may have little or no pain and little or no functional impairment with customary activities of daily living. The shoulder does, however, remain weak, and strenuous overhand activities, e.g., throwing or racquet sports, are likely to be at least somewhat painful or impaired, or both.

Others seem to do exceedingly poorly, having constant pain, especially night pain, and marked functional impairment. Typically, advanced glenohumeral degenerative changes can be confirmed on radiographic examination (Fig. 4–39).

The arthropathy seems to be related to functional instability of the shoulder, as opposed to the cuff tear per se. Instability from capsuloligamentous laxity, as discussed previously, can also lead to arthropathy over time.

In either case, treatment is surgical and ideally is carried out before marked symptomatic and functional deterioration and radiographically demonstrated degenerative changes occur.

A surgical caveat relates to decompression of the coracoacromial arch. If the torn cuff is reparable, then decompression to protect the repair is generally indicated. If, however, the cuff is not reparable, then decompression is contraindicated; it would render the functional acromiohumeral joint unstable, more likely exacerbate than alleviate activity-related pain, and limit future surgical (arthroplasty) options.

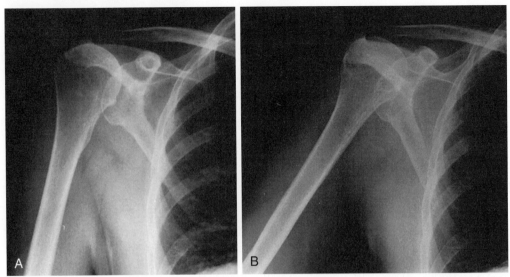

Figure 4–39. *A* and *B,* AP radiographs of the shoulder after an extensive, full-thickness rotator cuff tear. Note the superior subluxation of the humeral head relative to the glenoid fossa and marked glenohumeral osteophytosis.

REHABILITATIVE TREATMENT OF SHOULDER OVERUSE INJURIES

Most cases of shoulder overuse syndrome can be adequately treated with appropriate functional rehabilitation as presented later. This is true, within certain limits of severity of injury and demands to be placed on the shoulder, even for cases in which structural injuries, e.g., glenoid labral tears and partial- or small full-thickness rotator cuff tears, may be present.

Sequential objectives to be achieved are as follow:

Reduction of pain and inflammation
Restoration of scapular-stabilizing muscle function
Restoration of range of (glenohumeral) motion
Restoration of normal glenohumeral scapulothoracic patterns of motion
Restoration of (rotator cuff and long head of biceps) muscle endurance
Restoration of strength
Return to full function/shoulder-strenuous occupational and athletic activities

Experience has shown that carrying out rehabilitative treatment in the proper sequence is critical. For example, attempting strength training before a normal pattern of motion has been re-established simply reinforces the abnormal pattern. Our recommended treatment/rehabilitation sequence with specific treatment objectives and techniques for each step and criteria for advancement to the next step is presented in outline form in Table 4–4. Specific techniques and rehabilitation exercises are also illustrated in Figures 4–40 through 4–42.

In most cases of shoulder overuse syndrome, the single most important aspect of rehabilitative treatment is neuromuscular re-education—"unlearning" abnormal postures and patterns of motion and relearning proper mechanics. Most patients, even athletes with very good "body sense," do not

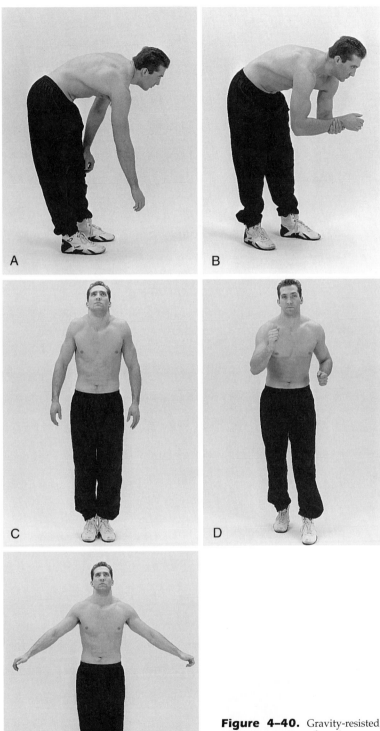

Figure 4–40. Gravity-resisted, endurance, range-of-motion exercises for the shoulder. *A* and *B,* Codman's pendulum exercises, unassisted *(A)* and assisted by the other limb *(B).* *C–E,* Additional "fungo" exercises ("shrugs," "saws," "swings," respectively).

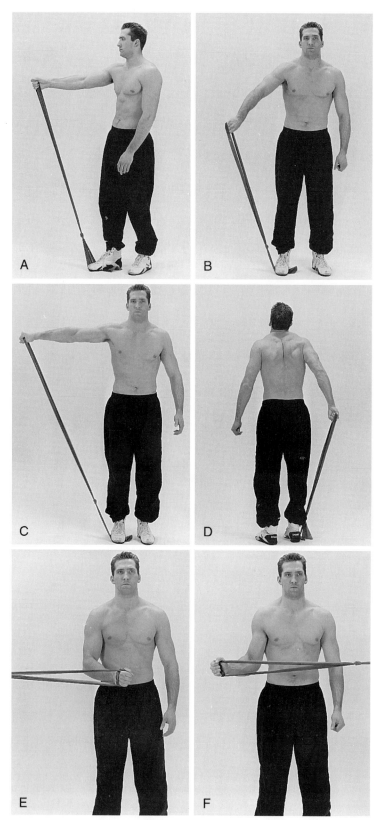

Figure 4–41. A–D, Specific Theraband exercises for the anterior deltoid, supraspinatus, and middle and posterior deltoid, respectively. E and F, Specific Theraband exercises for internal and external rotation.

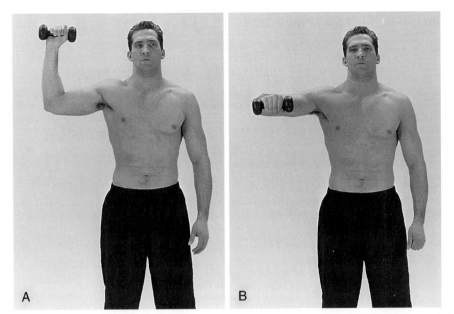

Figure 4–42. The "90/90" dumbbell resistance exercise for the rotator cuff, a recommended position- and muscle action–specific rehabilitation/"prehabilitation" exercise for throwing athletes. From a start position *(A)*, with the shoulder abducted 90 degrees and the elbow flexed 90 degrees, the dumbbell is lowered to horizontal *(B)* and raised back up. As the weight is lowered, internal rotation of the shoulder is resisted by eccentric action of the rotator cuff.

come by this easily. Hands-on motor skill coaching by a physical therapist has, in our experience, proved indispensable in this regard.

A caveat for the physician and therapist is that the frequency, duration, and intensity of rehabilitative exercise, as well as manipulative treatment and other activities, should be kept within the limits of relative rest. Attention should be paid to any symptoms during or following every session. The odd twinge of pain during activity is perhaps permissible but should be regarded with caution. Pain that persists for more than an hour afterward or is present the following day should be taken as an indication that the activity was excessive.

This is especially true regarding mobilization therapy. Any pain following treatment is probably indicative of an inflammatory response to tissue injury. The patient's response to increased pain will be limitation of active motion, and the net effect of treatment is more likely to be a further decrease rather than an increase in the range of motion.

Sport-specific functional drills are not begun until full and pain-free shoulder motion has been achieved. For a return to baseball pitching, the "fungo program" described by Kerlan is highly recommended. It can also be readily adapted to other overhand activities, e.g., serving in tennis or volleyball. The fungo program for throwers and a modified fungo program for tennis players are presented in outline form in Table 4–5.

Ideally, there is a gradually progressive return to full activity as symptoms permit. An absence of symptoms with an attempted level of activity is the criterion for advancement to that level of activity.

Table 4–5. "FUNGO" PROGRAMS

"Fungo" Return to Throwing Program[30]

The program derives its name from the fact that, as originally described, a baseball pitcher would throw to a fungo hitter, who in turn would hit the ball back to the pitcher. The essentials of the fungo program are as follows:

To minimize overuse, the throwing sessions are limited to 30 minutes, and a single ball is used. After each throw, the ball is hit or thrown back to the pitcher. The pitcher is instructed to throw with a full, easy, and painless motion. If there is any pain with attempted throwing, the pitcher refrains from throwing for 5 days. The sessions are preceded by stretching exercises and followed by stretching and ice massage.

Day 1 and 2. Pitcher in center field, throws ball so that it barely rolls to home plate.
Day 3. No throwing, continues other exercises.
Days 4 and 5. Pitcher between center field and second base, throws so ball arrives at home plate on third or fourth bounce.
Day 6. No throwing, continues other exercises.
Days 7 and 8. Pitcher at second base, throws so ball arrives at home plate on the fly (1–2 ft off ground).
Day 9. No throwing, continues other exercises.
Days 10 and 11. Pitcher on pitcher's mound, throws normal pitches.
Day 12. No throwing, continues other exercises.
Days 13 and beyond. Returns to normal activity.

Modified "Fungo" Program for Return to Tennis Serving

The player selects a court with a high backstop. Only one can of three balls is used. The balls must be hit and picked up before they are hit again. All serving is done from the service line. All other conditions noted previously pertain.

Days 1 and 2. Serves to hit backstop at eye level (5–6 ft off ground).
Day 3. Rest, continues other exercises.
Days 4 and 5. Serves to hit at or near junction of fence and ground.
Day 6. Rest, continues other exercises.
Days 7 and 8. Serves to hit backcourt boundary line.
Day 9. Rest, continues other exercises.
Days 10 and 11. Serves normally.
Day 12. Rest, continues other exercises.
Days 13 and beyond. Returns to normal activity.

N. OSTEOCHONDROSIS OF THE PROXIMAL HUMERAL EPIPHYSIS (LITTLE LEAGUER'S SHOULDER)

The differential diagnosis of "thrower's shoulder syndrome" in the skeletally immature includes injury (osteochondrosis) of the proximal humeral epiphysis, humeral stress fracture, glenoid osteochondrosis,[52] and elastofibroma,[25] all of which are rare.

Given the well-recognized and devastating problem of humeral capitellar osteochondrosis (Little Leaguer's elbow), there has been understandable concern about the possibility of similar injury to the shoulders of young throwing athletes. Indeed, overuse injury of the proximal humeral epiphysis, variously described in the literature as "epiphysitis," "epiphyseolyis," "false osteochondrosis," "fracture," "Little Leaguer's shoulder," "osteochondritis," and "stress fracture," has been reported. All appear to be the same entity and to be clinically quite similar to the other repetitive trauma-related osteochondroses, e.g., Little Leaguer's elbow, Osgood-Schlatter disease (traction apophysitis of the anterior tibial tubercle), or Sever's disease (traction apophysitis of the posterior calcaneus).

To put the problem in perspective, since it was first described by Dotter in 1953, there have been only 17 reported cases of Little Leaguer's shoulder in the English-speaking literature, and as late as 1990, a single case was considered reportable in a refereed journal.[1–3, 10, 17, 19, 55, 56] In contrast, Kibler reported that in his large series of young tennis players with shoulder overuse problems, 90% had the typical findings of "thrower's shoulder syndrome," as presented in the preceding section.[31]

In our experience, virtually all young athletes with throwing-related shoulder pain have essentially the same problems as do skeletally mature athletes. As discussed in the section on physical examination in [Structural] Glenohumeral Laxity/Contracture in part M, the finding of an increased range of external glenohumeral rotation and decreased range of internal rotation in the skeletally immature may be in part the result of bony torsion, as opposed to capsuloligamentous changes. The clinical significance of this is uncertain.

Our basic approach for young athletes with "thrower's shoulder syndrome" is the same as for older athletes, though we suggest that the possibility of bony or physeal injury be kept in mind. If after an appropriate trial of rehabilitative treatment, pain persists or promptly recurs with an attempted return to activity, further work-up, including radionuclide scintigraphy or MRI examination, is indicated.

One unique aspect of caring for young athletes is that there is appropriately a greater emphasis on injury prevention. Fortunately, there is a greater opportunity for this as well. Recommended measures for the prevention of "thrower's shoulder" problems in young athletes are as follow:

A preparticipation examination, in which treatable conditions such as posterior glenohumeral capsular contracture and rotator cuff insufficiency are sought

Rehabilitation of subclinical (asymptomatic) conditions identified on the preparticipation examination

Incorporation of "prehabilitation" stretching and strengthening exercises, identical to the rehabilitation exercises discussed previously, into the year-round training regimen

Keeping the frequency, duration, and intensity of all exercise within the limits of relative rest

Anticipating increased demands, e.g., the start of team practice, and allotting adequate time for preparation/adaptation

Limiting the total amount of pitching (especially individual practice in addition to games and team practice)

Learning and practicing proper throwing techniques

Emphasizing participation, fun, and motor skill learning over winning

Of all of these, parents' de-emphasizing winning is probably most important. If "Little League moms and dads" continually complain, "We lost because you put in Jimmy instead of Johnny," coaches will respond; Johnny will see more time on the mound. How does Johnny then continue to be the team's number 1 pitcher or Jimmy try to work his way back into the line-up? Beyond natural talent, it's "practice, practice, practice"—a set-up for overuse injury.

The effect of throwing different pitches probably also has more to do with competitiveness than technique. In order to be more competitive, a less talented young pitcher might try to learn to throw a curve ball or slider in addition to a fast ball and change-up. More pitches imply more practice required to perfect the pitches, which in turn implies a greater risk of overuse injury.

O. TRAUMATIC EXOSTOSIS OF THE HUMERUS ("BLOCKER'S NODULE")

In a small percentage of cases of chronic shoulder pain, radiographic examination may reveal new-bone formation on the lateral aspect of the humerus, in the area of the insertion of the deltoid or the origin of the brachialis. The new bone is the result of repetitive direct trauma, such as may occur with blocking in football, hence the term *blocker's nodule*. It may present as a painful or tender mass. If the deltoid muscle is involved, there may be pain and disability with shoulder abduction. If the brachialis is involved, there may be pain and disability with active elbow flexion, and elbow extension may be limited.

The major significance of this lesion is that it should not be confused with truly significant lesions, such as malignancies. Treatment is symptomatic. As for myositis ossificans, treatment should not include vigorous massage, painful passive stretching, and so forth, which may cause additional new-bone formation.

REFERENCES

1. Adams JE: Little League shoulder osteochondrosis of the proximal humeral epiphysis in boy baseball pitchers. Calif Med Assoc J 105:22, 1966.
2. Adams JE: Bone injuries in very young athletes. Clin Orthop 58:129–140, 1968.
3. Albert M, Drvaric DM: Little League shoulder: Case report. Orthopedics 13:779–781, 1990.
4. Allman FL Jr: Fractures and ligamentous injuries of the clavicle and its articulation. J Bone Joint Surg Am 49:774–784, 1967.
5. Arciero RA, Wheeler JH, Ryan JB, McBride JT: Arthroscopic Bankart repair versus nonoperative treatment for acute, initial anterior shoulder dislocations. Am J Sports Med 22:589–594, 1994.
6. Aronen JG: Problems of the upper extremity in gymnastics. Clin Sports Med 4(1):61–71, 1985.
7. Aronen JG: Anterior shoulder dislocations in sports. Sports Med 3(3):224–234, 1986.
8. Aronen JG, Regan K: Decreasing the incidence of recurrence of first time anterior shoulder dislocations with rehabilitation. Am J Sports Med 12:283–291, 1984.
9. Bankart ASB: The pathology and treatment of recurrent dislocation of the shoulder joint. Br J Surg 26:23–29, 1938.
10. Barnett LS: Little League shoulder syndrome: Proximal humeral epiphyseolysis in adolescent baseball pitchers. J Bone Joint Surg Am 67:495–496, 1985.
11. Bergfeld JA, Andrish JT, Clancy WG: Evaluation of the acromioclavicular joint following first- and second-degree sprains. Am J Sports Med 6:153–159, 1978.
12. Blazina ME, Satzman JS: Recurrent anterior subluxation of the shoulder in athletes—A distinct entity. J Bone Joint Surg Am 51:1037–1038, 1969.
13. Blom S, Dahlback LO: Nerve injuries in dislocations of the shoulder joint and fractures of the neck of the humerus. Acta Chir Scand 136:461–466, 1970.
14. Broström LA, Kronberg M, Nemeth G, Oxelback U: The effect of shoulder muscle training in patients with recurrent shoulder dislocations. Scand J Rehabil Med 24(1):11–15, 1992.
15. Buckerfield CT, Castle ME: Acute traumatic retrosternal dislocation of the clavicle. J Bone Joint Surg Am 66:379–385, 1984.
16. Cahill B: Osteolysis of distal part of clavicle in male athletes. J Bone Joint Surg Am 64:1053–1058, 1982.
17. Cahill BR: Little League shoulder: Lesions of the proximal humeral epiphyseal plate. J Sports Med 2:150–152, 1974.
18. Codman EA: The Shoulder. Boston, Thomas Todd, 1934.
19. Dotter WE: Little Leaguers' shoulder: A fracture of the proximal epiphyseal cartilage of the humerus due to baseball pitching. Guthrie Clin Bull 23:68–72, 1953.
20. Garrick JG, Requa RK: Medical care and injury surveillance in the high school setting. Physician Sportsmed 9:115–120, 1981.
21. Gerber C, Ganz R: Clinical assessment of instability of the shoulder, with special reference to the anterior and posterior drawer tests. J Bone Joint Surg Br 66:551–556, 1984.

22. Gilcreest EL: The common syndrome of rupture, dislocation, and elongation of the long head of the biceps brachii. An analysis of one hundred cases. Surg Gynecol Obstet 58:322–340, 1934.
23. Glick JM, Milburn LJ, Haggerty JF, Nishimoto D: Dislocated acromioclavicular joint: Follow-up study of 35 unreduced acromioclavicular dislocations. Am J Sports Med 5:264–270, 1977.
24. Glousman RE, Jobe FW, Tibone JE, et al: Dynamic EMG analysis of the throwing shoulder with glenohumeral instability. J Bone Joint Surg Am 70:220, 1988.
25. Haney TC: Subscapular elastofibroma in a young pitcher. A case report. Am J Sports Med 18:642–644, 1990.
26. Hawkins RJ, Kennedy JC: Impingement syndrome in athletes. Am J Sports Med 8:151–158, 1980.
27. Hill HA, Sachs MD: The grooved defect of the humeral head. A frequently unrecognized complication of dislocations of the shoulder joint. Radiology 35:690–700, 1940.
28. Imatani RJ, Hanlon JJ, Cady GW: Acute complete acromioclavicular separation. J Bone Joint Surg Am 7:328–332, 1975.
29. Jobe FW, Kvitne RS, Giangarra CE: Shoulder pain in the overhand or throwing athlete. The relationship of anterior instability and rotator cuff impingement [published erratum appears in Orthop Rev 18:1268, 1989]. Orthop Rev 18:963–975, 1989.
30. Kerlan RK, Jobe FW, Blazina ME, et al: Throwing injuries of the shoulder and elbow in adults. Curr Pract Orthoped Surg 6:41–48, 1975.
31. Kibler WB: The Sport Preparticipation Fitness Examination. Champaign, Ill, Human Kinetics Books, 1990.
32. Kocher T: Eine neue Reductionsmethode für Schulterverrenkung. Berlin Klin 7:101–105, 1870.
33. Kuriyama S, Fujimaki E, Katagiri T, Uemura S: Anterior dislocation of the shoulder sustained through skiing: Arthrographic findings and prognosis. Am J Sports Med 12:339–346, 1984.
34. Kvitne RS, Jobe FW: The diagnosis and treatment of anterior instability in the throwing athlete. Clin Orthop 291:107–123, 1993.
35. Matsen FA III, Zuckerman JD: Anterior glenohumeral instability. Clin Sports Med 2:319–338, 1983.
36. McLaughlin HL, MacLellan DL: Recurrent anterior dislocation of the shoulder. II: A comparative study. J Trauma 7:191–201, 1967.
37. Mumford EB: Acromioclavicular dislocation. J Bone Joint Surg 23:799–802, 1941.
38. Neer CS II: Displaced proximal humeral fractures. 1: Classification and evaluation. J Bone Joint Surg Am 52:1077–1089, 1970.
39. Neer CS II: Impingement lesions. Clin Orthop 173:70–77, 1983.
40. Nicol EE: Miners and mannequins. J Bone Joint Surg Br 36:171–172, 1954.
41. Pappas AM, Goss TP, Kleinman PK: Symptomatic shoulder instability due to lesions of the glenoid labrum. Am J Sports Med 11:279–288, 1983.
42. Protzman RR: Anterior instability of the shoulder. J Bone Joint Surg Am 62:909–918, 1980.
43. Rockwood CA Jr, Williams GR, Young CD: Injuries to the acromioclavicular joint. In Rockwood CA Jr, Green DP, Bucholz RW, Heckman JD (eds): Fractures in Adults, 4th ed, vol 2. Philadelphia, Lippincott-Raven, 1996, pp 1341–1413.
44. Rockwood CA Jr, Wirth MA: Injuries to the sternoclavicular joint. In Rockwood CA Jr, Green DP, Bucholz RW, Heckman JD (eds): Fractures in Adults, 4th ed, vol 2. Philadelphia, Lippincott-Raven, 1996, pp 1415–1471.
45. Rockwood CA Jr, Wirth MA: Subluxations and dislocations about the glenohumeral joint. In Rockwood CA Jr, Green DP, Bucholz RW, Heckman JD (eds): Fractures in Adults, 4th ed, vol 2. Philadelphia, Lippincott-Raven, 1996, pp 1193–1339.
46. Rokous JR et al: Modified axillary roentgenogram. A useful adjunct in the diagnosis of recurrent instability of the shoulder. Clin Orthop 82:84–86, 1972.
47. Rowe CR: The Bankart procedure: A long-term end-result study. J Bone Joint Surg Am 60:1–16, 1978.
48. Rowe CR: Acute and recurrent anterior dislocations of the shoulder. Orthop Clin North Am 11:253–270, 1980.
49. Rowe CR, Sakellarides HT: Factors related to recurrences of anterior dislocations of the shoulder. Clin Orthop 20:40–47, 1961.
50. Rowe CR, Zarins B: Recurrent transient subluxation of the shoulder. J Bone Joint Surg Am 63:863–871, 1981.
51. Selesnick FH, Jablon M, Frank C, Post M: Retrosternal dislocation of the clavicle. Report of four cases. J Bone Joint Surg Am 66:287–291, 1984.
52. Stanley DJ, Mulligan ME: Osteochondrosis dissecans of the glenoid. Skeletal Radiol 19:419–421, 1990.
53. Stimson LA: An easy method of reducing dislocations of the shoulder and hip. Med Record 57:356–357, 1900.
54. Strukel RJ, Garrick JG: Thoracic outlet compression in athletes. Am J Sports Med 6:35–39, 1978.
55. Torg JS: The Little League pitcher. Am Fam Physician 6:71–76, 1972.

56. Tullos HS, Fain RS: Little League shoulder: Rotational stress fracture of the proximal humeral epiphysis. J Sports Med 2:152–153, 1974.
57. Walsh WM, Peterson DA, Shelton G, Neumann RD: Shoulder strength following acromioclavicular injury. Am J Sports Med 13:153–158, 1985.
58. Warren RF: Subluxation of the shoulder in athletes. Clin Sports Med 2:339–354, 1983.
59. Yergason RM: Supination sign. J Bone Joint Surg 13:160, 1931.
60. Yoneda B, Welsh RP, MacIntosh DL: Conservative treatment of shoulder dislocation in young males. J Bone Joint Surg Br 64:254–255, 1982.

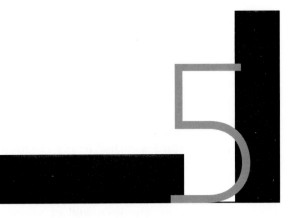

Elbow Injuries

Conditions to Be Referred

- Dislocations
- Radial head fractures with more than 5 mm of displacement
- Osteochondritis dissecans of capitellum
- Infected olecranon bursa
- Distal humerus fracture

Triage

Indications for Referral

- **Acute**
  History
    Neurological symptoms distal to elbow
    History consistent with dislocation
  Examination
    Any deformity (elbow or radial head)
  X-ray films
    Any fracture (but nondisplaced radial head)
    Dislocation
- **Gradual onset**
  History
  Examination
    Loose bodies
    Defect in capitellum (osteochondritis dissecans)

Indications for X-Ray Films

- **Acute**
  History
    Abrupt loss of motion
    Dislocation
  Examination
    Loss of motion
    Obvious deformity (dislocation, radial head)
- **Gradual onset**
  History
    Loose body sensation or locking
  Examination
    Tenderness at lateral joint line (capitellum)
    Loss of motion

Although not as complex as shoulder injuries, as glamorous as knee injuries, or as frequent as ankle injuries, elbow injuries in sports are nevertheless of great concern to athletes and their physicians. With any elbow injury, the use of the upper limb in sports is, at least temporarily, impaired. Certain injuries in certain sports, for example, osteochondrosis in a young gymnast, can be career ending, and no athlete is completely immune; even runners can trip and fall and injure their elbows.

Injuries to the elbow include two of the most commonly recognized sport-named injuries, tennis elbow and Little Leaguer's elbow. Common extensor tendinitis, or tennis elbow, may be considered the archetypal example of overuse injury and tendinitis. We discuss it and the medial tension/lateral compression syndromes, which include Little Leaguer's elbow, in some detail.

A complete discussion of fractures and dislocations about the elbow is clearly beyond the scope of this text. In this chapter we discuss mainly the sports medicine aspects of those injuries occurring frequently enough to be considered characteristic sports injuries—posterior and posterolateral elbow dislocations and radial head compression fractures.

We also briefly discuss the following less common sports injuries: olecranon bursitis (analogous to prepatellar bursitis at the knee [see Chapter 9, part H]), posterior impingement syndrome, and myositis ossificans (see also Chapter 8, part F).

Localization of signs and symptoms makes the diagnostic approach to these injuries rather straightforward, and we do not discuss it separately.

A. ANATOMY RELEVANT TO FRACTURES AND DISLOCATIONS

The radius and ulna are paired structures. With displaced fracture or dislocation of one, injury to the other must be sought. A classic example is Monteggia's lesion, a fracture of the proximal half of the ulna with dislocation of the radial head, produced either by a fall with forced pronation or by a direct blow over the posterior ulna.

The proximal aspect of the ulna articulates with the trochlea of the humerus, and the radial head articulates with the capitellum of the humerus and the radial notch of the ulna. In by far the majority of elbow dislocations, the joined radius and ulna dislocate together, posteriorly or posterolaterally with respect to the humerus.[7]

Three bony landmarks, the tip of the olecranon and the medial and lateral epicondyles, are in line when the elbow is extended and form an equilateral triangle when the elbow is flexed. With dislocation of the elbow, this relationship is lost, but it is maintained with supracondylar fractures, which can sometimes be mistaken for posterior dislocations.

The aphorism "A fracture is a soft tissue injury complicated by a broken bone" especially applies to elbow injuries. The typical posterior or posterolateral elbow dislocation involves, to a greater or lesser extent, tearing of the collateral ligaments, anterior joint capsule, and brachialis muscle. With severely displaced fractures or dislocations, the brachial artery and the median, radial, and especially the ulnar nerves are at risk.

In football and wrestling the "locker room diagnosis" of elbow hyperextension is often made. Many of these injuries are actually momentary subluxations of the elbow, and all involve sprains, particularly of the medial collateral ligament. The findings, prognosis, and treatment are similar to those of a reduced elbow dislocation.

B. POSTERIOR AND POSTEROLATERAL DISLOCATIONS OF THE ELBOW

HISTORY

MECHANISM OF INJURY. The usual mechanism of injury is a fall onto the outstretched hand with the limb abducted and the elbow extended. Relatively little force is required to dislocate the elbow—falling from a horse, falling from a gymnastic apparatus, or even falling from a standing height can produce the injury. A typical history is of slipping and falling backward onto the outstretched hand, as often occurs in skateboarding and roller skating.

SYMPTOMS. For the most part the symptoms are those usually associated with severe musculoskeletal injury, e.g., a snapping or cracking sensation at the time of injury, immediate pain, rapid swelling, limitation of motion, and an inability to continue activity. Pain is often localized mainly to the medial aspect of the elbow. With associated fracture of the medial epicondyle, crepitation may be noted.

PHYSICAL EXAMINATION

The injured arm is held with the elbow mildly flexed and supported, if possible, by the uninjured arm.

The hallmark finding is the striking and characteristic *deformity* of the elbow. The olecranon is prominent posteriorly or posterolaterally, and the skin is tented over it and indented between it and the arm. The normal triangular relationship of the olecranon and humeral epicondyles is lost (see part A).

Within a short while after injury, there is marked swelling, ecchymosis, and tenderness, usually most prominent medially. Neurovascular impairment is uncommon but must be ruled out (see part F and Chapter 6, part E).

RADIOGRAPHIC EXAMINATION

Radiographic examination is indicated to confirm the diagnosis and to rule in or out the presence of associated fracture of the medial epicondyle. Anteroposterior and lateral views are obtained "as is," without moving the elbow (Figs. 5–1 and 5–2).

Prereduction films are always preferred. However, if the clinical diagnosis of dislocation can be made with certainty and if a growth plate injury is unlikely (the athlete is high school age or older), gentle reduction may be

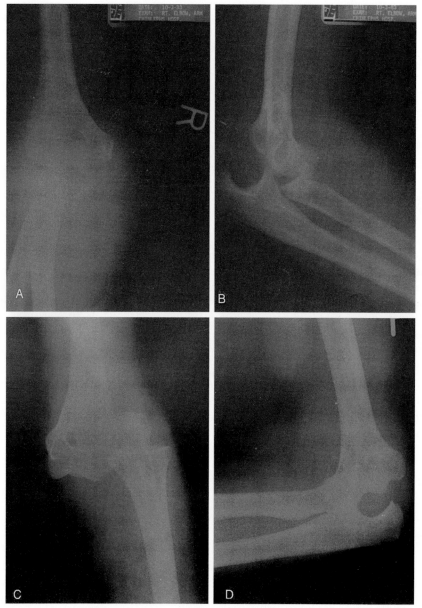

Figure 5-1. Anteroposterior (AP) and lateral radiographs of the elbow showing a typical posterior dislocation *(A and B)* and a lateral dislocation *(C and D)*.

attempted *by an experienced physician* on the playing field or in the locker room.[7] In all cases, postreduction films are indicated.

INITIAL TREATMENT

As with other major joint dislocations, dislocations of the elbow should be reduced as quickly, gently, and safely as possible. Early reduction minimizes the amount of muscle spasm that must be overcome to effect reduction and thereby minimizes discomfort and risk of further injury.

Judging only from the lateral radiograph, it would seem a simple matter

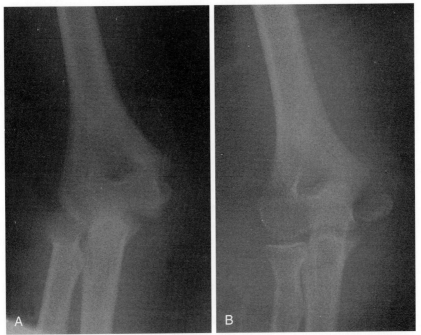

Figure 5–2. AP radiographs of the elbow demonstrating a posterolateral dislocation with associated avulsion fracture of the medial epicondyle. *A,* Prereduction. *B,* Postreduction. This injury is particularly common in the skeletally immature. An intra-articular fracture fragment may hinder closed reduction.

merely to extend the elbow and pull on the forearm. The temptation to do so, however, should be resisted, as it would only add to the anterior soft tissue injury.[7, 11] Rather, the elbow is kept in the "as-is" gently flexed position, and the coronoid process is disengaged from the olecranon fossa by gentle downward pressure on the proximal part of the forearm. With the use of the epicondyles and the olecranon as landmarks, mediolateral alignment is obtained. Then the forearm is brought forward to effect the reduction.

Within a few minutes after injury, reduction may be attempted without medication. If the reduction cannot be readily achieved, or if more time has elapsed since the injury, medication is required. Complete analgesia and muscle relaxation are necessary for atraumatic reduction. Usually this implies intravenous regional anesthesia (Bier's block), axillary nerve block, or general anesthesia.

After reduction, the neurovascular status of the limb is reassessed. The elbow is flexed and extended and the forearm pronated and supinated to confirm the reduction and to rule out mechanical block of normal joint motion. A posterior splint is applied, and radiographic examination is repeated.

An intra-articular fracture fragment may prevent closed reduction. Also, a clinically apparent "anatomical" reduction may not be—the radius and ulna may remain displaced laterally with the olecranon "articulating" with the groove between the trochlea and capitellum.

Because of the relative technical difficulty and the possibility of complications, we generally recommend that attempts at reduction be left to an orthopedist. Unreduced dislocations should be immobilized "as is" with sling and swathe. Intermittent icing is appropriate, whether or not reduction has been achieved.

REFERRAL

Orthopedic referral on an *urgent* basis is indicated for unreduced dislocations. Referral on an *emergent* basis is indicated if there is any neurovascular impairment. Even if reduction has been achieved, and especially in children, we recommend that an orthopedist be involved early in the management of this athletic career–threatening injury.

DEFINITIVE TREATMENT

As a rule, when closed reduction of the dislocated radius and ulna is carried out as described previously, associated avulsion fractures of the medial epicondyle are also reduced. However, if a fracture fragment remains in the joint or if closed reduction of the dislocation cannot be achieved, open reduction is indicated.

After reduction, posterior stability is assessed by gently extending the elbow; medial stability, by applying gentle valgus stress. If the reduction is unstable, as may be the case with grade III sprains of the medial collateral ligament or avulsion fractures of the medial epicondyle, and particularly if there is an anticipated return to activities such as throwing, gymnastics, and wrestling, operative treatment may be required.

After reduction or operation, the arm is placed in a posterior splint and sling. When swelling has stabilized, usually in 2 or 3 days, the splint is removed two or three times a day for pain-free, active range-of-motion exercises. Measures to reduce swelling, such as ice and electrogalvanic stimulation (EGS) treatments, may also be employed. If the elbow is stable, the use of the splint is generally discontinued altogether after a week or two, and only a sling is used for protection. Particularly in children, the sling serves as a reminder to the patient and others not to be too rambunctious.

Instability or extensive injury may necessitate using the splint for up to 4 weeks. However, if splinting is required for more than 1 week, the elbow should be immobilized in as much extension as its stability permits. Usually, immobilization in 45 degrees of flexion is possible. It is much easier to regain flexion than extension.

While the elbow is still in the splint, strength training is begun with gentle isometric exercises for the elbow flexors and extensors, and when the splint is removed, with antigravity flexion and extension. About the time that use of the splint is discontinued altogether, progressive resistance exercises with Theraband and contract/relax stretching are begun and advanced as tolerated. As the wrist flexors and extensors and pronator teres contribute to elbow stability, progressive resistance exercises for these muscles are also included (see parts E and F).

Under no circumstances are passive range-of-motion exercises employed. Carrying weights to promote extension is almost certain to enhance flexion contracture. Also, if there has been extensive soft tissue damage and any evidence of heterotopic calcification in the anterior soft tissues, then all but gentle, pain-free, active range-of-motion exercises are discontinued (see part H).

Loss of a few degrees of extension is not uncommon after any elbow dislocation. Because hyperextension is often present normally, loss of 5 or 10 degrees of extension may still allow the elbow to be held straight. If so, for support movements such as cartwheels in gymnastics, the elbow can still be "locked out." If not, longitudinal loading will produce flexion rather than compression forces at the joint, and the ability to resist elbow flexion will depend entirely on triceps strength. To compensate, the triceps must be superstrengthened and maintained that way.

Before complete healing and rehabilitation have occurred, the use of a small, hinged knee brace may provide sufficient mediolateral stability and permit sufficient flexion and extension that a conscientious athlete may safely resume some activities, such as limited gymnastics workouts. However, before the resumption of contact and collision sports, throwing, support moves in gymnastics, and so on, it is mandatory to have a pain-free, stable range of motion; full strength; and radiographic union of any fractures.

C. COMPRESSION FRACTURES OF THE RADIAL HEAD

HISTORY

MECHANISM OF INJURY. The usual mechanism of injury is a more or less vertical fall onto the outstretched hand with the elbow extended.

SYMPTOMS. The symptoms are those commonly associated with fractures, namely, immediate and well-localized pain, swelling, crepitation, increased pain on motion, and limitation of motion.

PHYSICAL EXAMINATION

The hallmark finding is *point tenderness* over the radial head. As with other intra-articular injuries, palpation may reveal a joint effusion (Fig. 5–3A). Elbow flexion and extension and forearm pronation and supination are variably limited and painful.

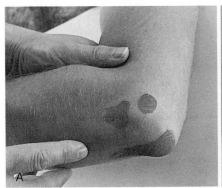 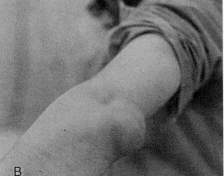

Figure 5–3. *A,* With distention of the elbow joint by blood or synovial fluid, the diffuse fluctuant swelling is most evident in the triangular space bounded by the radial head, lateral epicondyle, and tip of the olecranon. *B,* In contrast, with olecranon bursitis there is a discrete, sharply demarcated, fluctuant goose egg directly overlying the olecranon process.

RADIOGRAPHIC EXAMINATION

Radiographic examination is indicated mainly to assess displacement and comminution and to rule out physeal injury in the skeletally immature. With nondisplaced fractures, the fracture line may not be evident, but a positive fat pad sign (Fig. 5–4) is suggestive of the diagnosis.

INITIAL TREATMENT

The initial, mainly symptomatic, treatment comprises RICE (relative rest, ice, compression, and elevation), sling, analgesics, and the like. A splint may be employed for a few days, but as discussed in the previous section, prolonged immobilization of the elbow is not desirable.

REFERRAL

Orthopedic referral is indicated for unreduced displaced or severely comminuted fractures.

DEFINITIVE TREATMENT

With nondisplaced fractures, definitive treatment comprises early mobilization and rehabilitation of the muscles of the arm and forearm as symptoms permit (see part B). With clinical union of the fracture, activity may be resumed as tolerated.

Displaced fractures may require open reduction and internal fixation of

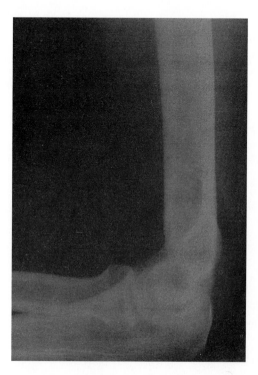

Figure 5–4. Lateral radiograph of the elbow showing a fat pad sign. Fluid within the joint displaces the anterior fat pad proximally and anteriorly, giving it a characteristic sail-shaped appearance.

the fracture fragment or, in the skeletally mature, excision of the radial head with or without prosthetic replacement. Even with operative treatment, however, there may be long-term complications, as typified by the medial tension/lateral compression and posterior impingement syndromes (see parts F and G).

D.   OLECRANON BURSITIS (MINER'S ELBOW, STUDENT'S ELBOW)

HISTORY

MECHANISM OF INJURY. Any direct trauma to the posterior aspect of the elbow can cause injury to the bursa, which lies between the skin and the olecranon. The typical injury is the result of *repetitive pressure and friction,* as is common in wrestling. A direct blow, as may occur in falling or diving for a ball, can produce acute, hemorrhagic bursitis. Abrasions (turf burns, road rash, and the like), lacerations, and puncture wounds (including those rendered by needle and syringe) can result in septic bursitis.

Once the condition becomes chronic, episodes of swelling occur with progressively less trauma. With each episode, the bursa tends to enlarge.

SYMPTOMS. The chief complaint is usually of the *swelling* itself. Pain, tenderness, and limitation of elbow flexion are variable, depending on the onset and cause.

Even when the bursa is not distended, the athlete may still notice some subcutaneous mass or irregularity overlying the olecranon. Although this actually represents the thickened, collapsed bursa, it is often perceived as being a loose body or "something broken off."

PHYSICAL EXAMINATION

Physical examination typically reveals a discrete, fluctuant, variably tender mass overlying the olecranon (Fig. 5–3B). Pressure over the mass brings the edges into sharp definition. Even when decompressed, the edges of the thickened bursa are usually readily palpable (see earlier). The mass may transilluminate, and elbow flexion may be limited by pain.

There may also be signs of infection—erythema, calor, "touch-me-not" tenderness, purulent exudate, cellulitis, lymphangitis, or lymphadenopathy, for example. Usually these are found in association with some disruption of the integument, such as abrasion or laceration.

RADIOGRAPHIC EXAMINATION

Radiographic examination is not required.

OTHER DIAGNOSTIC TESTS

Other diagnostic tests are not required unless there are symptoms or signs of infection, in which case aspiration of the bursa, with Gram's stain, and culture and sensitivity studies of the aspirate, is indicated.

INITIAL TREATMENT

Uncomplicated, *traumatic olecranon bursitis* can often be satisfactorily treated by rest (protection from further injury), ice, compression, and anti-inflammatory medication. Of these, compression and protection from further injury are most important.

Aspiration can be both diagnostic and therapeutic and is indicated if the clinical findings are consistent with acute hemorrhage, infection, or long-standing inflammation. The bursa is aspirated under sterile conditions, care being taken not to introduce the needle into the bursa through an area of skin abrasion (contamination) or infection. Unless there is evidence of infection, a snug compression wrap is then applied using 4×4s, ABDs, Tubi-Grip, and sometimes a neoprene sleeve. It is to be worn for a minimum of 1 week, and during the first 48 hours it is not to be removed even for icing.

If there is evidence of infection, additional treatment comprises warm soaks four times a day and administration of specific antibiotics. Pending the results of the culture and sensitivity studies, we usually begin antibiotic therapy with cephalexin 500 mg four times a day.

REFERRAL

Referral is indicated if infection does not respond promptly to treatment or if there is persistent inflammation, recurrent fluid accumulation, progressive enlargement of the bursa, and so on, despite appropriate initial treatment.

DEFINITIVE TREATMENT

If initial measures are unsuccessful, traumatic bursitis is next treated by repeat aspiration and corticosteroid injection. Under sterile conditions, fluid is aspirated, the needle is left in place, and a 1:1 mixture of betamethasone and 0.25% bupivacaine with epinephrine is instilled. A compression wrap is applied as previously described. The patient must understand that continuous compression not only is important but is critical. Bursectomy is the only remaining option for definitive treatment.

Septic bursitis may require incision and drainage. However, repeated aspiration, if successful, is preferable to wide incision, as the skin over the elbow is under tension, and healing by secondary intention is slow. Rarely, bursectomy may be required.

Elbow pads afford some protection during athletic activities such as football, indoor soccer, and skateboarding that entail a high risk of falling on the elbows. However, they are of decidedly limited utility in sports such as wrestling, in which constant rubbing, rather than direct blows, is the problem.

E. COMMON EXTENSOR TENDINITIS (TENNIS ELBOW, LATERAL EPICONDYLITIS)

Common extensor tendinitis, or tennis elbow, is clearly the most common cause of chronic elbow pain in athletes.

The term *tennis elbow,* though imprecise, has become a permanent part of the vocabulary of sports medicine. Some use the term to denote any elbow pain related to tennis playing or similar activities. Others, ourselves included, use the term specifically to denote the syndrome of lateral elbow and dorsal forearm pain related to use of the wrist extensor muscles.[5, 13–15]

The commonly used medical term for tennis elbow, *lateral (humeral) epicondylitis,* is anatomically precise but does not reflect the pathomechanics of the condition. We prefer the term *common extensor tendinitis,* which not only names the primarily involved structure but also suggests the mechanisms of injury, the signs and symptoms, the natural history, and the preferred therapy.

HISTORY

MECHANISM OF INJURY. Tennis elbow is the result of functional demands that exceed the strength, endurance, or flexibility of the wrist extensor muscles and tendons.[20] The cause of tennis elbow is multifactorial. Either prolonged repetitive use of the wrist extensors, as may occur in lifting parts off an assembly line, or sustained contraction, as may occur with gripping a hammer or a tennis racquet, can lead to overuse injury and tendinitis. Less commonly, tendinitis is simply the end result of a single acute injury.

Of the several etiological factors, the power grip seems to be most often implicated. Strong gripping requires synergistic action of the wrist extensors and the finger flexors (Fig. 5–5).

Impact and eccentric loading are other commonly implicated factors. Impact, which is transmitted via the grip to the wrist extensors, may be that of a racquet hitting a tennis ball or a hammer hitting a nail. Eccentric loading, in the case of tennis elbow, means that the wrist is forcibly (palmar) flexed or ulnar-deviated against the pull of the extensor muscles.

To the extent that an activity involves a power grip, impact, or eccentric loading of the wrist extensors, it is likely to cause tennis elbow. In racquet sports, any or all of the following risk factors may be contributory: gripping the racquet too tightly, an improper grip size, excessive string tension, an excessive racquet weight or stiffness, a faulty backhand technique ("leading-elbow backhand," "wristy backhand"), putting a top spin on backhand shots, hitting the ball off center.

It would appear that nearly all cases of acute second- or third-degree

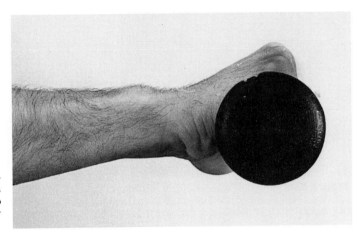

Figure 5–5. Power grip. Extension of the wrist affords greater mechanical advantage to the finger flexors and thereby permits a more powerful grip.

strains of the wrist extensors are the result of eccentric loading. Such injuries occasionally occur in racquet sports, e.g., with a mis-hit backhand shot, and in others, e.g., with a clean-and-jerk attempt in weight lifting. Tendinitis is the predictable sequela of incomplete recovery and rehabilitation of such injuries.

SYMPTOMS. The hallmark symptom is lateral elbow pain related to use of the wrist extensors.

With overuse injury there is often a characteristic onset and progression of symptoms. In most cases a careful history reveals some change—a new racquet, a different technique, increased playing time, and so on—preceding the onset of symptoms. At first athletes may be aware only of fatigue and spasm of the dorsal forearm muscles related to the unaccustomed activity. Then they may note the onset of aching lateral elbow pain after playing. Subsequently they may start to have sharp pain during play, especially with backhands and mis-hits. Eventually the pain may become so constant and severe as to preclude further playing and to interfere with activities of daily living, such as carrying a briefcase, wringing wet clothes, or even holding a cup of coffee.

Other possible symptoms (and signs) include crepitation related to the use of the inflamed tendon, and swelling and ecchymosis associated with acute strains.

PHYSICAL EXAMINATION

There are two hallmark signs of tennis elbow: *point tenderness over or just distal to the lateral humeral epicondyle* (the bony attachment of the common extensor tendon) *and pain with resisted wrist extension.*

Other possible physical findings include tenderness over the muscles of the dorsal forearm, pain with resisted finger extension, pain with resisted radial deviation of the wrist, and pain with passive stretching of the wrist extensors (Fig. 5–6).

With long-standing symptoms there is likely to be considerable atrophy and weakness of the extensor muscles and limitation of passive wrist flexion.

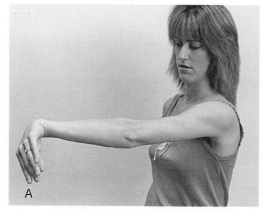 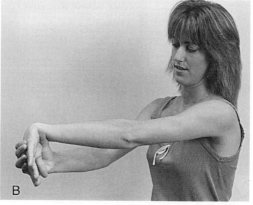

Figure 5–6. Stretching exercises for tennis elbow. The position of maximal stretch of the wrist extensors is with the elbow extended, the forearm pronated, and the wrist flexed. The stretching may be done actively *(A)* or passively *(B)*. The athlete stretches and holds for 10 seconds, then relaxes for 2 to 3 seconds. This is repeated 10 times.

RADIOGRAPHIC EXAMINATION

Elbow films may reveal calcification in the common extensor tendon. However, radiographic examination and other diagnostic tests are usually not required.

INITIAL TREATMENT

Initial treatment is symptomatic and anti-inflammatory.

With acute injury the principal aim is to prevent or reduce swelling. RICE is applicable. Ice and EGS treatments may also be appropriate.

With the more typical overuse injury, the aim is to reduce pain and inflammation. Relative rest is the most important aspect of treatment. Other treatment options include ice massage, friction massage, ultrasound therapy, and anti-inflammatory medication.

Relative rest implies avoidance of pain-producing athletic and nonathletic activities. The athlete who is advised to forgo tennis playing temporarily must also be cautioned with respect to gardening, housework, carpentry, carrying suitcases, and similar activities.

Athletes who have pain only on hitting backhand shots can continue to practice their forehand and overhead shots or perhaps even continue to play using a two-handed backhand stroke. Athletes who feel they must continue to play regardless of pain may find that the use of a tennis elbow forearm band permits them to do so with less pain.

The athlete who has pain even with "unavoidable" activities of daily living may require immobilization in the form of a sling or splint, or both. A volar splint with the wrist in 20 degrees of extension or a "gymnast's wrist splint" (see Chapter 6, part D) usually permits the functional use of the hand while preventing overuse of the wrist extensors.

Anti-inflammatory medication is one of the mainstays of initial treatment. We prefer to use an oral nonsteroidal anti-inflammatory drug (NSAID) (in appropriate anti-inflammatory doses) first.

If the response to initial therapy is inadequate; if further activity restriction, additional physical therapy, and so on are impractical; and if the physical findings are well localized, we would consider local corticosteroid injection. The risk and consequences of tendon rupture, a possible side effect of corticosteroid injection, are much less in the case of tennis elbow than in the case of tendons subject to weight-bearing loads. Of greater concern for some patients are the possible cosmetic side effects related to local skin atrophy or depigmentation. For the athlete seen within a few days of the onset of symptoms, an *initial*, successful corticosteroid injection may preclude the muscle weakness and thus appreciably shorten the rehabilitation period.

We prefer to use a mixture of a long-acting local anesthetic with the corticosteroid suspension. Prompt relief of pain and tenderness after injection lets both the athlete and the physician know that the medication was properly placed. It is important, however, to inform the athlete that the pain may later recur and last for a few hours to a few days. This reflects the fact that the effects of the local anesthetic are likely to wear off before the full effects of the corticosteroid are realized.

All concerned should understand that none of the foregoing measures are curative. Relief of pain and inflammation is not the "bottom line" of therapy but rather a first step that facilitates rehabilitation.

REHABILITATION

The aim of rehabilitation is to restore the strength, endurance, and flexibility of the wrist extensors. This can usually be accomplished with a home program, the key elements of which are static stretching exercises and progressive resistance Theraband exercises (see Figs. 5–6 and 5–7). Both the physician and the athlete should bear in mind that the longer the symptoms have been present, the longer the rehabilitative effort will take.

Stretching exercises are usually done as a warm-up before the resistance exercises. Isometric (manual resistance), isotonic (weights), or isokinetic exercises may be done instead of or in addition to the Theraband exercises. Heat or ultrasound therapy may be used before exercise. Ice in the form of ice packs or ice massage is used afterward.

It is important to inform the athlete that the prescribed therapeutic exercises have the potential to make the symptoms worse rather than better if done too vigorously or too soon. As with other activity, the concept of relative rest applies, i.e., the exercises should not produce immediate or delayed pain.

We have found that early in the course of rehabilitation the athlete is likely to tolerate limited-arc, fast-contraction, light-resistance Theraband exercises better than other resistance exercises (Fig. 5–7). The main purpose of the light-resistance exercises is to build muscular endurance. The athlete gradually works up to doing two and then three sets of these at a time before going on to heavier-resistance exercises.

Occasionally athletes are unable to do even light-resistance Theraband exercises without having pain. In this case, we recommend that they use an electrical muscle stimulator (EMS) unit until they are able to start doing the Theraband exercises (Fig. 5–8). EMS is time-consuming but usually well tolerated and effective.

REFERRAL

If symptoms persist or recur despite adequate nonoperative treatment, referral is indicated.

DEFINITIVE TREATMENT

In well over 90% of cases, all that is required for definitive treatment of tennis elbow is adequate rest, appropriate rehabilitation, correction of faulty technique, and gradual resumption of playing.

In tennis, elimination of the "leading-elbow backhand" may be the single most important factor in preventing recurrent symptoms. A larger grip size may lessen torque (eccentric loading) and thereby minimize the grip strength requirements.[4] Racquet stiffness and string tension must be consistent with the athlete's strength, muscular endurance, and playing ability. A competent coach can be invaluable in helping the athlete to sort out these considerations.

Return to tennis playing is accomplished by following a plan similar to the fungo program for shoulder injuries (see Table 4–5). Stretching exercises are done before and after practice. Ice is used after the final stretching. Only one can of balls is used to limit the number of strokes per session. Only

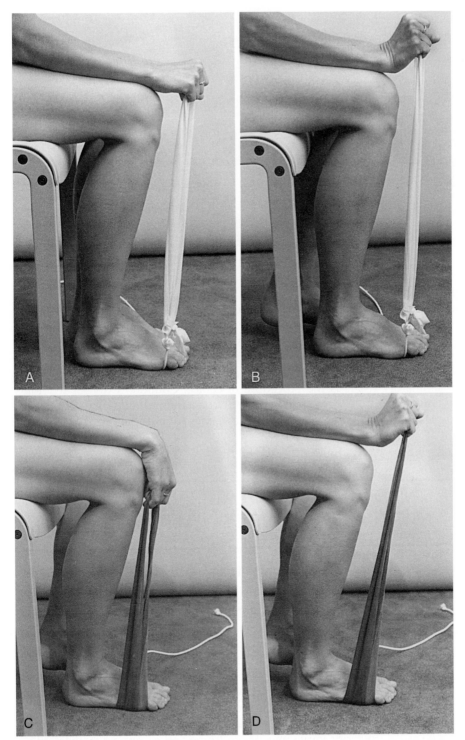

Figure 5–7. Theraband exercises for tennis elbow. *A* and *B,* Initially, limited-arc, fast-contraction, light-resistance exercises are best tolerated. The arc of motion is from neutral to about 30 degrees of extension. Repetitions are as rapid as possible and with very little tension on the Theraband. Muscular fatigue is the desired end point. The athlete stops when she can no longer maintain rapid, rhythmic contractions. She may experience a mild burning sensation in the dorsal forearm muscles but should have no elbow pain during or after the exercises. *C* and *D,* Subsequently the athlete advances as tolerated to heavy-resistance exercises. The arc of motion is then from full (palmar) flexion to full extension, and the repetitions are slower.

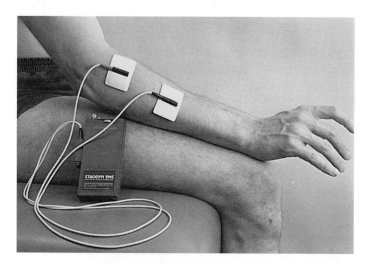

Figure 5–8. Use of an electrical muscle stimulator for tennis elbow. Excessive tension in the muscle and tendon should be avoided. Quick, rhythmic contractions are preferable to sustained contractions. As with Theraband exercises, the athlete may experience a mild burning sensation in the muscles but should have no elbow pain during or after the exercises.

painless strokes are practiced (usually forehands first, then serves, then backhands). Practice time is gradually increased until the athlete is able to resume playing.

In our experience, operative treatment of tennis elbow is required in less than 2% of cases. Extensor tenotomy (release of the common extensor tendon or just the origin of extensor carpi radialis brevis) with débridement of chronic inflammatory tissue is the procedure of choice. Common extensor tenotomy is sometimes done percutaneously.[3] All concerned should understand that surgical treatment is sometimes a necessary adjunct to, and not a substitute for, all of the foregoing measures.

F. MEDIAL TENSION/LATERAL COMPRESSION SYNDROMES (FLEXOR/PRONATOR TENDINITIS, MEDIAL EPICONDYLITIS, LITTLE LEAGUER'S ELBOW, PITCHER'S ELBOW, CAPITELLAR OSTEOCHONDROSIS)

The elbow injuries produced by excessive medial tension/lateral compression (valgus) forces are characteristic of throwing athletes and are certainly of great concern, particularly in young throwing athletes.

Little Leaguer's elbow and *pitcher's elbow* seem to have become permanent terms in the vocabulary of sports medicine. Neither term, however, is diagnostically precise. Several different medial tension/lateral compression injuries, as well as the posterior impingement syndrome and triceps mechanism injury, can cause elbow pain in throwing athletes. Moreover, other athletes, such as golfers, gymnasts, tennis players, wrestlers, and weight lifters—and even violinists—are susceptible to the same kinds of elbow injuries as are throwers. Occasionally, medial elbow symptoms are referred—a reflection of a thoracic outlet syndrome rather than a local problem.

The most common of the medial tension/lateral compression syndromes consists of medial elbow and volar forearm pain related to use of the wrist flexor and pronator teres muscles. The commonly used medical term for this syndrome is *medial (humeral) epicondylitis*, but we prefer the term *flexor/pronator tendinitis*, which not only names the primarily involved structure but also suggests the mechanisms of injury, signs and symptoms, natural history, and preferred therapy. Fortunately such ambiguous terms as "golfer's elbow," "curler's elbow," and "reverse tennis elbow," have not become so ingrained in the parlance of sports medicine that anyone needs to feel compelled to use them.

The most serious of these syndromes is traumatic avascular necrosis of the humeral capitellum. In the literature and in common usage, both the terms *osteochondrosis* and *osteochondritis dissecans* have been used to describe this syndrome; however, *osteochondrosis* is the more correct term.[18]

HISTORY

MECHANISM OF INJURY. *Repetitive valgus stress* at the elbow is the most common mechanism of injury. In baseball and javelin throwing, for example, the elbow is subject to marked valgus stress as the arm is brought forward in the throwing motion. In gymnastics the elbows are subject to valgus stress when weight is borne by the upper limbs with the elbows locked. In violin playing, the left elbow is subject to nearly continuous valgus stress.

Medial tension overload typically produces extra-articular injury, e.g., flexor/pronator strain or tendinitis, ulnar collateral ligament sprain, ulnar traction spurring, or ulnar neuritis (Fig. 5–9A–C).[2, 6, 10] The cause of flexor/

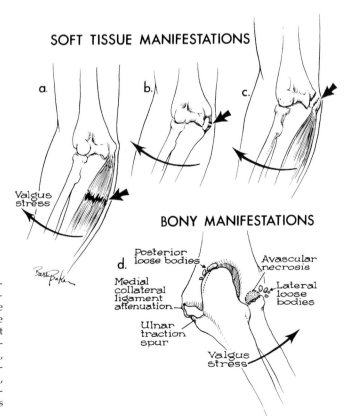

Figure 5–9. Composite of the various bony and soft tissue manifestations of repetitive valgus stress at the elbow. *a,* Flexor/pronator muscle strain; *b,* medial collateral ligament sprain; *c,* medial epicondylar avulsion fracture; *d,* lateral loose bodies, posterior loose bodies, capitellar osteochondrosis. (From Barnes DA, Tullos HS: An analysis of 100 symptomatic baseball players. Am J Sports Med 6:62–67, 1978.)

SOFT TISSUE MANIFESTATIONS

a.

b.

c.

Valgus stress

BONY MANIFESTATIONS

Posterior loose bodies

d.

Medial collateral ligament affenuation

Avascular necrosis

Lateral loose bodies

Ulnar traction spur

Valgus stress

pronator tendinitis is multifactorial, analogous to that of common extensor tendinitis discussed in the previous section. The tendinitis is the end result of functional demands that exceed the strength, endurance, or flexibility of the wrist flexor and pronator teres muscles and tendons.

Lateral compression overload typically results in intra-articular injury, e.g., capitellar osteochondrosis, radial head deformity, loose body formation, and degenerative joint disease (Fig. 5–9D). Osteochondrosis is a condition of the skeletally immature. It is thought to be "a disorder of endochondral ossification caused by vascular insufficiency and induced by repetitive micro-trauma to a vulnerable epiphysis."[18]

Injury in throwers appears to be related both to the method of delivery and to the total amount of throwing. The more sidearm the delivery, the greater the valgus stress at the elbow and the greater the likelihood of injury.[1] Beyond that, implication of certain pitches, such as the curve ball, probably reflects the fact that to throw any pitch well, one must throw it frequently.[19] The more pitches in one's repertoire, the more throwing required to perfect them all. The symptomatic young pitcher is usually one who, in addition to throwing in regular practice, also throws daily to a parent, sibling, or coach.

Among elite tennis players, flexor/pronator tendinitis seems to be more common than extensor tendinitis. Serving and overhead shots (which are not unlike throwing) and putting top spin on forehand shots are commonly implicated.

In our experience, flexor/pronator tendinitis is a fairly common weight-training ailment, whereas tennis elbow is not. Curls with heavy weights and few repetitions are commonly implicated. (In doing curls, the elbow flexors are the prime movers, but the wrist flexors must also resist the force of gravity throughout the lift.)

Acute medial tension/lateral compression injuries, such as flexor/pronator strains, ulnar collateral ligament sprains, and radial head compression fractures, do occur, especially in wrestling and gymnastics.[8, 16, 17] As with tennis elbow, chronic problems may be sequelae of such injuries.

Not infrequently, thrower's elbow problems appear to be complications of, or at least associated with, thrower's shoulder problems. The athlete may get trapped in a vicious circle of favoring one at the expense of the other, with the result that both get progressively worse.

SYMPTOMS. The hallmark symptom of flexor/pronator tendinitis is *medial elbow pain* related to use of the wrist flexor and pronator teres muscles. As with common extensor tendinitis (see part E), there is often a characteristic onset and progression of symptoms.

The usual presenting symptoms of ulnar neuritis are medial elbow pain and sensitivity, radiation of pain to the ulnar forearm and hand, and *paresthesias*, particularly of the ulnar two digits of the hand.

Pain, which may or may not be well localized laterally, is the usual presenting symptom of the lateral compression syndromes. With degenerative changes, and particularly with loose body formation, there may also be crepitation, swelling, and *locking*.

Stiffness of the elbow after activity is a common but nonspecific symptom. The limitation of motion caused by pain, swelling, or muscle spasm must be differentiated from true locking, which is caused by mechanical impingement. True locking occurs abruptly and definitely blocks further motion. When this occurs, the athlete typically "fiddles with the elbow" until motion is just as abruptly unblocked. Further history may reveal that the athlete sometimes feels something moving around inside the joint. Such findings imply *an osteochondral loose body* until proved otherwise (see also Chapter 9, parts A and B).

PHYSICAL EXAMINATION

There are two hallmark signs of flexor/pronator tendinitis: *point tenderness over or just distal to the medial humeral epicondyle* (the bony attachment of the flexor carpi and pronator teres tendons) *and pain with resisted wrist flexion or forearm pronation.* Other possible physical findings include medial soft tissue swelling, tenderness over the muscles of the volar forearm, painful limitation of elbow extension, and pain with passive stretching of the wrist flexors (Fig. 5–10).

Physical examination may or may not confirm a history consistent with ulnar neuritis, as the athlete may be seen before frank neurological deficits can be demonstrated. *Tinel's test* is a specific provocative test for neuropathy. Light percussion over the nerve at the site of injury/regeneration may produce a tingling sensation in its distribution. Impaired *two-point discrimination* over the palmar surfaces of the small finger and ulnar half of the ring finger is the most sensitive and specific sign of ulnar nerve sensory dysfunction. Motor function of the ulnar nerve is readily assessed by resisted abduction and adduction of the fingers. Subtle weakness of first dorsal interosseous or abductor digiti quinti muscles may sometimes be observed (see also Chapter 6, part E).

The lateral compression syndromes are typically evidenced by lateral joint line tenderness and provocation of lateral elbow pain as the elbow is flexed and extended with valgus stress applied. Other possible findings include flexion or valgus deformity of the elbow, effusion (see Fig. 5–3*A*), crepitation, and demonstration of true locking.

With posterior impingement syndrome, pain and tenderness are usually well localized posteriorly or posteromedially. Resisted elbow extension is not painful, but the range of extension is usually limited, and abrupt passive

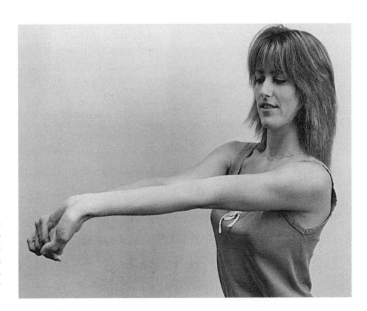

Figure 5–10. Stretching exercises for flexor/pronator tendinitis. The position of maximal stretch of the wrist flexors is with the elbow extended, the forearm supinated, and the wrist dorsiflexed.

extension typically reproduces the impingement pain (see part E). In contrast, with triceps tendinitis, resisted extension is painful and passive extension is not.

RADIOGRAPHIC EXAMINATION

If the clinical findings alone are sufficient to make the diagnosis of flexor/pronator tendinitis in a skeletally mature athlete, radiographic examination is not required; otherwise, it is recommended. Symptoms or signs of lateral compression syndrome or persistence of any symptoms in the skeletally immature are indications for radiographic examination.

Radiographs of the elbow of the throwing arm often show cortical thickening, hypertrophy of the medial epicondyle, and alteration of the trabecular pattern. These changes probably reflect the physiological adaptation of bone to repetitive valgus stress and must be differentiated from the pathological changes associated with medial tension or lateral compression overload.

Displacement (avulsion fracture) or fragmentation of the medial epicondyle, widening of the apophyseal line, or traction spurs of the coronoid process of the ulna may be seen with medial tension overload.

The findings associated with lateral compression overload are more ominous. The hallmark signs of osteochondrosis are *radiolucent areas*, *fragmentation*, and *deformity of the capitellum*. Plain films may also demonstrate loose bodies or deformity of the radial head.

OTHER DIAGNOSTIC TESTS

A complete diagnostic work-up may include a radionuclide bone scan, computed tomography, or magnetic resonance imaging, for example, to identify or localize loose bodies or articular defects (Fig. 5–11). The decision to order such studies, however, may generally be deferred to the consulting orthopedist.

INITIAL TREATMENT

Initial treatment is symptomatic and anti-inflammatory.

With acute injury the principal aim is to prevent or to reduce swelling. RICE is applicable. Ice and EGS treatments may also be appropriate.

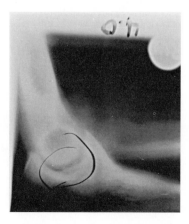

Figure 5–11. Arthrotomogram of the right elbow of a competitive tennis player demonstrating an intra-articular osteochondral loose body.

With the more typical overuse injury, the aim is to reduce pain and inflammation. Relative rest, which implies avoidance of pain-producing athletic and nonathletic activities, is the most important aspect of treatment. The athlete who has pain even with "unavoidable" activities of daily living may require immobilization in the form of a sling.

Anti-inflammatory medication is one of the mainstays of initial treatment of flexor/pronator tendinitis. We prefer to use an NSAID (in appropriate anti-inflammatory doses). We consider local corticosteroid injection only in the skeletally mature, and then only if the response to initial therapy was inadequate; if further activity restriction, additional physical therapy, and so on were impractical; and if the physical findings were well localized. Other treatment options include ice massage, friction massage, ultrasound therapy, and contrast baths. All concerned should understand that none of the foregoing measures are curative.

We have found that ulnar neuritis often responds well to a "burst" of oral corticosteroid medication. For adults we usually prescribe prednisone in divided daily doses of 60 mg per day for 2 days, then 40 mg per day for 2 days, then 20 mg per day for 2 days, and then 10 mg per day for 2 days.

REHABILITATION

Rehabilitation principally aims to restore or to enhance the strength, endurance, and flexibility of the wrist flexors and pronator teres. This can usually be accomplished with a home program, the key elements of which are static stretching exercises and progressive resistance exercises (Fig. 5–12; see also Fig. 5–10).

As with tennis elbow, early in the course of rehabilitation the athlete is likely to tolerate limited-arc, fast-contraction, light-resistance Theraband exercises better than other resistance exercises. The main purpose of the light-resistance exercises is to build muscular endurance. The athlete gradually works up to doing two and then three sets of these at a time before going on to heavier-resistance exercises.

If there is associated posterior impingement, short-arc progressive resistance exercises for the elbow flexors are included (see part E). If triceps tendinitis (elbow extensor overload) is a factor, rehabilitation is directed specifically at stretching and strengthening the triceps mechanism.

REFERRAL

Most cases of lateral compression syndrome probably merit orthopedic consultation or referral. An exception might be in the skeletally mature athlete with normal radiographs and no symptoms or signs of loose body formation. Certainly *any evidence of loose body formation, osteochondrosis, radial head deformity, or other intra-articular injury* is an indication for referral.

Most cases of medial tension syndrome do not require referral. Notable exceptions are *acute avulsion fractures* of the medial epicondyle or *apophyseal injuries* in the skeletally immature. The presence or absence of other extra-articular radiographic changes, e.g., ulnar traction spurring, does not usually alter the initial management. Referral is mainly indicated if symptoms persist or recur despite adequate nonoperative treatment.

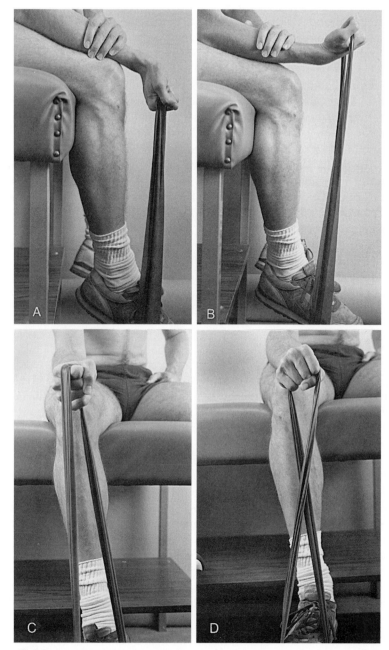

Figure 5–12. Theraband exercises for flexor/pronator tendinitis. Initially, limited-arc, fast-contraction, light-resistance wrist flexion exercises may be best tolerated. Subsequently the athlete advances as tolerated to heavy-resistance wrist flexion *(A and B)* and forearm pronation *(C and D)* exercises.

DEFINITIVE TREATMENT

In most cases of soft tissue injury, all that is required for definitive treatment is adequate rest, appropriate rehabilitation, correction of faulty technique, and gradual resumption of activity. Return to throwing or serving in tennis is accomplished in a manner similar to that of the fungo program for shoulder injuries (see Table 4–5). In our experience, operative treatment of flexor/pronator tendinitis is very seldom required.

Operative treatment is indicated for symptoms or signs of mechanical impingement. Arthroscopy may be diagnostically useful, but arthrotomy is usually necessary for the extraction of intra-articular loose bodies. The results are generally gratifying.

Osteochondrosis generally requires operative treatment. If there is no disruption of the articular cartilage, it is sometimes treated expectantly, i.e., by protection from pain-producing activity and reassessment several weeks later. Operative treatment ranges from simple drilling of an intact fragment to enhance its blood supply, to removal of a loose, deformed fragment and débridement and drilling of the underlying crater. Once intra-articular changes have occurred, however, the prognosis is not good for return to symptom-free, high-level activity such as baseball pitching.

Clearly the best treatment for osteochondrosis is *prevention*. In general, we recommend limiting the number of pitches thrown by young ball players, coaching them to throw safely, having them warm up properly, "prehabilitating" the flexor/pronator muscles, and, most importantly, paying attention to any symptoms.

G. POSTERIOR IMPINGEMENT SYNDROME

HISTORY

MECHANISM OF INJURY. The typical mechanism of injury is repetitive, rapid, forceful extension of the elbow, as may occur with throwing, punching, swinging a racquet or bat, or doing handstands.* Repetitive valgus stress at the elbow, with impingement of the medial aspect of the olecranon against the medial edge of the olecranon fossa, has also been implicated.[10, 22] Thus, baseball players, handball players, tennis players, javelin throwers, gymnasts, and so on, i.e., the same athletes liable to medial tension/lateral compression injury, are also liable to posterior impingement.

SYMPTOMS. The onset of symptoms is most likely to occur early in the season, with resumption of activity after a layoff. The hallmark early symptom is *sharp pain as the elbow snaps into extension* during activity. The pain is usually well localized to the posterior or posteromedial aspect of the elbow.

The athlete may also complain specifically about limitation of motion. Gymnasts, for example, may say they have difficulty "locking the elbows out" in full extension.

Other symptoms include stiffness and diffuse, aching pain (usually associated with joint effusion), tenderness, crepitation, and a loose body sensation. There may also be symptoms of associated medial tension/lateral compression injury, especially ulnar neuritis (see part E).

---

*Extension overload may also result in one of several triceps mechanism injuries, i.e., strain, tendinitis, apophyseal injury, or olecranon stress fracture. As discussed later, differentiation from posterior impingement is rather straightforward. Apophyseal injury is quite analogous to Osgood-Schlatter disease of the quadriceps mechanism (see Chapter 9, part J). Diagnosis and management of triceps mechanism injuries follow the general plan for management of musculotendinous injuries presented in Chapters 2 and 3.

PHYSICAL EXAMINATION

The hallmark signs are *point tenderness over the posterior or posteromedial aspect of the olecranon and provocation of pain with abrupt passive extension of the elbow.* Valgus stressing of the elbow during the terminal 5 to 10 degrees of extension often reproduces impingement pain. In contrast to triceps tendinitis, resisted elbow extension is not pain producing.

Palpation may reveal osteophyte formation, particularly on the postero-medial aspect of the olecranon. Painful limitation of elbow extension or actual flexion deformity, crepitation, and joint effusion are nonspecific findings.

RADIOGRAPHIC EXAMINATION

Radiographs are indicated to determine the extent of bony impingement and the presence or absence of loose body formation. Bony impingement is perhaps best characterized by large osteophyte formation on the posteromedial aspect of the olecranon. Cortical thickening of the olecranon fossa can often be demonstrated even in asymptomatic athletes and probably represents a physiological adaptation of bone to repetitive stress.

INITIAL TREATMENT

Initial treatment consists of relative rest and other measures to reduce pain, swelling, and inflammation. NSAIDs, ice massage, contrast baths, ice and EGS treatments, and so on are routinely used. Taping to limit extension and valgus stress may permit continuation of some athletic activities without pain.

REHABILITATION

The aim of rehabilitation is to strengthen the elbow flexors (biceps, brachialis, and brachioradialis) to enhance their action as decelerators of elbow extension. This can best be accomplished with short-arc (avoiding full extension), progressive-resistance exercises (curls and reverse curls), using relatively heavy weights or stiff Theraband. Vigorous stretching of the elbow flexors is avoided.

REFERRAL

Unless there is evidence of loose body formation or evidence of bony impingement and persistence of symptoms despite adequate nonoperative treatment, referral is not required.

DEFINITIVE TREATMENT

In the majority of cases of posterior impingement, all that is required for definitive treatment is adequate rest, appropriate rehabilitation, and gradual resumption of activity. Operative treatment of bony impingement (débridement, osteophytectomy, osteotomy of the olecranon tip) can provide good short-term symptomatic relief, but symptoms are likely to recur.[22] Arthrotomy for the extraction of loose bodies in the olecranon fossa is technically straight-forward and generally yields good results.

H. MYOSITIS OSSIFICANS

In the context of sports medicine, myositis ossificans refers to the heterotopic formation of bone in traumatized soft tissues, especially muscle. The muscles of the anterior aspect of the arm (notably brachialis) share with those of the anterior aspect of the thigh (quadriceps) a particular liability for this to occur (see also Chapter 8, part F).

The clinical significance of myositis ossificans is threefold. (1) Soft tissue trauma about the elbow, even a bruise, cannot be dismissed as "just a bruise." (2) The usual sports medicine rehabilitation approach to soft tissue injury does not apply. (3) Myositis ossificans is usually "season ending" and may very well preclude any athletic use of the limb for several months to a year, or even longer if operative treatment is required.

HISTORY

MECHANISM OF INJURY. Myositis ossificans is a complication of acute soft tissue injuries about the elbow and anterior aspect of the arm. The initial injury may be a contusion, strain, sprain, fracture, or dislocation. A typical injury in football, for example, is a contusion resulting from a direct blow to the anterior aspect of the arm delivered by an opponent's helmet, shoulder pads, or forearm. Characteristically there is a *re-injury*, e.g., another contusion, before the original injury has resolved.[9] The re-injury may be iatrogenic; all of the following have been implicated: passive stretching, massage therapy, ultrasound therapy, traumatic reductions, and early operative treatment.[7, 9, 11, 12, 21]

SYMPTOMS. The symptoms associated with the initial acute injury are quite variable, as the injury may be anything from "just a bruise" to an obvious fracture or dislocation. In general, the more extensive the swelling, ecchymosis, and disability, the greater the risk of myositis ossificans.

Unusually prolonged pain and swelling after the initial injury, undue difficulty regaining lost motion, particularly extension of the elbow, or excessive pain on motion raise the index of suspicion for myositis ossificans. However, the usual presenting symptom is *a painful "lump" in the front of the arm.*

PHYSICAL EXAMINATION

By and large, the physical examination correlates with the history. At 2 or 3 weeks after injury, one typically finds variably tender, indurated swelling of the anterior aspect of the arm. Somewhat later, palpation may define a *discrete, woody mass.* Limited elbow extension and pain and disability with active elbow flexion are common but nonspecific findings.

RADIOGRAPHIC EXAMINATION

If the clinical findings are suggestive of the diagnosis, radiographic examination is indicated. Evidence of heterotopic bone formation may be found as early as 3 weeks after injury. The initial radiographic appearance is of diffuse, amorphous, fluffy calcification in the soft tissues anterior to the humerus. As the lesion is followed radiographically, it may be seen first to enlarge, then to condense, with its margins becoming increasingly better defined as it "matures" (Fig. 5–13).

OTHER DIAGNOSTIC TESTS

Radionuclide bone scans are routinely employed to assess the maturity of the lesion. The course of myositis ossificans is usually followed clinically and

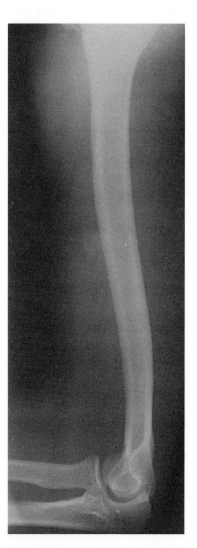

Figure 5–13. Lateral radiograph of the arm showing the heterotopic bone formation anterior to the distal third of the humerus typical of myositis ossificans traumatica. In this case, the patient, a high school football wide receiver, had ignored his trainer's and physician's admonitions to protect his contused arm from further injury.

radiographically. When two radiographs taken 1 month apart show no change in the lesion, a bone scan is obtained. A negative, or "cold," scan confirms that the lesion has matured.

We have also found that myositis ossificans may be clearly demonstrated on a bone scan before there is any radiographic evidence of the lesion (see Fig. 8–10). As with stress fractures, bone scanning appears to be the more sensitive indicator of an active process. We recommend that a bone scan be obtained early to confirm the clinical diagnosis of myositis ossificans if initial radiographic examination fails to do so.

INITIAL TREATMENT

The initial treatment of the acute (precursor) injury is aimed at minimization of swelling and protection from further injury. It comprises essentially RICE and the injury-specific measures discussed in previous sections. Gentleness to tissues is of paramount importance. For a return to collision sports, adequate padding is mandatory.

REHABILITATION

Early, vigorous rehabilitation, as is the rule for most sports injuries, is contraindicated if there is a risk of developing myositis ossificans. Passive stretching, massage therapy, and ultrasound therapy are specifically contraindicated. If there is no evidence of heterotopic bone formation, pain-free active range-of-motion exercises and pain-free isometric and concentric progressive resistance exercises are permitted.

If there is evidence of active myositis ossificans, any potential gains from rehabilitation must be weighed against the risk of exacerbating the lesion. We differ from some authors in not always immobilizing the elbow. Because lost motion can be so devastating to the athlete and so difficult to regain, we permit cautious, pain-free, active motion before the lesion has matured. For the athlete, this implies complete avoidance of any and all painful activities. As strength deficits are relatively quickly and easily reversed, resistance exercises are not begun until the lesion has matured. With radiographic and bone scan evidence that the lesion is no longer active, a full elbow rehabilitation program, as discussed in previous sections, is instituted.

REFERRAL

Referral may be considered should the athlete, parent, or coach question the diagnosis and proposed treatment, particularly the need to restrict activity for such a long while. Otherwise, referral is mainly indicated for surgical excision of a *mature* mass of bone large enough to interfere with normal elbow function.

DEFINITIVE TREATMENT

Time may not heal all wounds, but it is the only thing that heals myositis ossificans. The aim of treatment is thus to *prevent the condition* or, once it has occurred, to *prevent its exacerbation*. The key elements of successful treatment are patience, a high index of suspicion, and effective patient education.

Operative treatment is seldom required and is contraindicated until the lesion has matured. Usually the bony mass regresses in size over time. A large mass causing persistent pain or limitation of motion may need to be excised.

REFERENCES

1. Albright JA et al: Clinical study of baseball pitchers: Correlation of injury to the throwing arm with method of delivery. Am J Sports Med 6:15–21, 1978.
2. Barnes DA, Tullos HS: An analysis of 100 symptomatic baseball players. Am J Sports Med 6:62–67, 1978.
3. Baumgard SH, Schwartz DR: Percutaneous release of epicondylar muscles for humeral epicondylitis. Am J Sports Med 10:233–236, 1982.
4. Bernhang AM et al: Tennis elbow: A biomechanical approach. J Sports Med 2:235–260, 1974.
5. Curwin S, Stanish WD: Tendinitis: Its Etiology and Treatment. Lexington, Mass, DC Heath, 1984.
6. DeHaven KE, Evarts CM: Throwing injuries of the elbow in athletes. Orthop Clin North Am 4:801–808, 1973.
7. Delee JC et al: Fractures and dislocations of the elbow. *In* Rockwood CA Jr, Green DP (eds): Fractures in Adults, 2nd ed. Philadelphia, JB Lippincott, 1984, pp 559–654.
8. Garrick JG, Requa RK: Epidemiology of women's gymnastics injuries. Am J Sports Med 8:261–264, 1980.
9. Jackson DW, Feagin JA: Quadriceps contusion in the young athlete: Relation of severity of injury to treatment and prognosis. J Bone Joint Surg Am 55:95–105, 1973.
10. Kerlan JK et al: Throwing injuries of the shoulder and elbow in adults. Curr Pract Orthop Surg 6:41, 1975.
11. Loomis LK: Reduction and aftertreatment of posterior dislocation of the elbow. Am J Surg 63:56–60, 1944.
12. Mohan K: Myositis ossificans traumatica of the elbow. Int Surg 57:475–478, 1972.
13. Nirschl RP: The etiology and treatment of tennis elbow. J Sports Med 2:308–309, 1974.
14. Priest JD et al: Elbow and tennis. I: An analysis of players with and without pain. Physician Sportsmed 8:81–91, April 1980.
15. Priest JD et al: Elbow and tennis. II: A study of players with pain. Physician Sportsmed 8:70–85, May 1980.
16. Requa RK, Garrick JG: Injuries in interscholastic wrestling. Physician Sportsmed 9:44–51, April 1981.
17. Roy SP: Intercollegiate wrestling injuries. Physician Sportsmed 7:83–94, November 1979.
18. Singer KM, Roy SP: Osteochondrosis of the humeral capitellum. Am J Sports Med 12:351–360, 1984.
19. Sisto DJ et al: An electromyographic analysis of the elbow in pitching. Am J Sports Med 15:260–263, 1987.
20. Strizak AM et al: Hand and forearm strength and its relation to tennis. Am J Sports Med 11:234–239, 1983.
21. Thompson HC III, Garcia A: Myositis ossificans (aftermath of elbow injuries). Clin Orthop 50:129–134, 1967.
22. Wilson FD et al: Valgus extension overload in pitching elbow. Am J Sports Med 11:83–88, 1983.

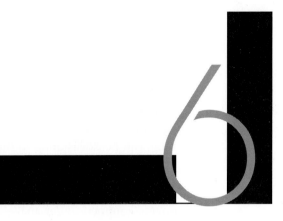

Hand and Wrist Injuries

The athlete's hand and wrist are vulnerable to injury in virtually all sports.[1, 3, 4, 7, 9, 11, 17, 25] Contact and collision sports, skiing, and gymnastics account for most of these injuries, but even a runner may fall onto an outstretched hand or a swimmer "jam a finger" on a turn.

Although a comprehensive review of hand and wrist injuries is beyond the scope of this text, a brief discussion of certain injuries is in order. In this chapter we mainly discuss those injuries that occur commonly or principally in sports. However, we also include some injuries that, although relatively uncommon, can be devastating to the athlete whose sport requires use of the hand. The specific injuries discussed are scaphoid fracture, sprains of the ulnar collateral ligament of the metacarpophalangeal joint of the thumb (gamekeeper's thumb, skier's thumb), injuries about the interphalangeal joints of the fingers (jammed finger, mallet finger, coach's finger, and so on), dorsal (radiocarpal) impingement syndrome (gymnast's wrist), and activity-related neuropathies (carpal tunnel syndrome, cyclist's palsy, and the like).

A. SCAPHOID FRACTURE

Scaphoid (carpal navicular) fracture is not an especially common sports injury but, if unrecognized or undertreated, can be career ending. As discussed later, there are several diagnostic and therapeutic pitfalls to be avoided.

The most egregious diagnostic error is to dismiss the fractured scaphoid as "just a sprain." If the athlete says, or has been told, that a wrist is sprained, a red flag should be raised in the examiner's mind. We agree with Flatt that wrist sprain is all too often "a catchall misdiagnosis."[9]

HISTORY

MECHANISM OF INJURY. The usual mechanism of injury is a *fall onto the outstretched hand* with the wrist dorsiflexed and radially deviated. Biomechanical studies have shown that the classic scaphoid fracture is produced when the wrist is fully dorsiflexed, whereas a fracture of the distal part of the radius is produced when the wrist is only slightly dorsiflexed.[6] Thus, falling vertically from a height, e.g., falling off a balance beam in gymnastics, is especially likely to result in a scaphoid fracture, whereas falling more or less horizontally is perhaps more likely to result in a Colles' fracture.

Scaphoid fracture may also be produced by *striking an object or an opponent with the heel of the hand,* as may occur in football or other collision sports.

SYMPTOMS. The hallmark symptom is *pain,* which is usually localized to the base of the thumb and radial aspect of the wrist. The pain may be rather mild but is accentuated by motion of the wrist or forearm. The use of the hand in general, and grip strength in particular, is impaired. Swelling may be minimal.

PHYSICAL EXAMINATION

The hallmark sign of a scaphoid fracture is *point tenderness* over the bone (Fig. 6–1). This is a consistent finding, not likely to become obscured by soft tissue swelling.

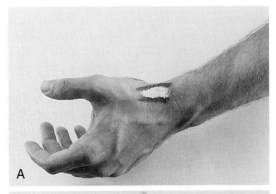

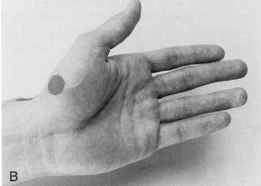

Figure 6–1. Surface anatomy of the radial aspect of the carpus. *A,* The scaphoid is palpable dorsally in the anatomic snuff box, i.e., just distal to the radial styloid between the tendons of extensor pollicis longus and brevis. *B,* The scaphoid tuberosity is palpable volarly as a rounded bony prominence at the base of the thenar eminence.

A sensitive, though nonspecific, sign of a scaphoid fracture is pain localized to the radial aspect of the carpus with motion of the wrist, especially at the limits of palmar flexion, dorsiflexion, and radial deviation. A sensitive and somewhat more specific sign is provocation of pain by longitudinal compression of the thumb against the carpus (Fig. 6–2).

RADIOGRAPHIC EXAMINATION

Standard and special scaphoid views of the wrist are indicated if the clinical findings are suggestive of the diagnosis. Radiographic examination may dif-

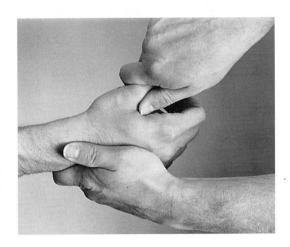

Figure 6–2. The examiner grips the thumb and gently compresses the metacarpus against the carpus. Provocation of pain by this maneuver is a reliable sign of scaphoid fracture.

ferentiate other fractures about the wrist, e.g., Colles' fracture of the distal radius, radial styloid fracture, and Bennett's fracture/dislocation of the thumb, from scaphoid fracture. Radiographic examination may also confirm a scaphoid fracture. However, initial *"negative x-rays" do not rule out a scaphoid fracture.*

It cannot be overemphasized that initial radiographic findings may be normal in as many as 15% of the cases of acute scaphoid fracture. With nondisplaced fractures, radiographic findings may become abnormal only when some resorption of bone has occurred at the fracture site. Thus the fracture line might not become apparent until 2, 4, or 6 weeks or longer after injury. Acute scaphoid fracture is thus a clinical, not a radiographic, diagnosis.

The delayed appearance of a thin fracture line is not a poor prognostic sign. Some resorption of bone must take place before healing occurs. However, a widened, smooth fracture line with subchondral sclerosis and degenerative changes—often cystic in nature—indicates delayed union or an old, ununited fracture. Complete sclerosis and collapse of the proximal fragment indicate that aseptic necrosis has occurred.

OTHER DIAGNOSTIC TESTS

A radionuclide bone scan can be used to resolve the dilemma of whether to continue immobilization when the physical findings are equivocal and radiographic examination is negative. In patients younger than 65 years, 95% of fractures are noted on bone scans within 24 hours of injury.[13-15] Unfortunately the traumatic synovitis associated with wrist trauma results in "interference" during the first 48 hours resulting in difficulties in interpretation.[24] Murphy and associates[21] have demonstrated that a bone scan done at 4 days after injury accurately *rules out* a scaphoid fracture. However, even at 4 days after injury, false-positives occur, tolerable when one considers that scanning identified an appreciable number of other unsuspected fractures. Thus in many athletic situations, it may be appropriate to order a bone scan 4 days after injury.

INITIAL TREATMENT

Any athlete who has sustained an acute wrist injury and has any tenderness in the region of the scaphoid should be treated as though the injury were a scaphoid fracture until that possibility is ruled out by radiographic examination at 2 and 4 weeks after injury or by bone scan at 4 or more days after injury.[6, 9, 21] If one chooses the 4-day bone scan option, rather than casting of the wrist, the application of a simple wrist splint and the avoidance of athletic activities will probably provide sufficient protection.

The mainstay of treatment is adequate *immobilization*, which implies at the very least a cast or splint that extends from the level of the interphalangeal joint of the thumb to just below the elbow. Some authors recommend also incorporating the index and middle fingers or all fingers to the level of the proximal interphalangeal joints and extending the cast above the elbow sufficiently to control pronation and supination.[6]

Our usual practice is to use a thumb spica splint initially (Fig. 6–3*A* and *B*). The thumb, hand, wrist, and forearm are padded as for a cast, and then a plaster splint is applied to the volar aspect of the thumb and forearm and

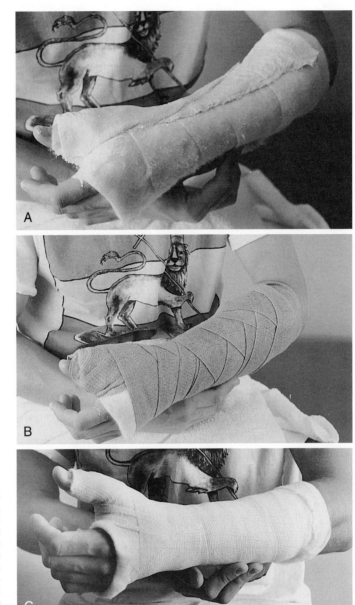

Figure 6–3. Immobilization for scaphoid fracture. *A* and *B,* Initially a noncircumferential thumb spica/volar forearm splint is used. *C,* After the swelling has resolved, a circumferential cast is used. A thumb spica/short arm cast provides sufficient immobilization for most nondisplaced fractures of the distal and middle thirds of the scaphoid.

held in place with an elastic wrap. This immobilizes as well as a thumb spica/short arm cast, yet will accommodate any swelling that might occur. When the swelling has resolved, usually in a week or so, the splint can be replaced with an appropriate circumferential cast (Fig. 6–3C). For nondisplaced fractures of the distal and middle thirds of the scaphoid, a thumb spica/short arm cast will usually suffice.

As with any injury requiring immobilization, the usual precautions about swelling are given, and, of course, any rings must be removed.

RICE (rest, ice, compression, elevation) is appropriate, as are anti-inflammatory and analgesic medications. Rest and compression are provided by the immobilization. Ice packs are applied over the elastic wrap. Elevation may mean simply using a sling or may require keeping the hand propped up on pillows.

REFERRAL

Because of the high risk of complications, such as delayed union, nonunion, and avascular necrosis, all displaced scaphoid fractures, all fractures of the proximal third, and all fractures not immediately recognized and treated as such should be referred for orthopedic evaluation and treatment.

Orthopedic referral is also indicated for any complications of treatment, such as delayed union. It should be appreciated, however, that the healing time depends on the fracture site. A scaphoid tuberosity fracture may heal in as little as 4 weeks, whereas because of the diminished blood supply proximally, a fracture of the proximal pole may require 20 weeks or longer to heal.[6] The diagnosis of delayed union is best made radiographically (see earlier).

Orthopedic consultation or referral may also be appropriate if a scaphoid fracture is suspected clinically but cannot be confirmed radiographically at 4 or more weeks after injury.

DEFINITIVE TREATMENT

Acute fractures, identified early and treated uninterruptedly by any of the standard closed techniques, can be expected to heal without complication in at least 90% of cases.[6] In such cases, some radiographic evidence of healing is usually apparent by 6 weeks. Immobilization is continued until there is complete radiographic union. Appropriate rehabilitation then completes the definitive treatment.

Athletes, coaches, and parents readily appreciate that the standard recommended treatment will at least temporarily interfere with or preclude continued sports participation. They may very well question the necessity of a cast up to the elbow (or beyond) "just for a crack in that little wrist bone," especially if the fracture cannot be demonstrated radiographically. The physician must be able to convince them that the risks and consequences of complications with undertreatment far outweigh any disadvantages of overtreatment.

Even with delayed diagnosis and treatment, or with radiographic evidence of delayed union, some fractures eventually heal with closed treatment. Thus, the physician should not accept an argument that the fracture "need not be treated till the end of the season, because it's not going to heal anyway."

Acute operative intervention is required only if closed reduction of a displaced fracture cannot be achieved. Otherwise, operative intervention is required mainly for chronic pain and disability as a result of nonunion or aseptic necrosis, or both. If a decision has been made to operate for an established nonunion, it may be reasonable to delay the operation to allow the athlete to finish the competitive season.

Some orthopedists have reported satisfactory results using custom-made "soft" (Silastic) casts for the treatment of acute, uncomplicated fractures.[23] Some athletes have thus been allowed to continue participation in collision sports while their fractures were healing; however, the average healing time was longer than that usually reported. We believe that the decision to use a nonstandard treatment such as this is best left to an orthopedist or hand surgeon.

OTHER CARPAL FRACTURES

Fractures of the lunate are less common but pose diagnostic and therapeutic problems similar to those of scaphoid fractures.[6, 9, 26] The approach to diagnosis and treatment is essentially the same as discussed previously. Dorsal avulsion chip fractures, especially of the triquetrum, are not uncommon in sports. However, in contrast to the situation with complete fractures of the scaphoid and lunate, diagnosis is readily confirmed radiographically, and treatment is essentially symptomatic.[9]

B. SPRAINS OF THE ULNAR COLLATERAL LIGAMENT OF THE METACARPOPHALANGEAL JOINT OF THE THUMB (GAMEKEEPER'S THUMB, SKIER'S THUMB)

Sprains of the ulnar collateral ligament (UCL) of the metacarpophalangeal (MCP) joint of the thumb can occur in any sport but are especially common in skiing. To both the athlete and the examiner, the acute injury may seem rather inconsequential. However, the tendency to dismiss it as "just a sprain" should be avoided. Unrecognized or inappropriately treated grade III sprains are likely to result in chronic pain and disability. Even grade II sprains can be temporarily painful and disabling, more so than might be expected from the apparent severity of injury.

The commonly used term *gamekeeper's thumb* was first used in reference to chronic sprains of the UCL incurred by British gamekeepers who killed wounded rabbits by snapping their necks.[2] Although subsequently sometimes used to denote acute ligamentous injury, the term is perhaps best used to describe chronic symptomatic UCL insufficiency. Some authors have used the term *skier's thumb* to denote the acute injury, reflecting the fact that UCL sprain is the second most common injury sustained by skiers.[3, 19]

ANATOMY

The UCL underlies the aponeurosis of the adductor pollicis, which inserts onto the dorsoulnar aspect of the proximal phalanx. With rupture of the UCL (or avulsion of its distal bony attachment), the proximal end of the ligament can be folded back on itself and the aponeurosis can become interposed between the torn ends.[28] If this happens, immobilization, no matter how prolonged, will not result in healing. With insufficiency of the UCL, contraction of the adductor pollicis tends to cause subluxation rather than normal adduction of the MCP joint. Thus, the key pinch grip, the chuck grip, and the power grip all may be impaired.

HISTORY

MECHANISM OF INJURY. Injury is the result of *forcible abduction and extension of the thumb*, as may occur in falls onto the outstretched hand, collision with an object or opponent, and catching a ball. In football defensive line play, "catching" the thumb on the opponent's clothing or pads can produce the injury. It would appear, however, that falling onto the outstretched hand while holding a ski pole is by far the most common mechanism of injury.

The abduction forces on the MCP joint, and hence the severity of UCL injury, clearly seem to be increased by the added leverage provided by the tightly held ski pole. Looping a wrist strap around the wrist and under the thumb obviously invites injury. We are not convinced, however, that strapless poles are the key to injury prevention. Indeed, they may predispose to other injury, e.g., interphalangeal joint dislocation and extensor tendon rupture, as well as fail to prevent UCL tears.[22] Being able to discard the poles and remembering to do so when falling would seem to be the best way of avoiding injury.

SYMPTOMS. The hallmark symptom of acute injury is *pain* localized to the dorsoulnar aspect of the MCP joint. At first, the pain may be rather mild, and the athlete may be underwhelmed by the injury. However, the pain is accentuated by abduction of the thumb, as may occur in catching a ball. There is disability in such activities, as well as in those requiring a strong pinch or power grip. Subsequent swelling and ecchymosis generally correspond to the severity of injury.

The symptoms of chronic UCL insufficiency are chronic "arthritic" pain and disability in gripping (see earlier).

PHYSICAL EXAMINATION

The hallmark sign of acute injury is *point tenderness* over the injured structure or structures. With grade II sprains, tenderness may be limited to the ulnar aspect of the MCP joint, just over the UCL (Fig. 6–4A). With grade III sprains, the tenderness may extend over the dorsum of the joint, reflecting associated tearing of the capsule. With avulsion fracture of the base of the proximal phalanx, as opposed to tearing of the ligament, there is likely to be well-localized bony tenderness. With either a grade III sprain or a fracture, there is likely to be associated swelling and ecchymosis, but not so much as to obscure the localization of the physical findings.

Pain elicited when the MCP joint is gently valgus stressed confirms the diagnosis of acute UCL injury (Fig. 6–4B). The demonstration of a definite end point of motion as the ligament becomes taut confirms the diagnosis of a grade II sprain. With acute injury, however, no attempt should be made to demonstrate abnormal motion or the absence of a definite end point. The diagnosis of a grade III sprain can best be confirmed by other means (see later).

RADIOGRAPHIC EXAMINATION

Unless the physical findings permit the diagnosis of a grade I or II sprain, anteroposterior and lateral views of the thumb are indicated to differentiate an avulsion fracture from a grade III sprain and to assess the apposition of fracture fragments.

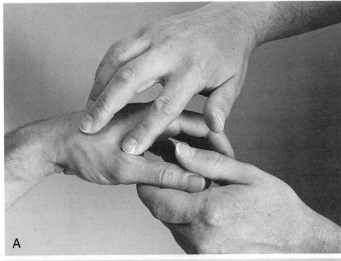

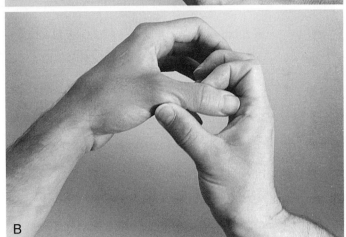

Figure 6–4. Physical findings in acute injury of the ulnar collateral ligament of the metacarpophalangeal joint of the thumb. *A,* Maximal point tenderness is elicited along the ulnar aspect of the joint. *B,* Applying slight valgus (abduction) stress to the metacarpophalangeal joint elicits pain. It may also demonstrate a definite end point of motion indicating that the ligament is intact. The examiner uses only the thumb and index finger to apply the stress. The examiner has first stress tested the metacarpophalangeal joint of the uninjured thumb and does not attempt to open the injured joint more than the uninjured joint opens. Applying greater stress to demonstrate abnormal motion or the absence of an end point is contraindicated.

OTHER DIAGNOSTIC TESTS

LIGAMENTOUS STRESS TESTING. Ideally, valgus (abduction) stress testing can differentiate grade III from grade II sprains. However, doing so essentially means reproducing the mechanism of injury, which, in the case of a grade III injury, risks a loss of apposition of the torn ends of the ligament, or fracture fragments as the case may be, and interposition of the adductor aponeurosis. Thus if a grade III sprain or an avulsion fracture can be demonstrated by other means, vigorous stress testing is contraindicated.[19]

As discussed earlier, in the setting of acute injury, gentle stress testing is usually done to confirm the presence of UCL injury and to confirm the diagnosis of a grade I or II sprain, but not to confirm the diagnosis of a grade III sprain. In the setting of chronic symptoms, stress testing can more readily be performed to assess ligamentous insufficiency, as there is no risk of causing further injury. In either setting, however, vigorous stress testing, stress testing under local anesthesia, or radiographic documentation of the findings is seldom, if ever, necessary.

ARTHROGRAPHY. Arthrography of the MCP joint can reliably and atraumatically confirm or rule out the diagnosis of a grade III sprain of the UCL.[8]

Also, whether the torn ends of the ligament are in apposition can usually be determined.[12, 19] This permits a logical decision to be made about closed versus open treatment of the torn UCL. Arthrography is thus routinely indicated unless physical examination permits the diagnosis of a grade II sprain, or standard radiographic examination reveals an avulsion fracture.

INITIAL TREATMENT

With either a grade III sprain or an avulsion fracture, initial treatment is much the same as that previously described for a scaphoid fracture. Immobilization and compression are provided by a thumb spica/volar forearm splint (see Fig. 6–3).

With a grade II sprain, it may be appropriate to use a thumb spica splint for a while if there is much pain and swelling. However, early mobilization with relative rest, contrast baths, ice, electrogalvanic stimulation (EGS) treatments, and so on usually lessen the athlete's "downtime." The injured UCL can be adequately protected for most activities by abduction-limiting adhesive taping (Fig. 6–5).

REFERRAL

Prompt referral to an orthopedist or hand surgeon is indicated if a grade III injury with adductor interposition cannot be ruled out on the basis of physical, standard radiographic, and arthrographic examination.

Referral may also be considered for symptomatic chronic ligamentous insufficiency if nonoperative measures are found to be unacceptable.

DEFINITIVE TREATMENT

With grade III injury, open reduction is required if there is loss of apposition of the torn ends of the ligament or fracture fragments and interposition of the adductor aponeurosis. Otherwise, closed treatment usually suffices.

In either case, apposition must be maintained by continuous immobilization for at least 4 to 6 weeks. Initially a noncircumferential thumb spica splint can be used. After the swelling has resolved, a circumferential thumb spica/short arm cast is applied. Immobilization is continued until clinical and radiographic union has been achieved.

After immobilization is no longer required, the MCP joint must still be protected until normal motion and strength have been restored. Adequate protection and support for most activities are provided by abduction-limiting adhesive taping (see Fig. 6–5).

Taping is also appropriate for grade II sprains and symptomatic chronic ligamentous insufficiency. In most cases, it is the only specific treatment required.

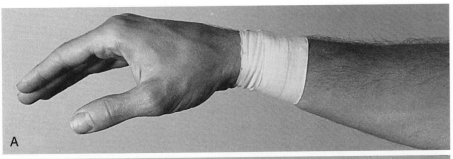

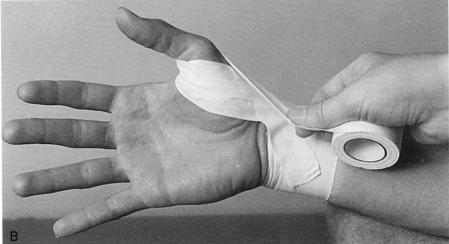

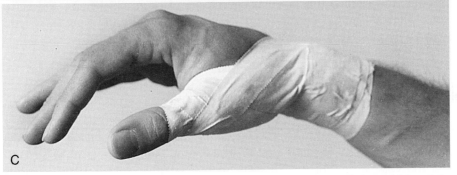

Figure 6–5. Abduction-limiting taping for support of the metacarpophalangeal joint of the thumb.

C. INJURIES ABOUT THE INTERPHALANGEAL JOINTS OF THE FINGERS (JAMMED FINGER, MALLET FINGER, COACH'S FINGER)

Injuries about the interphalangeal (IP) joints of the fingers are ubiquitous in sports, especially in those that involve catching or striking a ball with the hand.[4, 7, 9–11, 16, 17] The most common specific injuries are disruption of the extensor mechanism at the distal interphalangeal (DIP) joint, disruption of the volar plate of the proximal interphalangeal (PIP) joint, and sprains or posterior (dorsal) dislocation of either joint.

The nonspecific locker room terms *jammed finger* and *coach's finger* refer, respectively, to the mechanism of injury and the usual initial treatment (see later). The terms *mallet finger*, *baseball finger*, and *cricket finger* all refer specifically to disruption of the extensor mechanism at the DIP joint.

HISTORY

MECHANISM OF INJURY. Injury typically occurs when the outstretched finger is "jammed" backward by a *direct blow to the fingertip*. If the jamming force causes hyperflexion of the DIP joint, disruption of the extensor mechanism may occur. If it causes hyperextension of the PIP joint, volar plate injury may result. Hyperextension of either joint may produce posterior dislocation. Dislocation usually involves complete disruption of at least one of the ligaments.[10, 17]

SYMPTOMS. *Pain, swelling, and disability* are common to all these injuries. The athlete is usually aware of any associated *deformity*. With extensor mechanism disruption, athletes usually have noticed that they cannot actively extend the DIP joint. With dislocation, more often than not, reduction has been attempted and usually achieved by the athletes themselves, or by a spectator, trainer, or coach, hence the term *coach's finger*.

It is important to appreciate that even after the acute symptoms have subsided and normal function has been restored, some thickening and stiffness of the joint may persist indefinitely, particularly with the more severe injuries.

PHYSICAL EXAMINATION

Generally physical examination confirms the history. There is *point tenderness* over the dorsum of the DIP joint with extensor mechanism disruption and over the volar aspect of the PIP joint with volar plate injury. With extensor mechanism disruption, there is also flexion deformity of the DIP joint and an inability to extend the joint actively. With unreduced posterior dislocations, there is the obvious deformity of dorsal displacement of the more distal bone. Swelling and ecchymosis generally correspond to the severity of injury.

RADIOGRAPHIC EXAMINATION

Radiographic examination of the injured finger is indicated to rule in or out associated avulsion fractures and to rule out displaced fracture as opposed to dislocation. Avulsion fractures are usually best demonstrated on the individual lateral view. With disruption of the extensor mechanism, there may be an avulsion fracture of the dorsal aspect of the base of the distal phalanx. With volar plate injury or posterior dislocation, there may be an avulsion fracture of the volar aspect of the base of the more distal bone.

OTHER DIAGNOSTIC TESTS

Other diagnostic tests are not required.

INITIAL TREATMENT

Dislocations should be reduced as quickly and atraumatically as possible. As alluded to previously, closed reduction of dislocations of the IP joints is usually readily achieved with gentle in-line traction on the finger, often without any anesthesia. In some cases, digital nerve block may be required. A single attempt at reduction on the playing field or in the locker room may be reasonable. However, there is usually not so much urgency involved that the physician cannot wait for appropriate radiographic examination before attempting the reduction. Occasional difficulty is encountered in obtaining full reduction because of soft tissue interposition between the joint surfaces. In this case, further attempts at closed reduction are contraindicated.

Immobilization is indicated for the more severe acute injuries. As a general rule, to prevent soft tissue contractures the injured hand should be immobilized with the MCP joints of the fingers nearly fully flexed and the IP joints nearly fully extended, a position in which the ligaments and intrinsic muscles are under maximal tension (Fig. 6–6). There are, however, some injury-specific exceptions. With volar plate injuries and posterior dislocations, the involved joint should be immobilized in about 30 degrees of flexion. The objective is to bring the torn soft tissues, or fracture fragments as the case may be, into apposition. Often, adequate immobilization is provided by simply taping the injured finger to an adjacent finger (see later). With an

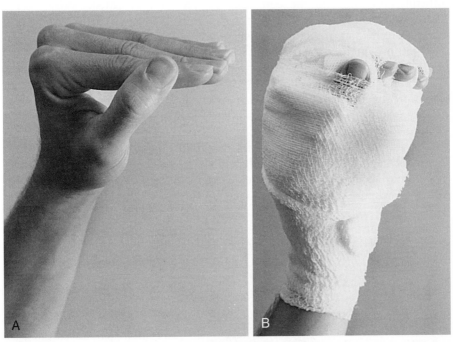

Figure 6–6. Immobilization of the entire hand may be required in the case of severe injury. The generally preferred position is with the wrist in neutral position, the thumb widely abducted, the metacarpophalangeal joints of the fingers in nearly 90 degrees of flexion, and the interphalangeal joints of the fingers in 5 to 10 degrees of flexion.[9]

acute mallet finger injury, the DIP joint is immobilized in full extension, again so as to bring the injured tissues into apposition.

RICE is applicable to all injuries.

REFERRAL

Referral on an urgent basis to an orthopedist or hand surgeon is indicated for open fractures and dislocations and for irreducible dislocations. Prompt referral is also indicated for avulsion fractures that involve 25% or more of the joint surface and for those in which the avulsed fragment is widely displaced and rotated out of position. Otherwise, referral is mainly indicated for complications or failures of closed treatment.

DEFINITIVE TREATMENT

In most cases, adequate immobilization, protection, and rehabilitation are all that is required.

In the case of volar plate injury, the PIP joint should be immobilized in 30 degrees of flexion for 3 weeks. Active flexion is then permitted, but extension should be blocked at 15 degrees of flexion for an additional 2 or 3 weeks. In the well-supervised situation, this can be accomplished with adhesive taping, thus permitting the athlete to continue playing. In the less well supervised situation, a malleable splint would be preferable (Fig. 6–7).

With extensor mechanism disruption, closed treatment requires immobilization of the DIP joint in extension, usually for 4 weeks or more. This is usually best accomplished with a Smillie cast.[27] Cast application may be difficult, however, and the compliant patient may be satisfactorily treated with a malleable splint. In either case, both extreme hyperextension and inadvertent flexion of the joint must be avoided.

Not infrequently the athlete with mallet finger injury is not seen by the physician immediately after injury. If radiographic examination reveals an avulsion fracture of the distal phalanx, there is a good chance of success with closed treatment, even if delayed. However, if instead the injury involves rupture of the tendon, the chances of success are poor if closed treatment is delayed for more than a few days.

Operative treatment for mallet finger injury may be considered if closed treatment has failed or is deemed unlikely to succeed. However, the trade-offs should be appreciated. The flexion deformity is largely of cosmetic significance, whereas any limitation of active flexion, as might occur as a result

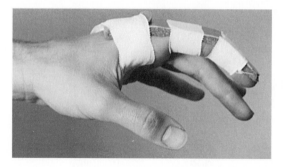

Figure 6–7. Dorsal extension block splint for treating volar plate injuries of the proximal interphalangeal joint. It is especially important to secure the proximal phalanx to the splint so that flexion of the metacarpophalangeal joint does not allow inadvertent extension of the proximal interphalangeal joint.

of operative treatment, is likely to be functionally significant. This is especially true for the ring and small fingers, whose primary use is for power grip. In general, operative treatment does not offer any advantage over closed treatment.[29]

D. DORSAL (RADIOCARPAL) IMPINGEMENT SYNDROME (GYMNAST'S WRIST)

Dorsal impingement syndrome is a unique cause of wrist pain in gymnasts. Its clinical significance is twofold. It can be absolutely disabling, and it must be differentiated from other causes of wrist pain, especially carpal fracture.

HISTORY

MECHANISM OF INJURY. The mechanism of injury is *repetitive dorsiflexion loading of the wrist*, as occurs especially in the vault, floor exercise, and balance beam events.

SYMPTOMS. The hallmark symptom is activity-related *pain* localized to the dorsum of the wrist. With long-standing symptoms, the athlete is also likely to complain of limited as well as painful wrist extension.

PHYSICAL EXAMINATION

The hallmark signs are *point tenderness* along the dorsum of the radiocarpal joint, *provocation of pain* with abrupt dorsiflexion of the wrist, and eventually painful *limitation* of the range of dorsiflexion.

RADIOGRAPHIC EXAMINATION

Radiographic study of the carpus with special scaphoid views is routinely indicated to rule out carpal fracture, even though the athlete does usually not recall any specific antecedent injury. The physician and athlete can ill afford to overlook a significant carpal fracture (see part A). Also, injuries of the distal radial epiphysis and aseptic necrosis of the carpal bones in gymnasts have been reported.[20, 25] Lateral views of the carpus in neutral and full dorsiflexion may (rarely) reveal either lunate subluxation or actual bony impingement that blocks dorsiflexion.

OTHER DIAGNOSTIC TESTS

Radionuclide bone scan to rule out a stress fracture or an occult carpal fracture should be considered if radiographic examination is unenlightening and if symptoms persist for more than 2 weeks or so despite adequate rest and therapy.

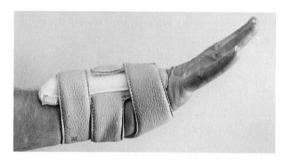

Figure 6–8. A dorsiflexion-limiting splint may allow the gymnast with impingement symptoms to continue training.

INITIAL TREATMENT

Initial treatment comprises essentially relative rest; measures to reduce swelling, e.g., contrast baths, ice, and EGS treatments; and anti-inflammatory medication. Relative rest may imply simply using a dorsiflexion-limiting gymnast's wrist splint while training is continued (Fig. 6–8). Adhesive taping may also be used for this purpose.

REFERRAL

Referral is required only if radiographic examination or a bone scan reveals a more serious problem or if symptoms do not respond to standard therapy.

DEFINITIVE TREATMENT

In most cases, adequate rest, symptomatic treatment as discussed previously, and appropriate rehabilitation are all that is required, and indeed are all that is usually effective.

Rehabilitation is primarily aimed at increasing the strength and endurance of the wrist flexors to provide a dynamic dorsiflexion-limiting splint. Stretching exercises to regain lost motion may or may not be effective.

E. ACTIVITY-RELATED NEUROPATHIES (CARPAL TUNNEL SYNDROME, CYCLIST'S PALSY)

Numbness of the hand is a fairly common complaint of athletes, particularly cyclists. The possible causes range from simple exposure to cold and wet conditions to various pressure neuropathies to vascular impairment.

The term *carpal tunnel syndrome* is well known to most physicians. It refers specifically to symptoms produced by entrapment of the median nerve at the wrist. *Ulnar tunnel syndrome* is a similar term used to describe entrapment of the ulnar nerve at the wrist. It is important to remember, however, that entrapment neuropathies producing symptoms in the hand can occur elsewhere in the course of the nerves from the cervical spine to the hand.

The terms *cyclist's palsy* and *handlebar palsy* have been used specifically to denote ulnar neuropathy in cyclists, ostensibly the result of direct pressure on the nerve in the hand.[1] In our opinion the choice of words is unfortunate, as it suggests that this is the most common cause of cyclists' complaints and that motor rather than sensory impairment is the more common problem, neither of which appears to be true.

HISTORY

MECHANISM OF INJURY. In some instances the exact pathomechanics can be surmised. For example, overuse of the finger flexor muscles, as might occur in training for the rings or parallel bars in gymnastics, can cause sufficient inflammation and swelling of the tendons in the unyielding carpal tunnel to compress the vulnerable median nerve and produce a carpal tunnel syndrome.

In other cases the examiner may be unable to discern the exact mechanism of injury. It is nevertheless important to characterize as precisely as possible the circumstances in which the symptoms occur. For example, what are the positions of the cyclist's shoulders, elbows, wrists, and hands when symptoms occur? Are symptoms more likely to be produced when the hand position cannot be varied, as while riding a mountain bike as opposed to a bicycle with conventional dropped handlebars? Are the gloves and handlebars too sparsely padded? Is the bicycle too long or the handlebars too low for the cyclist, causing excessive weight to be placed on the hands? Careful direct questioning, as well as actual observation of the cyclists on their own bicycles, is not only helpful, but usually essential. Similar sport-specific considerations apply to athletes in other sports.

SYMPTOMS. Paresthesias (*numbness and tingling*) in the distribution of the affected nerve are the most common symptoms of neuropathy. Pain is a somewhat less common symptom. With median neuropathy, symptoms are characteristically localized to the thumb, index, and middle fingers; with ulnar neuropathy, to the ring and small fingers. A glovelike distribution of symptoms is more typical of vascular insufficiency than neuropathy.

Paresis is a distinctly less common complaint. Occasionally, however, an athlete may describe what appears to be diminished muscular endurance. For example, gymnasts with carpal tunnel syndrome may state that there is a progressive loss of grip strength as they proceed through a workout.

PHYSICAL EXAMINATION

Physical examination may or may not confirm the history, as the athlete typically appears for treatment before frank neurological deficits can be demonstrated.

Impaired *two-point discrimination* is the most sensitive and specific sign of sensory nerve dysfunction.[5, 18] Two-point discrimination is readily assessed with a paper clip, a ubiquitous, small, inexpensive, and painless, albeit "low-tech," diagnostic instrument. The fingertip is touched with one or two ends of the paper clip at varying distances apart. An inability to discriminate two points 5 mm apart probably implies some neurological deficit, even in the individual with thick calluses. An inability to discriminate two points 10 mm apart implies complete loss of protective sensation.

Motor function of the median nerve is readily assessed by resisted opposition of the thumb; that of the ulnar nerve, by resisted abduction and adduction of the fingers; and that of the radial nerve, by extension of the MCP joints of the thumb and fingers. Muscle or skin atrophy is rarely observed.

Phalen's test is a specific provocative test for carpal tunnel syndrome. Holding the wrist in full palmar flexion may reproduce pain or paresthesias in the radial three digits.

Tinel's test is a specific provocative test for neuropathy. Light percussion over the nerve at the site of injury/regeneration may produce a tingling sensation in the distribution of the nerve. Sites at which a positive Tinel's sign is commonly elicited are the volar aspect of the wrist (median and ulnar nerves), posteromedial aspect of the elbow (ulnar nerve), and axilla (brachial plexus).

Other signs of neuropathy as well as signs of vascular insufficiency are discussed under thoracic outlet syndrome (see Chapter 7, part C).

RADIOGRAPHIC EXAMINATION

If osteophyte encroachment on the carpal tunnel is suspected, radiographic examination may be indicated.

OTHER DIAGNOSTIC TESTS

Electromyography and nerve conduction studies may be indicated if frank neurological deficits are demonstrated, or if neuropathy cannot be confirmed or ruled out on the basis of physical examination.

INITIAL TREATMENT

Initial treatment comprises relative rest; measures to reduce swelling, e.g., contrast baths, ice, and EGS treatments; and anti-inflammatory medication. Relative rest may sometimes imply immobilization. Anti-inflammatory medication usually means an initial trial of oral NSAIDs. Occasionally local corticosteroid injection may be required.

REFERRAL

If disabling symptoms persist or if frank neurological deficits are demonstrated and do not resolve with appropriate nonoperative treatment, referral is indicated.

DEFINITIVE TREATMENT

In most cases the most important aspect of treatment is modification of activity to eliminate the mechanism or mechanisms of injury; hence the importance of the history (see previous). Occasionally operative intervention will be required for decompression of an entrapped nerve.

REFERENCES

1. Burke ER: Ulnar neuropathy in bicyclists. Physican Sportsmed 9:53–56, April 1981.
2. Campbell C: Gamekeeper's thumb. J Bone Joint Surg Br 37:148–149, 1955.
3. Carr D et al: Upper extremity injuries in skiing. Am J Sports Med 9:378–383, 1981.
4. Dawson WJ, Pullos N: Baseball injuries to the hand. Ann Emerg Med 10:302–306, 1981.
5. Dellon AL: The moving two-point discrimination test: Clinical evaluation of the quickly adapting fiber/receptor system. J Hand Surg 3:474–480, 1978.
6. Dobyns JH, Linscheid RL: Fractures and dislocations of the wrist. *In* Rockwood CA Jr, Green DP (eds): Fractures in Adults, 2nd ed. Philadelphia, JB Lippincott, 1984, pp 412–510.
7. Ellsasser JC, Stein AH: Management of hand injuries in a professional football team: Review of 15 years of experience with one team. Am J Sports Med 7:178–182, 1979.
8. Engel J et al: Arthrography as a method of diagnosing tear of the ulnar collateral ligament of the metacarpophalangeal joint of the thumb ("gamekeeper's thumb"). J Trauma 19:106–109, 1979.
9. Flatt AE: The Care of Minor Hand Injuries, 4th ed. St Louis, CV Mosby, 1979.
10. Green DP, Rowland SA: Fractures and dislocations in the hand. *In* Rockwood CA Jr, Green DP (eds): Fractures in Adults, 2nd ed. Philadelphia, JB Lippincott, 1984, pp 313–411.
11. Hikosaka K et al: Athletic injuries of the hand. Orthopedics 30:622–628, 1979.
12. Linscheid RL: Arthrography of the metacarpophalangeal joint. Clin Orthop 103:91, 1974.
13. Martire JR: The role of nuclear medicine bone scans in evaluating pain in athletic injuries. Clin Sports Med 6:713–737, 1987.
14. Matin PM: Appearance of bone scans following fractures including immediate and long term studies. J Nucl Med 20:1227–1231, 1979.
15. Matin PM: Bone scintigraphy in the diagnosis and management of traumatic injury. Semin Nucl Med 12:104–122, 1983.
16. McCue FC III et al: Athletic injuries of the proximal interphalangeal joint requiring surgical treatment. J Bone Joint Surg Am 52:937–956, 1970.
17. McCue FC III et al: Hand and wrist injuries in the athlete. Am J Sports Med 7:275–286, 1979.
18. Moberg E: Objective methods of determining functional value of sensitivity in the hand. J Bone Joint Surg Br 40:454–466, 1958.
19. Mogan JV, Davis PH: Upper extremity injuries in skiing. Clin Sports Med 1:295–308, 1982.
20. Murakami S, Nakajima H: Aseptic necrosis of the capitate bone in two gymnasts. Am J Sports Med 12:170–173, 1984.
21. Murphy DG et al: Can a day 4 bone scan accurately determine the presence or absence of scaphoid fracture? Ann Emerg Med 26:434–438, 1995.
22. Primiano GA: Skier's thumb injuries associated with flared ski pole handles. Am J Sports Med 13:425–427, 1985.
23. Riester JH et al: A review of scaphoid fracture healing in competitive athletes. Am J Sports Med 13:159–161, 1985.
24. Rolfe IJ et al: Isotope bone imaging in suspected scaphoid trauma. Br J Radiol 54:762–767, 1981.
25. Roy S et al: Stress changes of distal radial epiphysis in young gymnasts. A report of 21 cases and review of the literature. Am J Sports Med 13:301–308, 1985.
26. Ryan JR: Fracture and dislocation about the carpal lunate. Ann Emerg Med 9:158–160, 1980.
27. Smillie IS: Mallet finger. Br J Surg 24:439–445, 1937.
28. Stener B: Displacement of the ruptured ulnar collateral ligament of the metacarpophalangeal joint of the thumb. J Bone Joint Surg Br 44:869–879, 1962.
29. Wehbe MA, Schneider LH: Mallet fractures. J Bone Joint Surg Am 66:658–669, 1984.

7

Neck, Back, and Nerve Injuries

Conditions to Be Referred

- ◆ Acute spinal fractures
- ◆ Stress fracture/stress reaction of bone
- ◆ Acute herniated intervertebral disc
- ◆ Chronic herniated intervertebral disc with neurological deficit or intractable pain
- ◆ Cervical spinal stenosis
- ◆ Thoracic or lumbar spinal stenosis with neurological deficit or intractable pain
- ◆ Spinal cord or nerve root compression
- ◆ Brachioplexopathy
- ◆ Cauda equina syndrome
- ◆ Thoracic outlet syndrome

T r i a g e

Indications for Referral

- **Acute**
  History
    Loss of sensation
    Numbness, tingling
    Loss of strength
    Sudden onset, severe neck or back
    pain
    Loss of bowel or bladder control
  Examination
    Sensory neurological deficit
    Motor deficit (strength or muscular
    endurance)
    Hyporeflexia
  X-ray films
    Fracture
    Dislocation
    Intervertebral segmental instability
- **Gradual Onset**
  History
    Loss of sensation
    Numbness, tingling
    Loss of strength
    Loss of bowel or bladder control
    Radiating limb pain, e.g., sciatica
    Intractable neck or back pain
    Neck or back pain in patients
    younger than 20 years (especially
    lumbar extension–related low-back
    pain)
    Neck or back pain in patients older
    than 60 years
    Painful limitation or impairment of
    activity
  Examination
    Sensory neurological deficit
    (especially saddle distribution
    anesthesia)
    Motor deficit (strength or muscular
    endurance)
    Hyporeflexia
  X-ray films
    Fracture
    Dislocation
    Intervertebral segmental instability
    Spondylolysis with
    spondylolisthesis
    Spondylolysis with positive
    radionuclide scintigraphy ("hot
    bone scan")

Indications for X-ray Films

- **Acute**
  History
    Trauma-related neck, back, or
    radiating limb pain
    Sudden onset, severe neck or back
    pain
    Loss of sensation
    Numbness, tingling
    Loss of strength
    Loss of bowel or bladder control
    Examination
    Sensory neurological deficit
    Motor deficit (strength or muscular
    endurance)
    Hyporeflexia
- **Gradual Onset**
  History
    Intractable neck, back, or radiating
    limb pain
    Neck or back pain in patients
    younger than 20 years (especially
    lumbar extension–related low-back
    pain)
    Neck or back pain in patients older
    than 60 years
  Examination
    Sensory neurological deficit
    Motor deficit (strength or muscular
    endurance)
    Hyporeflexia

Acute and overuse injuries of the neck and back are among the most ubiquitous and disabling of human afflictions. They are also perhaps among the most challenging problems for clinicians, sports physicians included. Although a comprehensive discussion of these problems is beyond the scope of the text, we would be remiss not to highlight, at least, certain topics of particular importance to the primary sports physician. These include the prevention and initial management of severe injury, brachial plexus injuries, thoracic outlet syndrome, low-back pain, spondylolysis, sciatica, and Scheuermann's disease, each of which we discuss briefly below.

A.   SEVERE SPINAL INJURY

Although rare, spinal fractures, dislocations, and cord injuries do occur in sports. In fact, sports account for some 10% to 15% of all severe spinal injuries.[50, 58] American football has received much of the bad press regarding these injuries, but it is by no means the worst offender.[2–4, 8, 9, 11, 28–30, 34, 35, 48–50, 64, 66–69] All studies from this and other countries implicate recreational water sports as the cause of most sports-related severe spinal injuries.[31, 44, 50, 59] Other sports that have been implicated are hang gliding, trampolining, horseback riding, rodeo, downhill skiing, wrestling, gymnastics, rugby, ice hockey, and mechanical bull riding.[8, 9, 24, 37, 39, 42, 45–47, 50–52, 58, 60, 63]

INITIAL ASSESSMENT AND MANAGEMENT

If anything in sports is more tragic than catastrophic spinal injury, it is the severe injury made catastrophic by improper treatment. This is not just a theoretical concern. In one series of spinal cord injuries, some 10% of patients had the onset or worsening of neurological deficit after the original injuries had occurred.[41] There are numerous accounts of patients who became quadriplegic after having been able to ambulate or to move their limbs at the scene of the accident. In our own practices, we have had a patient walk in with an unstable neck fracture some 2 weeks after having been bucked off his horse and landing on his head. Another appeared with a complaint of neck pain several hours after a bicycle accident in which he had landed on his head with sufficient force to break his helmet in two. He had actually been referred from the emergency department for another problem without immobilization or radiographic examination of his cervical spine.

The caveats remain. An apparent absence of neurological deficit does not rule out spinal injury. *Anyone who has sustained substantial trauma to the head or neck is presumed to have an unstable injury of the cervical spine until that possibility has been ruled out.*[56] To do so clinically, one must demonstrate sequentially that the patient is fully alert, has no neck pain or tenderness, has no neurological deficit, and, finally, has a full and pain-free range of active neck motion. If any one of these criteria is not met, then immobilization and radiographic examination are required.[56, 70, 71]

As with any emergent situation, the keys to optimal management are being prepared and attending to priorities. Before the fact, local medical resources, transportation resources, and definitive care/referral resources must be identified, and protocols for utilization of those resources must be established. Essential equipment, ideally standardized and exchangeable within the local emergency medical service (EMS) system, must be assembled and maintained. All personnel, including team physicians, trainers, and coaches, having responsibility for the care of athletes must be appropriately oriented to all the protocols and to their specific responsibilities in the event of injury.

It is not possible to provide a complete list of essential equipment applicable to every sports situation. However, consideration of the treatment priorities discussed later, the unique aspects of each sport, and the capabilities of the health care providers determine which equipment is essential for a given situation.

Of paramount importance is to have an efficient plan for carrying out, according to priorities, the initial assessment and management of the injured athlete. In a critical situation, the standard approach to patient care—take a history, do a physical examination, make an assessment, come up with a treatment plan—is obviously inappropriate. We employ the approach recommended by the Committee on Trauma of the American College of Surgeons—*primary survey, resuscitation, secondary survey, and definitive care.*[56]

The primary survey is simply a rapid assessment of vital functions. The idea is to find out what is about to kill the patient. Resuscitation is what is done to prevent that from happening. It is begun simultaneously with identification of any airway, breathing, or circulatory problems in the primary survey (see later). The secondary survey is a head-to-toe assessment of the patient. The idea is to identify all the problems that will eventually require definitive treatment of some sort. Providing such treatment may require referral to a specialist or transportation to a trauma center, or both.

The mnemonic 1ABCDEH represents the assessment/treatment priorities, i.e., the order in which the primary survey/resuscitation is to be carried out. (We have slightly modified the standard Advanced Trauma Life Support ABCs[56] to make them more applicable to situations on the field or on the court, as well as in the hospital.)

1. *First, do no harm.* Ascertain that the cervical spine is protected until spinal injury has been ruled out. Do not permit any unnecessary manipulation of the neck, such as removal of a helmet. When it is necessary to turn or move the athlete, use the proper logrolling technique (Fig. 7–1).

A. *Airway.* As the highest treatment priority, airway patency must either be confirmed or obtained. Simply asking the athlete a question ("Annie, Annie, are you OK?") is a useful way to begin assessing both the airway and the level of consciousness (see later). In the athlete with an apparent airway problem, use the jaw-lift maneuver and a suction device first. Do not use a head-tilt–neck-lift maneuver (see Fig. 7–1).

   If unsuccessful in clearing the airway, proceed quickly to nasotracheal intubation or cricothyroidotomy. In children, orotracheal intubation may be attempted with an assistant carefully immobilizing the head and neck. Do not attempt tracheostomy as an emergency procedure.

B. *Breathing.* Next, adequate ventilation must be ensured. Provide positive-pressure ventilation if indicated. Relieve tension pneumothorax if present.

   Under ideal circumstances, the chest would be completely exposed to permit proper inspection, palpation, and auscultation. By simple palpation, one should be able to ascertain whether the thorax expands and contracts appropriately with respiration and be able to detect a gross flail chest or marked subcutaneous emphysema.

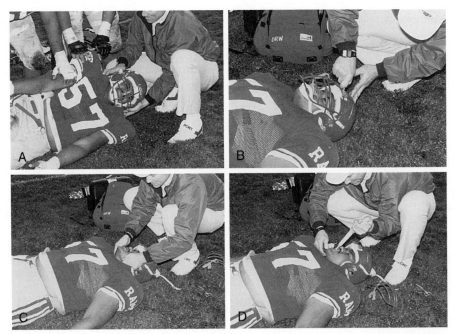

Figure 7–1. Proper technique for establishing a patent airway in an unconscious football player. *A*, Logrolling the athlete to the supine position. *(It takes only a few extra seconds to protect the spine, whereas cord injury last a lifetime.)* Four persons are required. The leader controls the head and neck and directs the other three, who are positioned at the shoulders, hips, and legs. The leader's hands are crossed initially and unwind as the athlete is turned by the three assistants. The objective is to roll the athlete's body as a unit, keeping the spine immobile. Thereafter an assistant maintains secure immobilization of the head and neck throughout all subsequent maneuvers. *B*, If breathing is inadequate or impaired, access to the airway is gained by removing the mask, not the helmet. The mask is removed entirely. Cage-type masks are removed by cutting the plastic hinges with a scalpel or, preferably, a sharp knife. The cuts are made on the side of the hinge away from the face. Older bar-type masks are removed with a bolt cutter. *C*, The athlete's mouth guard is removed, and the airway is opened with a chin-pull or jaw-thrust maneuver. (If immediate access to the airway is not required, i.e., if cervical-spine protection is the only concern, the chin strap is not unfastened.) A head-tilt–neck-lift maneuver to open the airway is contraindicated. *D*, The airway is cleared of any secretions, vomitus, blood, and so on, that may be present. A cook's basting syringe can be used for this purpose. This item, which can probably be filched from most kitchens, is the portable suction device par excellence. Thereafter the position of the jaw is maintained and the suctioning repeated as necessary.

   C. *Circulation*
      1. Identify and control external hemorrhage. Use direct pressure over the wound.
      2. Assess the adequacy of cardiac output by checking the pulse or pulses, the skin color, and capillary refill. Palpable radial, femoral, and carotid pulses imply systolic pressures of at least 80, 70, and 60 mm Hg, respectively. Thumbnail capillary refill in the time it takes to say "capillary refill" suggests normovolemia.
   D. *Disability.* Carry out a brief, baseline neurological (disability) assessment. Check the size and reactivity of the pupils. Use the *AVPU* mnemonic, which follows, to describe the level of consciousness:
      A = Alert
      V = Responds to verbal stimuli
      P = Responds to painful stimuli
      U = Unresponsive

E. *Exposure.* The aphorism in the emergency department, "Undress to assess," reflects the importance of a thorough examination so as not to miss anything important. This obviously has limited at-the-scene applicability in some winter and water sports situations, in which too much exposure may already be a major problem. Still, a judicious look at a particular injury may be appropriate. For example, one does not want to wait until blood has soaked through 4 in. of down clothing before perceiving the need to control the hemorrhage associated with an open fracture.

H. *Help.* On completion of the primary survey, the extent of the life-threatening injuries and the requirements for further management of those injuries should be apparent. Obtain help and arrange for transportation as appropriate.

Fundamental as these concepts are, they are sometimes forgotten or ignored in the "heat of battle." If indeed there are no life-threatening problems, following the protocol described takes only a few seconds. If, however, there is a life-threatening problem, following the protocol can avoid unnecessary trouble and may help save the patient's life.*

PREVENTION

As there is no satisfactory definitive treatment for spinal cord injury, prevention must be a paramount concern for all sports physicians. Understanding the epidemiology and mechanisms of injury is a necessary prerequisite.

Some authors have called attention to the occurrence of severe injury in ectomorphic ("goose-necked") individuals and have suggested that strength training may be a key to injury prevention.[12, 29, 30, 38, 48, 49, 52, 58, 60] We agree with those who have shown that appropriate rehabilitation may reduce the probability of subsequent nonsevere injury,[3] but we are skeptical that muscular development or lack thereof has any direct effect on the risk of sustaining severe injury. The slightly built defensive back attempting an open-field tackle of a larger opponent, with the crowd yelling "Stick him! Stick him!" may indeed be a set-up for severe injury. However, his risk derives not from insufficient neck girth, but from the likelihood that he will try something unsafe, namely, head-down or spear tackling.

Case report and epidemiological studies have helped clarify the pathomechanics of severe spinal injury in sports.[11, 24, 29, 31, 44, 45, 47–49, 51, 58–60, 63, 64, 67–69] Axial loading is by far the most common mechanism. When the neck is slightly flexed, the normal cervical lordosis is lost, and the cervical spine becomes a straight column. Impact to the crown of the head can then produce axial loading of the cervical spine with excessive energy absorption, fracture or dislocation, and cord injury. This is the mechanism of spinal injury with head-down blocking and tackling (sticking or spearing) in football. It is also the mechanism by which diving into shallow water and striking the bottom or a submerged object can produce spinal injury.

These studies suggest that elimination of those practices that cause axial

---

*A more complete discussion of the resuscitation and subsequent evaluation and treatment of the severely injured athlete is beyond the scope of this text. We refer the interested reader to Torg's text *Athletic Injuries to the Head, Neck, and Face*,[64] and we highly recommend the American College of Surgeons' Advanced Trauma Life Support Course for Physicians[56] to all physicians who are in positions to care for severely injured athletes.

loading of the cervical spine could result in fewer severe injuries. Subsequent epidemiological studies have revealed that, for football at least, this is indeed the case.[3, 11, 34, 35, 64] In 1975, the use of the helmet or face mask in blocking and tackling was outlawed. In 1977 and 1980, other rule changes were made that allowed offensive players more liberal use of the hands and arms for blocking. Since these rule changes, the incidence of catastrophic spinal injuries in football has dropped to an all-time low.

These and other studies[24, 39, 42, 46, 47, 63, 65, 66] reveal that imprudent or illegal practices are the major causes of severe spinal injury in recreational and organized sports. It seems, therefore, that safety education and appropriate modification and strict enforcement of the rules of play are the keys to injury prevention. Torg states, "It is not sufficient for coaches to refrain from teaching techniques utilizing the top or the crown of the helmet as a primary point of contact. Coaches must teach the players not to use such techniques."[64] We agree and add that sports physicians must help get the message across to coaches, parents, fans, and athletes.

B. BRACHIAL PLEXUS INJURIES (BURNERS, STINGERS)

Although they have not received much attention in the literature, brachial plexus injuries are very common in collision sports.[3, 6, 7, 40, 51] It has been reported that more than 50% of collegiate football players have sustained such injuries in the course of their playing careers.[7, 40]

The usual presentation is transient, burning upper limb pain and paresthesias following a block or tackle. The locker room terms for these symptoms, *burner* and *stinger,* connote, but are not precisely synonymous with, brachial plexus injury. Burning upper limb pain may represent spinal cord injury,[28] and brachial plexus injury may be noted simply as weakness, without the typical antecedent pain.[40]

Most brachial plexus injuries appear to be neurapraxias. That is, there is temporary disruption of nerve function, with full recovery in a matter of minutes, and with no subsequent signs of axonal degeneration. In some cases, however, weakness persists for weeks, and electromyography is consistent with axonal degeneration. As a rule, substantial recovery occurs by 6 weeks, which indicates that these injuries are probably mixed neurapraxias and axonotmeses. Very rarely, there is no recovery of nerve function even after 6 or more months, indicating that neurotmesis, or complete axonal disruption, had occurred.[6]

In theory, perhaps, any of the roots, trunks, divisions, cords, or peripheral nerves that make up the brachial plexus might be injured. It appears, however, that in fact it is the upper trunk that is most commonly injured. Clinical and electromyographic examination of athletes with persistent weakness characteristically reveals involvement of the upper-trunk–supplied muscles, namely, deltoid, supraspinatus, infraspinatus, and biceps.[7, 40] Although isolated spinal accessory, suprascapular, axillary, and long thoracic peripheral nerve injuries do occur in sports, they are typically produced by different mechanisms of injury.[6]

In the evaluation of the athlete with upper limb pain, paresthesias, or paresis, the detection of spinal cord injury is of paramount concern. Also of concern are the differentiation of brachial plexus injury from thoracic outlet syndrome and the differentiation of neurapraxia from more severe brachial plexus injury.

HISTORY

MECHANISM OF INJURY. Injury is produced when the upper trunk of the brachial plexus is stretched by *forcible depression of the ipsilateral shoulder*, as may occur during blocking or tackling in which the shoulder is the primary point of contact. Usually there is also lateral flexion of the neck to the contralateral side, but there may be hyperextension or lateral flexion of the neck to the ipsilateral side.

There was some concern that the football rule changes of 1975, which prohibited the use of the helmet and face mask in blocking and tackling, would result in an increased incidence of brachial plexus injury. Such epidemiological evidence as is available does not support this hypothesis.[10] In fact, there is some suggestion that since the subsequent rule changes permitting greater use of the hands and arms for blocking, the incidence of this type of injury has decreased.[3]

SYMPTOMS. The hallmark symptoms of the burner or stinger are *severe, burning, unilateral upper limb pain associated with paresthesias and weakness*. Typically the *pain starts at the shoulder and radiates distally to the hand*. Neck pain is not a typical feature. The intense pain usually lasts for a few seconds and is followed by numbness, tingling, and weakness, which usually lasts for a few minutes.

Complete resolution of symptoms is the rule, although, as noted previously, some athletes have residual weakness for several weeks or more. Uncommonly, an athlete may have characteristic weakness without ever having had a typical stinger.

Red flags that should alert the examiner to *possible spinal cord injury* are loss or alteration of consciousness, neck pain, and bilateral limb involvement.

PHYSICAL EXAMINATION

The acutely injured athlete is most likely to be seen coming off the playing field or off the mat vigorously shaking an arm to get the sensation back. Regardless of the presentation, the examiner's attention is first directed toward ruling out spinal cord injury (see part A). If there are no signs or symptoms of spinal cord injury, then specific testing of the neck, shoulder girdle, and upper limb muscles is carried out. Of particular significance are abduction and external rotation of the shoulder and flexion of the elbow. Return of full strength within a few minutes of injury is characteristic of neurapraxias and may reasonably be considered the criterion for a return to play.

The athlete is re-examined after the game and again the following day. There may be palpable tenderness of the trapezius that persists for a few days;[6] however, with neurapraxia only, there is no demonstrable motor deficit.

With more severe injury, the hallmark finding is *persistent weakness of the deltoid, supraspinatus, infraspinatus, and biceps muscles*. (See Chapter 4, part A and Figs. 4–13 and 4–14 for techniques of specifically testing these muscles.) Other upper-trunk–supplied muscles, namely, brachioradialis, pronator teres, and the wrist extensors, may also be involved. Sensory deficits have not been reported.[6, 7, 40]

These findings are different from the neurological findings associated with thoracic outlet syndrome. With compression, as opposed to stretching, of the brachial plexus, it is the lower trunk that is characteristically affected, and sensory deficits, especially of the ulnar aspect of the forearm and hand, are not uncommon.[23]

RADIOGRAPHIC EXAMINATION

When persistent paresis is found on physical examination, it seems prudent to obtain radiographs of the cervical spine. However, in the reported series of brachial plexus injuries, the clinical findings were diagnostic and the cervical spine films were all within normal limits.[7, 40]

OTHER DIAGNOSTIC TESTS

Electromyographic examination is indicated when physical examination at 3 weeks after injury is equivocal or unreliable. We do not believe that it is mandatory at that time, unless the clinical findings are not diagnostic. It seems to be more useful when there is no apparent recovery of nerve function by 6 weeks after injury. It also seems that in the primary care setting, isokinetic testing is a more practical way to assess muscle function quantitatively.

INITIAL TREATMENT

Other than time and rest, initial treatment is not required.

REFERRAL

Although not necessarily required, referral may be appropriate in those cases in which significant paresis persists longer than 6 weeks and intensive, ongoing physical therapy is required.

REHABILITATION

Rehabilitation is specific for the involved muscles (see Chapter 4, part A). When paresis is either profound or prolonged, electrical muscle stimulation may be useful for maintaining muscle tone until voluntary muscle action is possible.[62]

RETURN TO SPORTS PARTICIPATION

Athletes who have suffered a stinger should be advised that they are at increased risk for recurrent injury[3, 6] and that they are probably at increased risk for more severe brachial plexus injury.[6] No return to contact situations is permitted until there is complete resolution of symptoms and full restoration of muscle strength. At Iowa, coach Haden Fry's system of automatic demotion of position after any time-loss injury seems to be a prudent means of gradual return to collision sports.[3] Before resuming contact, the football player should have his equipment rechecked for proper fit and should be provided with a neck roll that limits lateral flexion.[6, 7, 62] Most of the neck rolls worn by football players do not satisfactorily limit neck motion.

C.   THORACIC OUTLET SYNDROME

Thoracic outlet syndrome is an uncommon cause of activity- or position-related upper-limb pain and paresthesias in athletes.[23, 55] Symptoms are produced by compression of the brachial plexus or the subclavian vessels in their course from the neck and thorax to the upper limb. Such compression may occur even in the absence of abnormal structures such as a cervical rib. In these instances it appears that the plexus is stretched by excessive protraction of the scapula; a common finding is a weakened shoulder.

HISTORY

MECHANISM OF INJURY. Symptoms are not related directly to acute injury but rather to position and activity, particularly *repetitive or prolonged overhead use of the upper limb.* A swimmer, for example, may complain of a hand's "going to sleep" after a few minutes of freestyle swimming. Thoracic outlet syndrome, rather than direct pressure on the median or ulnar nerves, may account for cyclist's palsy. Throwing, rowing, weight lifting, serving in tennis, and grooming horses are other reported symptom-producing athletic activities.[23, 55] Nonathletic activities such as long hours at a computer keyboard can also provoke the paresthesias, probably the result of chronic scapular protraction. Not uncommonly, patients complain of being awakened at night by symptoms as a result of sleeping with their arms overhead.

SYMPTOMS. Symptoms are quite variable. In our experience, *paresthesias*, particularly in the hand and forearm, are the most common presentation. However, *pain* in the neck, chest, shoulder girdle, or upper limb, or combinations of these, may be the presenting symptom. Much less commonly, *weakness* may be the primary complaint.[23]

PHYSICAL EXAMINATION

Protraction or drooping of the shoulder girdle, associated with either an ectomorphic body type or overdevelopment of the pectoral musculature, is a common, but nonspecific, finding. Protraction (forward positioning) of the shoulder is best identified while taking the history, *before* the actual shoulder examination, because once the patient realizes the shoulder is to be examined, the patient inevitably "sits up straight" and retracts the shoulder girdle.

With compression, as opposed to stretching, of the brachial plexus, it is the lower trunk that is characteristically affected, and sensory deficits, especially of the ulnar aspect of the forearm and hand, are not uncommon.[23] Diminished two-point discrimination on the ring and small fingers is the most reliable sign of lower trunk or ulnar nerve sensory deficit. A positive Tinel's sign at the elbow or wrist might indicate that the problem is peripheral nerve entrapment rather than thoracic outlet syndrome, but hyperirritability from a more proximal stretch might produce these same signs.

With arterial compression the paresthesias do not conform to a particular neurological pattern. Instead, just the hand, the hand and forearm, or the entire limb feels numb. Various provocative tests have been described. Of these, the overhead exercise test involving rapidly opening and closing the hand with the shoulder fully abducted, and Wright's test, i.e., combined abduction of the shoulder, rotation of the neck to the opposite side, and Valsalva maneuver, are the most reliable. The criteria for a positive test are diminution or abolition of the radial pulse and the reproduction of symptoms. Auscultation of a subclavian artery bruit at the same time is further evidence of arterial compression.

Isolated venous compression is quite rare. The symptoms are vague, and the only findings are likely to be postexercise swelling and cyanosis of the affected limb. With severe impairment of venous outflow, there may be engorgement of the superficial limb and collateral veins.

RADIOGRAPHIC EXAMINATION

Radiographic study is indicated to rule out cervical rib, cervical spinal stenosis, and pulmonary tumor. Bony encroachment on the neuroforamina is best demonstrated with oblique views of the cervical spine. Pulmonary tumors that may account for brachial plexus compression are best demonstrated with apical lordotic chest films.

OTHER DIAGNOSTIC TESTS

In the primary care setting the clinical diagnosis of thoracic outlet syndrome should suffice in most cases. Confirmatory tests, such as nerve conduction studies, Doppler studies, and angiography, are mandatory only if surgical treatment is being considered.

INITIAL TREATMENT

Initial treatment consists of relative rest and anti-inflammatory medication. If protraction of the shoulder is pronounced, a trial of a figure-of-eight clavicle support is often indicated.

REFERRAL

Specialty referral is indicated if there is no response to symptomatic treatment, activity modification, and rehabilitation. Symptoms consistent with arterial compression, auscultation of a subclavian bruit, and the presence of a long cervical rib on radiographic examination are reasonable indications for consultation with or referral to a vascular surgeon.

DEFINITIVE TREATMENT

In most cases, activity modification and rehabilitation constitute the definitive treatment. If the history and physical examination have accurately defined the positions or motions of the neck and upper limb that reproduce symptoms, even competitive athletes may be able to avoid symptoms by slightly altering their technique or by eliminating certain training practices. Recreational or fitness athletes can even more easily find alternative activities that are not symptom producing. Particularly if symptoms are attributable to pectoral hypertrophy and protraction of the shoulder girdle, athletes should avoid exercises such as push-ups and bench presses and concentrate on scapular retraction exercises.

Rehabilitation simply comprises progressive resistance strengthening exercises for the elevators and retractors of the shoulder girdle.

Surgical treatment may be required if severe or substantially disabling symptoms persist. The specific treatment depends on the specific underlying problem.

D.   LOW-BACK PAIN

CLASSIFICATION

Perhaps the most honest way of dealing with the subject of low-back pain would be to admit some limitations from the outset. We do not purport to have a quick and infallible method of sorting out the myriad causes of low-back pain. We hope to provide here only some guidelines for differentiating those causes of low-back pain that are amenable to simple treatment and rehabilitation from those that may require definitive treatment of some sort, and that would therefore merit a more complete diagnostic work-up or specialty referral. We believe this task is made a little easier by broadly classifying low-back pain as mechanical, structural, or extrinsic, after McKenzie.[27]

Mechanical Pain

Mechanical pain is that which is produced by excessive or prolonged mechanical deformation of structures containing nociceptive nerve endings. The involved structures may be either normal or inflamed.

Evaluation for possible mechanical causes of the athlete's low-back pain seems to be of obvious importance. There is probably some element of mechanical pain in most cases of low-back pain in athletes, and in some cases the pain appears to be purely mechanical. Moreover, the definitive treatment of mechanical low-back pain is rather straightforward.

The *hallmark symptoms* of mechanical pain are its *intermittency* and its clear *correlation with certain postures or positions*. It is neither as easy nor as important to identify which of many possible structures are involved as it is to determine which posture or position produces the pain.

We emphasize that mechanical or postural low-back pain is not synonymous with lumbar hyperlordosis. Indeed, any postural abnormality or excess can produce pain. We also emphasize that what constitutes *excessive* for a given individual depends in part on that individual's muscular endurance and range of motion. For example, if there has been an unrehabilitated prior injury with resultant contracture, some positions within the normal limits of motion may be excessive and pain producing.

Historical attention is focused on the circumstances in which pain occurs. Pain with relaxed or prolonged sitting, working at a desk, gardening, and so on implicates sustained lumbar flexion as its cause. Pain with relaxed standing, walking, or running tends to implicate hyperextension.

With more complex activities the athlete may be able to isolate the positions or motions that are pain producing. The gymnast, for example, may describe pain with moves such as back walkovers, or a dancer may state that doing arabesques is painful, both of which would implicate hyperextension. Competitive shooters may complain of pain with shooting a rifle from a standing position, which might implicate combined extension, rotation, and lateral bending.[16]

Physical examination seeks to confirm the presence of any mechanical abnormality. The athlete is observed while sitting and standing. Is there reduced or accentuated lumbar lordosis? Is there a lateral shift? (We use the term *lateral shift* synonymously with the terms *list* and *scoliosis* to refer to any deviation of the spine from the midline.) Any of these may be the cause or the effect, or both, of the low-back pain.

When standing, the athlete is asked to place the hands on the thighs and then run them down the front of the legs, moving as far as possible into a position of lumbar flexion. Any limitation of motion, lateral shift, or pain produced is noted.

Positional pain should be differentiated from that produced by muscular action. If there has been a paraspinous muscle strain, lumbar flexion with the torso unsupported by the hands may cause painful spasm of the involved muscle, whereas gentle flexion with the torso supported by leaning on the examining table may actually be pain relieving.

The athlete is also asked to place the hands in the small of the back and to lean backward as far as possible, and to twist and bend to the side or, alternatively, to shift the torso from side to side.[27] Again, any limitation of motion or pain produced is noted.

If accentuated lordosis is noted, the range of hip motion should be assessed. Tightness of the hip flexors, iliopsoas, or rectus femoris is not uncommon in gymnasts and bicyclists.[14] It can produce anterior tilt of the pelvis and secondarily hyperlordosis and apparent hamstring tightness. Hip flexor and hamstring tightness can be demonstrated with the Thomas and straight-leg–raising tests, respectively (Fig. 7–2).

Assessment of hip motion is particularly important in dancers with low-back pain (Fig. 7–3; see also Fig. 7–2). The turned-out (en dehors) position of the lower limb in dance requires extreme external rotation of the hip. A dancer with femoral anteversion or even "normal" hips will obviously have difficulty with this position. Sometimes, however, the dancer has learned to "cheat" by flexing the hip, which permits more external rotation. Standing with the hip flexed means standing with the pelvis tilted anteriorly and the lumbar spine hyperextended. Arabesques require both external rotation and

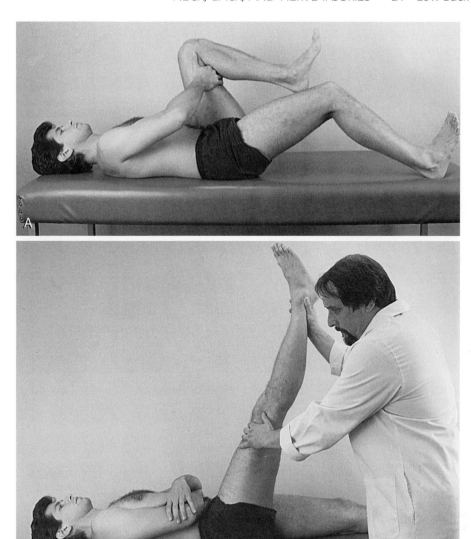

Figure 7–2. Tests for assessing hip flexor and hamstring tightness. With the contralateral hip flexed, the pelvis is tilted posteriorly and the effect of lumbar hyperlordosis on hip motion is canceled. *A,* Tightness of the hip flexors is revealed by involuntary flexion of the ipsilateral hip, a positive Thomas test. *B,* Hamstring tightness is revealed by limitation of straight-leg raising. This is a more specific test for hamstring flexibility than toe touching is.

extension of the hip of the working (raised) leg. The dancer may also have learned to cheat at these by flexing the hip of the support leg, tilting the pelvis anteriorly, and hyperextending the spine. Low-back pain and even spondylolysis is often the price the dancer pays for habitual cheating.

If weight-bearing activities, i.e., standing, walking, or running, seem to be pain producing, then examination should include assessment of the possible relationship of the pain to a discrepancy in lower-limb length.[57] Perhaps for scientific purposes, lower-limb length is best determined radiographically. We have found, however, that for practical purposes, lower-limb length can be adequately assessed by physical examination. The most reliable and clinically useful way of doing this is to determine whether the pelvis is level during neutral standing (Fig. 7–4). The athlete stands with the feet slightly apart, legs parallel, knees straight ahead, and arms hanging loosely at the sides. The

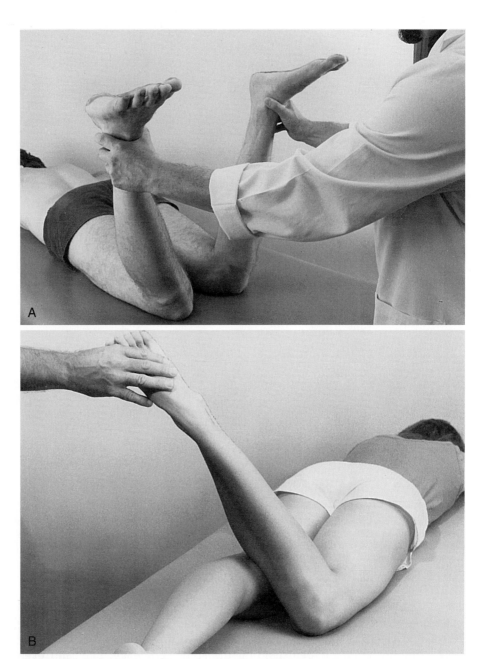

Figure 7–3. Assessment of the range of hip rotation. The athlete is prone. The examiner ascertains that the pelvis is kept flat on the examining table so that any effect of hip flexion is eliminated. *A,* Internal rotation of both hips is assessed by holding the knees together and flexed to. 90 degrees and then letting the feet fall apart. *B,* External rotation of each hip is assessed by positioning the patient with the contralateral knee extended and then letting the ipsilateral foot fall across the midline. Normally there is about 90 degrees of total hip rotation. With femoral anteversion, most of this motion consists of internal rotation, whereas with femoral retroversion, most of the motion consists of external rotation. At least 45 degrees of external rotation is required for proper turnout in ballet.

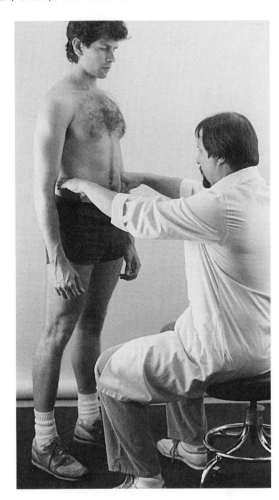

Figure 7–4. Assessment of lower limb length—palpation of the anterior superior iliac spines. The athlete stands with feet slightly apart, legs parallel, knees straight ahead, arms hanging loosely at the sides.

examiner palpates the anterior superior iliac spines, the iliac crests, the posterior superior iliac spines, and the greater trochanters, noting the relative heights of each. If these landmarks are all higher on one side than the other, there is at least a functional limb-length discrepancy. If there is pronation (arch collapse) of the foot of the apparently shorter limb, the effect of correcting the pronation should be noted (Fig. 7–5).

Many asymptomatic individuals have detectable limb-length discrepancies. To help judge whether an apparent limb-length discrepancy is clinically significant, we use the magazine test. This simply has the athlete stand first with one foot and then the other on a magazine. Standing with the shorter limb on the magazine, the athlete should feel better or more balanced, whereas standing with the longer limb on the magazine the athlete should feel unbalanced. If these criteria are satisfied, a trial of correcting the discrepancy is indicated. This may involve lifting the heel or taping the foot, or both, to control pronation.

If the pain is clearly related to a specific activity, it is desirable to observe the athletes during that activity. Have them bring their athletic clothing, footwear, equipment, and so on with them. Observe runners as they run in the hallway or on a treadmill. Is there any lumbar hyperlordosis or lateral shift? Observe cyclists in their usual riding position on their own bicycle, preferably on a training stand (see Chapter 3, part D and Fig. 3–3). Is there

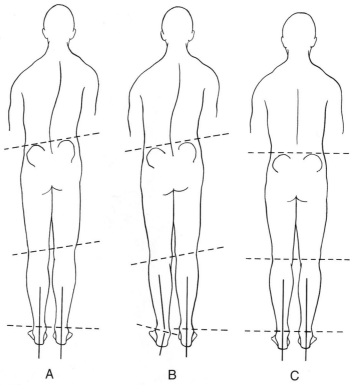

A   B   C

Figure 7–5. Assessment of lower-limb length—effect of pronation (arch collapse) of the foot. *A*, Anatomical limb-length discrepancy. *B*, Functional limb-length discrepancy secondary to arch collapse on the "short" side. *C*, Disappearance of functional limb-length discrepancy with orthotic correction of the arch collapse. (Modified from Subotnick SI: Limb length discrepancies of the lower extremity [the short leg syndrome]. J Orthop Sports Phys Ther 3:11–16, 1981. Courtesy of Marianna Amicarella, artist.)

excessive flexion of the lumbar spine? Observe dancers attempting the positions or motions that cause pain. Is the pelvis tilted anteriorly and the spine hyperextended to compensate for limited hip motion?

Structural Pain

Structural pain is that which is produced by actual derangement of the bony components of the vertebral column or related structures. A synonymous term is *spondylogenic pain*. The derangement may be traumatic, degenerative, rheumatological, infectious, neoplastic, and so on.

Regardless of the cause, there is an inflammatory response of the involved structures to the derangement. Accordingly, there is likely to be at least an element of *constant pain*, which serves to differentiate structural from purely mechanical pain. Of course, there is also likely to be a mechanical component of the pain, i.e., *exacerbation of the pain with certain motions or positions of the spine*, which serves to differentiate intrinsic from extrinsic low-back pain.

Diagnostic accuracy is obviously more important with structural than with purely mechanical pain but may be just as difficult to achieve. As discussed later, clinical attention is directed to the onset, duration, and *localization* of the pain.

In our experience, the most frequent causes of structural low-back pain in athletes seem to be strains of the lumbar paraspinous muscles and sprains of the interspinous, iliolumbar, and sacroiliac ligaments. As with sprains and strains in general, there is usually a history of (acute or repetitive) antecedent trauma, localized tenderness at the site of injury, and pain reproduced with increased tension (passive stretch or resisted action) of the involved structure or structures. Treatment is symptomatic and rehabilitative. The aim is to prevent residual loss of motion, strength, and muscular endurance and thereby to minimize the risk of recurrent injury and mechanical low-back pain.

Tenderness over the sacroiliac joint in most cases probably represents a strain of the erector spinae muscle at its insertion on the posterior superior iliac spine. True sacroiliac pain can best be reproduced with iliac compression or Patrick's tests (Fig. 7–6). The differentiation is probably of greatest importance when pain has persisted despite adequate rest, in which case rheumatological disease, such as ankylosing spondylitis, should be ruled out.

An important cause of structural pain in the skeletally immature athlete is stress reaction or fracture of the pars interarticularis of the vertebral arch. If the stress fracture is detected early enough, it is potentially reversible.[19–21, 32] *Red flags* that should alert the examiner to the likelihood of this diagnosis are the persistence of pain despite adequate rest; participation in dance, football (especially linemen), gymnastics, and weight training; the production of pain with hyperextension; and a hyperlordotic posture with apparent hamstring shortening.[13, 14, 19–21, 54, 61, 62] The diagnosis and its implications are discussed in greater detail in part E.

Obviously athletes are not immune to disease of the intervertebral disc. Although degeneration and subsequent bulging or herniation of the nucleus pulposus are a common cause of low-back pain in the middle-aged, frank herniation may actually be more common in adolescent and young adult athletes.[53] Jackson reports that disc disease is implicated in some 10% of skeletally immature athletes with persistent low-back pain.[19]

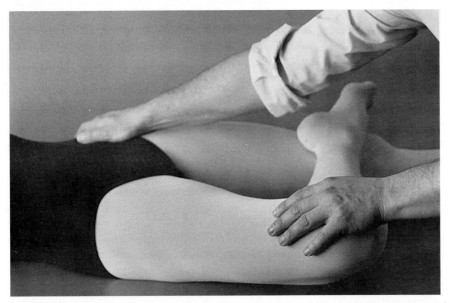

Figure 7–6. Patrick's test. The patient's lower limbs are placed in a figure-four position with one hip abducted and externally rotated, the knee flexed, and the heel resting on the opposite knee. The examiner applies downward pressure on the flexed knee. If the ipsilateral sacroiliac joint or iliolumbar ligament is inflamed, pain will be produced and localized to that site.

Disc disease may occur as low-back pain with or without sciatica. Discogenic low-back pain not associated with sciatica may be treated essentially as mechanical low-back pain. Even when sciatica is present, the pain is often amenable to mechanical (rehabilitative) treatment.[25, 27, 62] The differential diagnosis and treatment of sciatica are discussed in part F.

Other causes of structural low-back pain are much less common. Osteoporosis and jumps or falls from heights or other vertical-loading mechanisms can produce compression fractures of the lumbar vertebrae that are noted as acute pain. Neoplasm, infection, or rheumatological disease can occur as chronic pain.

Extrinsic Pain

Extrinsic pain is that which is referred to the back from other structures. The terms *viscerogenic, vasculogenic,* and *neurogenic* describe the possible etiologic factors. For the most part, extrinsic disease can be differentiated from intrinsic disease by the fact that it is usually *not associated with activity or relieved by rest*. Rarely, however, infections and neoplasms involving the spinal cord or cauda equina may mimic disc herniation.[43]

The caveat is that when low-back pain persists for more than a few weeks and cannot be attributed to pars interarticularis or disc disease, then work-up is indicated to rule out the less common causes of intrinsic or extrinsic pain such as neoplasm, infection, or rheumatological disease.

INITIAL TREATMENT

It should be clearly understood that acute low-back pain is almost always a self-limited process. Regardless of the treatment, some 50% of patients are better within 1 week, 85% within 1 month, and more than 90% within 2 months.[27] The efficacy of any pharmacological, manipulative, physical, or other therapy should be judged within that context.

Clearly, time and relative rest are the most important aspects of successful treatment. The postures and activities that are pain producing are identified by the history and physical examination. They should be avoided until the acute pain subsides. To the extent that rest must sometimes be compromised, some simple mechanical aids may be useful. These may include a lumbar roll to limit lumbar flexion in sitting, a corset to help limit either flexion or extension, a hip-hugger corset to support the sacroiliac joint, and a heel lift to correct limb-length discrepancy.

Purely mechanical pain need not be treated by other than mechanical means. To the extent that structural derangement, inflammation, and constant pain are present, pharmacological treatment may be appropriate. We commonly use analgesics or nonsteroidal anti-inflammatory medications in this setting.

Some patients may welcome the sedative effects of the minor tranquilizers, euphemistically referred to in this setting as "muscle relaxants." Other patients, particularly those who have to drive, go to work, or go to school, may find the sedation unwelcome. For actually relieving muscle spasm, ice and electrogalvanic stimulation (EGS) treatments are our treatment of choice.

Gentle manipulation, or preferably therapist-directed self-manipulation, can sometimes provide dramatic relief of symptoms. This is perhaps most evident with sciatic scoliosis, the marked muscle spasm and lateral shift sometimes associated with a bulging disc. Manipulative therapy is further discussed in part F.

We are, of course, pleased when we are able to help make our patients more comfortable. However, especially with back pain, we think that it is important to teach the patient that the acute pain is self-limited, that symptomatic treatment of any kind is not curative, and that the real trick is preventing recurrent or chronic pain. We believe that we do athletes no great service by fostering their dependence on us to resolve their episodes of low-back pain.

REFERRAL

Time and the severity of symptoms are the key diagnostic tests. *Pain that is constant, severe, and not alleviated at all by positional changes* is a reasonable indication for specialty referral. As mentioned previously, pain that *persists for more than a few weeks despite appropriate treatment* is also an indication for referral. Ideally, referral is made to a back specialist.

More specifically, cases of purely mechanical pain and lumbosacral sprains and strains need not be referred. Certainly, disc space infections, unstable fractures, neoplasms, and the like should be referred. The extent to which primary physicians may reasonably choose to manage pars interarticularis, disc, and rheumatological disease varies considerably. Consultation, if not referral, is probably appropriate.

REHABILITATION

The role of exercise in the prevention and treatment of low-back pain is not without controversy. Abdominal strengthening has long been advocated for the correction of accentuated lumbar lordosis,[72] and more recently, paraspinous strengthening has been advocated for the correction of reduced lumbar lordosis,[27] although there is no evidence that any strengthening exercise actually alters posture.[17] The most commonly recommended abdominal exercise, the sit-up, as it was conventionally performed with the feet held down by a partner, is predominantly a hip flexor exercise. The training effect, if any, of doing sit-ups in this manner would be to increase, rather than decrease, anterior pelvic tilt. Moreover, the acute effect of doing sit-ups is to double intradiscal pressure,[36] obviously less than desirable when back pain is related to disc disease.

On the other hand, postural abnormality may be the result of soft tissue contracture, which can be corrected by specific stretching exercises. Furthermore, the severity and duration of low-back pain have been shown to be correlated with decreased strength of the trunk muscles.[1, 17] It has also been shown that workers who do not possess adequate strength relative to their job demands suffer a higher incidence of back injury.[17, 36] It is in this context that we advocate flexibility and strength training for athletes with low-back pain.

If examination reveals limited lumbar motion, then rehabilitation is appropriately directed at restoring that motion. For example, limitation of flexion is particularly likely to occur after unrehabilitated strains of the paraspinous muscles. Subsequently, activities requiring a normal range of lumbar flexion

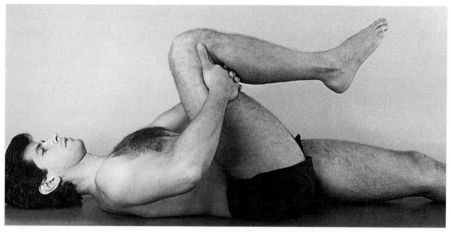

Figure 7–7. Lumbar paraspinous muscle stretching. This is a modification of one of the four original Williams flexion exercises.[72]

may be pain producing. Treatment consists of paraspinous stretching exercises, as seen in Figure 7–7. Limitation of extension is particularly common with disc disease. Treatment is as shown in Figure 7–8. If examination reveals lumbar hyperlordosis and limited hip extension, then attention is also directed at stretching the hip flexors (Fig. 7–9).

Strength training is clearly indicated to restore any deficits that may follow muscle injury. Abdominal strengthening is a mainstay of treatment for back pain associated with lumbar hyperextension; and paraspinous strengthening, for pain associated with lumbar flexion. The aim is not to effect a dramatic postural change, but rather to allow the extension and flexion

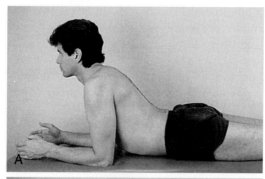

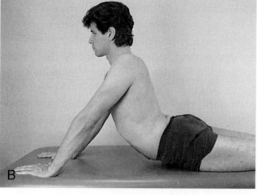

Figure 7–8. Extension in lying (A) and stretching (B) for restoration of lumbar extension. (After McKenzie RA: The Lumbar Spine: Mechanical Diagnosis and Therapy. Waikan, NZ, Spinal Publications, 1981.)

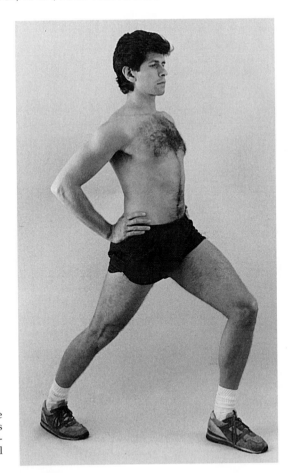

Figure 7–9. Stretching exercise for the (right) hip flexors (iliopsoas and rectus femoris). This is a modification of one of the four original Williams flexion exercises.[72]

activities, respectively, to be performed with greater muscular control, and thereby without pain. We believe that complete back rehabilitation (or "prehabilitation" of the uninjured athlete) should include strengthening of the entire torso—rectus abdominis, abdominal obliques, and paraspinous muscles. Again, the aim is not to change the athlete's posture, but rather to make the torso a strong muscular cylinder capable of supporting in large part the loads that would otherwise have to be borne by the spinal column. This is a particularly important consideration for strength athletes such as football players, wrestlers, weight lifters, and field athletes. The preferred techniques for abdominal and paraspinous strengthening are seen in Figures 7–10 and 7–11.

Pelvic-tilt–shoulder-lift sit-ups (crunches, curl-ups, half sit-ups) are the safest and most effective abdominal strengthening exercises (see Fig. 7–10). The knees are kept flexed, and the feet are not held down. The pelvis is tilted posteriorly, eliminating the hollow under the back. The posterior pelvic tilt is maintained by isometric action of the lower part of the rectus abdominis. Both shoulders are then slowly lifted off the floor, the position is held for a count of 6, and then the shoulders are slowly lowered to the floor. Sit-ups done in this manner selectively exercise the rectus abdominis muscle.[15] A variation that involves greater activity of the oblique abdominal muscles is to lift alternately one shoulder, then the other, off the floor.[15, 18] The end point of these exercises is muscle fatigue to the extent that the posterior pelvic tilt

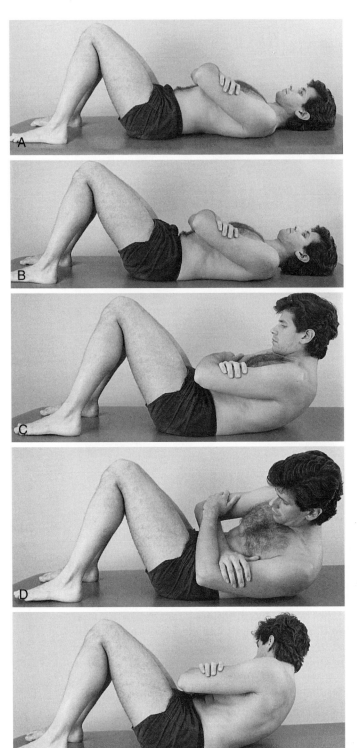

Figure 7–10. Pelvic-tilt–shoulder-lift sit-ups (crunches). *A,* Starting position—knees flexed, feet not held down. *B,* To exercise the lower rectus abdominis, the pelvis is tilted posteriorly, eliminating the hollow under the back. *C,* To exercise the upper rectus, both shoulders are slowly lifted off the floor, the position is held for a count of six, and then the shoulders are slowly lowered to the floor. *D* and *E,* To exercise the oblique abdominal muscles, alternately one shoulder and then the other is lifted off the floor.

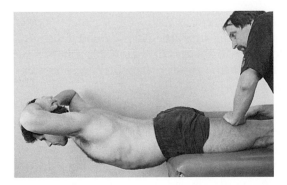

Figure 7–11. Trunk extensor strengthening. The torso is lifted from a flexed to a neutral position. Active hyperextension (extension past neutral) is associated with high intradiscal pressures and is not recommended. (Redrawn after Teitz CC, Cook DM: Rehabilitation of neck and low back injuries. Clin Sports Med 4:455–476, 1985.)

cannot be maintained. Compared with conventional sit-ups, lumbar flexion and rotation, and consequently intradiscal pressures, are minimized.[15, 18]

Paraspinous (trunk extensor) strengthening exercises can be done from either the prone or the supine position. Hip lifting from a supine position is recommended for the injured athlete. Exercise is then advanced as tolerated to trunk extension against gravity from a prone position (see Fig. 7–11). The torso is lifted from a flexed to a neutral position. Active hyperextension (extension past neutral) is associated with high intradiscal pressures and is not recommended.[18]

Flexion exercises are contraindicated in acute disc disease manifested by sciatica, flexion-induced pain, or a lateral shift. They are also contraindicated immediately after prolonged rest, when the disc is hyperhydrated and more susceptible to injury.[18] Extension exercises are contraindicated in symptomatic pars interarticularis disease.

Maintenance of posture is more a function of muscular endurance than of muscular strength.[17] Probably the most effective training for sport-specific muscular endurance is the sport activity itself, performed with proper technique. If postural correction is desired, it is more likely to be achieved through flexibility training, motor learning, or bracing than through strength training.

In addition to specific stretching and strengthening exercises, treatment of mechanical low-back pain may involve sorting out certain sport-specific mechanical problems, e.g., orthotically correcting a runner's foot pronation, adjusting a bicycle to fit a cyclist, teaching a dancer to avoid forced turnout. A knowledgeable coach, instructor, or trainer can help a great deal with this.

E. PARS INTERARTICULARIS STRESS FRACTURE, SPONDYLOLYSIS, AND SPONDYLOLISTHESIS

Stress fracture of the pars interarticularis of the vertebral arch is an important cause of structural low-back pain in the skeletally immature athlete. The terminology is admittedly a bit cumbersome, but it does accurately describe the pathomechanics.

The term *spondylolysis* correctly refers to a radiographically demonstrable defect of the pars interarticularis. Such defects may represent sequelae of stress fractures or may simply represent developmental defects. The latter appears to be more common.[5] Spondylolysis may or may not be symptomatic.

The term *spondylolisthesis* refers to anterior displacement of one vertebral body on another. The displacement may occur as the result of either spondy-lolysis or abnormal elongation of the pars interarticularis. Spondylolisthesis also may or may not be symptomatic. To the extent that displacement may occur acutely, there may be a rather acute onset of symptoms, sometimes referred to as *spondylolisthetic crisis*.[5]

HISTORY

MECHANISM OF INJURY. To the extent that any of the conditions are the result of injury, the mechanism of injury appears to be *repetitive extension loading of the lumbar spine*, such as may occur in dancing, football (especially line play), gymnastics, and weight training.[5, 13, 14, 19–21, 54, 61, 62]

SYMPTOMS. The hallmark symptom is activity-induced or -exacerbated low-back pain. The pain is usually unilateral and fairly well localized. The pain is characteristically produced by hyperextension of the lumbar spine, and the athlete may very well be able to identify one or more specific pain-producing activities, such as back walkovers in gymnastics or blocking in football.

With spondylolisthesis the athlete may also be aware of posture or gait disturbances, the onset of which may be rather acute.

PHYSICAL EXAMINATION

The hallmark physical finding is reproduction of pain with lumbar hyperex-tension. The one-leg–standing lumbar extension test seen in Figure 7–12 is a reasonably sensitive, though rather nonspecific, test. It usually reproduces the pain associated with pars interarticularis stress fracture. If the stress fracture is unilateral, standing on the ipsilateral leg produces more pain.

With stress fractures the signs typically associated with sciatica are nota-bly absent. Moderate hyperlordosis and hamstring tightness are not uncom-mon, but marked hyperlordosis and hamstring tightness are more typical of spondylolisthesis (Fig. 7–13). Severe spondylolisthesis may be associated with sciatica (see part F).

RADIOGRAPHIC EXAMINATION

Radiographic study of the lumbosacral spine is indicated to rule out spondy-lolysis and spondylolisthesis. Defects of the pars interarticularis are best demonstrated with oblique views (Fig. 7–14). The extent of spondylolisthesis is best demonstrated with a standing lateral view.

OTHER DIAGNOSTIC TESTS

If radiographic examination is normal but symptoms have persisted despite appropriate treatment, a radionuclide bone scan is indicated to confirm or rule out a stress fracture. If radiographic examination reveals spondylolysis, a bone scan is indicated to determine whether the pars defect is acute.

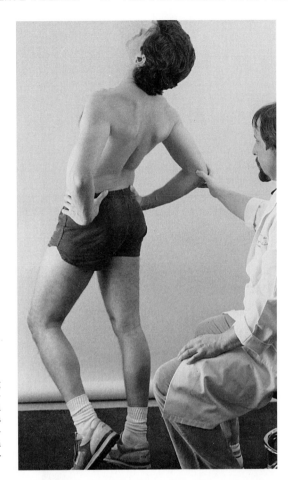

Figure 7–12. One-leg–standing lumbar extension test for pars interarticularis stress fracture. (Redrawn after Ciullo JV, Jackson DW: Pars interarticularis stress reaction, spondylolysis, and spondylolisthesis in gymnasts. Clin Sports Med 4:95–110, 1985.)

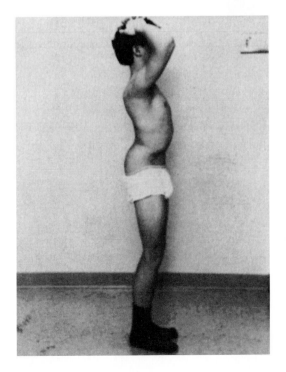

Figure 7–13. Typical features of spondylolisthesis include marked hyperlordosis with apparent shortening of the torso and flattening of the buttocks. Associated spasm and marked tightness of the hamstrings may produce gait disturbances. (From Ciullo JV, Jackson DW: Pars interarticularis stress reaction, spondylolysis, and spondylolisthesis in gymnasts. Clin Sports Med 4:95–110, 1985.)

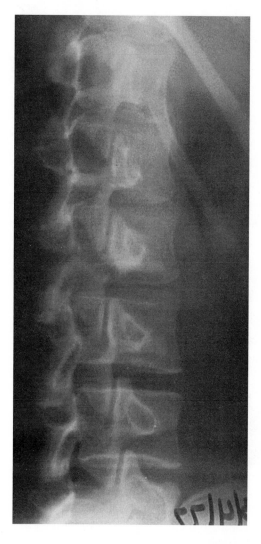

Figure 7–14. So-called Scottie dog sign of spondylolysis. The dog's ear, snout, and foreleg represent, respectively, the superior articular facet, the lateral process, and the inferior articular facet. Spondylolysis (L2) is represented by the dog's wearing a radiolucent collar.

INITIAL TREATMENT

Initial treatment consists primarily of *relative rest*, which in most cases amounts to avoidance of lumbar hyperextension. Simple measures such as ice and EGS treatments to reduce muscle spasm may be appropriate but should not be used to permit continued sports participation despite pain.

REFERRAL

Orthopedic referral is indicated if symptoms do not respond to the conservative treatment discussed later or if there is spondylolisthesis in which vertebral displacement is greater than 25% of the width of the vertebral body.

DEFINITIVE TREATMENT

If detected early enough, *stress fractures are potentially reversible.*[19–21, 32] The aim of treatment is to facilitate healing and to prevent progression to spondylolysis and spondylolisthesis. Whether or not radiographic examination reveals a defect, if the bone scan is abnormal, treatment as for stress fracture is indicated.

The mainstay of treatment is *strict avoidance of pain-producing activity.* Usually this implies discontinuance of sports participation for a matter of weeks to months. In our practice, bed rest or antilordotic bracing is rarely required. However, bracing may sometimes be appropriate for an elite athlete in that it may permit continued sports participation without pain.[5, 19, 32]

We believe that rehabilitation is an important adjunct to relative rest in the treatment and prevention of stress fractures. Abdominal strengthening exercises and hamstring stretching exercises (see part D) may be started early. Paraspinous strengthening exercises are contraindicated until symptoms have resolved.

The end point of treatment is a normal bone scan and complete resolution of symptoms. This may or may not correlate with resolution of the spondylolysis on radiographic examination, as pars defects may heal by bony or fibrous union.

Whether or not they have symptoms, until their growth is completed, athletes with spondylolysis are at some risk for developing spondylolisthesis. The risk is greatest between the ages of 9 and 14 years and is greater in girls than in boys. Any child with spondylolysis should be followed radiographically until vertebral growth is completed. We recommend spot lateral radiographs at 6-month intervals in asymptomatic children and as necessary if symptoms occur.

Athletes with spondylolisthesis are permitted to participate in sports provided the vertebral displacement is less than 25% of the width of the vertebral body and the athlete is without symptoms. Less-than-promising athletes in high-risk sports, such as football and gymnastics, are encouraged to consider alternative athletic pursuits.

Surgical treatment of spondylolysis or spondylolisthesis is rarely required.

F. SCIATICA

The term *sciatica* refers to pain in the distribution of the sciatic nerve, i.e., the buttock, posterior aspect of the thigh, leg, and foot. The pain may or may not be associated with low-back pain, paresthesias, or frank neurological deficits.

DIFFERENTIAL DIAGNOSIS

The most common cause of sciatica is impingement of L4, L5, or S1 nerve roots by a bulging or herniated lumbar intervertebral disc. However, sciatica is by no means synonymous with disc disease. As discussed previously, a bulging disc may produce low-back pain without sciatica. Conversely, sciatica may be the presenting symptom of other disease processes. The differential diagnosis also includes lumbar spinal stenosis, piriformis syndrome, facet syndrome, and neoplasm.[22, 33, 43, 53]

Spinal stenosis refers to bony encroachment on the spinal canal or neuroforamina. The bony abnormality may be developmental, degenerative, spondylolisthetic, post-traumatic, or postoperative. If sufficiently severe, it can produce nerve root impingement and sciatica. Characteristically, the pain is induced or exacerbated by exercise and relieved by rest.

Piriformis syndrome refers to sciatica associated with overuse of the piriformis muscle, one of the external rotators of the hip. As the sciatic nerve leaves the pelvis, its peroneal division either directly underlies, pierces, or directly overlies the belly of the piriformis muscle. Injury, inflammation, and spasm of the muscle can result in impingement and inflammation of the nerve. Characteristically the pain is induced or exacerbated by activities that require repetitive external rotation of the hip, such as running or dancing.

Facet syndrome refers to sciatica associated with degenerative or inflammatory conditions of the intervertebral facet joints. Mooney and Robertson have presented experimental and clinical evidence that facet joint disease can appear as typical sciatica.[33] However, as there is no actual impingement of the sciatic nerve or its roots, the sciatica represents referred pain and is not associated with paresthesias or neurological deficits.

HISTORY

With disc disease there is typically a history of nagging low-back pain; however, the athlete often first appears for medical evaluation after an episode of acute, severe low-back pain and sciatica. The sciatica may be unilateral or bilateral, which correlates, respectively, with lateral or central bulging or herniation of disc material.

The acute pain is characteristically produced or exacerbated by conditions that increase intradiscal pressure. These include coughing, sneezing, Valsalva maneuvers, and lumbar flexion. The pain is not uncommonly relieved by lumbar extension. If indeed the athlete has been able to find a position of comfort during the acute painful episode, there is a better prognosis for successful treatment by mechanical means.[27]

In athletes with discogenic pain there is often a history of repetitive loading of the flexed spine. For example, weight lifters and body builders admit to dead lifts, bent-over rowing, incline sit-ups, and the like as being part of their usual routines.

With lumbar spinal stenosis, the back pain and sciatica are much more likely to be related to activity than to a particular static posture. The pattern of abrupt onset and discontinuance of symptoms with initiation and cessation of exercise can closely resemble intermittent claudication due to peripheral arterial occlusive disease and has been referred to as *neurogenic claudication*. As with disc disease, the sciatica may be unilateral or bilateral.

With piriformis syndrome the pain is also more likely to be activity than posture related. The symptoms are usually unilateral. A dancer with piriformis syndrome will probably admit to having had difficulty with turnout of the symptomatic leg.

With facet syndrome the symptoms are likely to be induced or exacerbated by lumbar extension and relieved by lumbar flexion.

With any of the syndromes caused by nerve root or nerve impingement, paresthesias and hypesthesias may be part of the clinical picture. The athlete, however, is unlikely to have noted any weakness.

PHYSICAL EXAMINATION

Maneuvers for reproducing sciatica by stretching the sciatic nerve are probably as well known to patients with chronic or recurrent pain as to their physicians. Some variations of Lasègue's straight-leg–raising test that may help to confirm abnormal test results are shown in Figure 7–15.

With any of these maneuvers, the criterion for abnormal findings is the reproduction of sciatica or paresthesias, rather than reproduction of low-back pain. As straight-leg raising may be limited in patients with facet syndrome, abnormal test results should best be considered suggestive of, rather than conclusive for, nerve root or nerve impingement and inflammation.[33]

With acute discogenic pain, there is likely to be a loss of the normal lumbar lordosis. Lumbar extension while standing is likely to be limited but not pain producing, whereas lumbar flexion is likely to reproduce both back pain and sciatica. *Sciatic scoliosis*, i.e., a lateral shift of the lumbar spine away

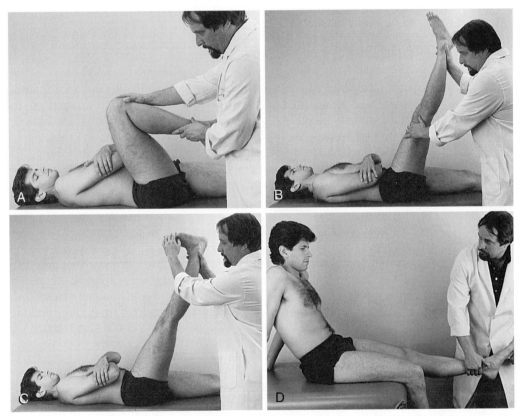

Figure 7–15. Tests for sciatica. *A,* With the patient supine, passive flexion of the hip while simultaneously flexing the knee does not appreciably stretch the sciatic nerve. Although this maneuver may increase intradiscal pressure by reversing lumbar lordosis, it is less likely than straight-leg raising to reproduce sciatica. *B,* Passive flexion of the hip with the knee extended, i.e., straight-leg raising, does indeed stretch the sciatic nerve. Reproduction of sciatica with straight-leg raising in the absence of symptoms with simple hip flexion constitutes a positive Lasègue test. Further evidence of sciatic nerve or nerve root involvement is provided by the following test: *C,* After the limit of straight-leg raising has been reached, the leg is lowered slightly to reduce tension on the nerve. With the leg held in that position, dorsiflexion of the ankle increases tension on the nerve and should again produce symptoms. *D,* With the patient seated, passive extension of the knee is anatomically quite similar to straight-leg raising. Even if the patient is distracted, for example, by testing the plantar reflexes, lifting the foot should reproduce the sciatica or cause the patient to lean backward to reduce tension on the nerve.

from the symptomatic side and unrelated to lateral pelvic tilt, is a highly specific finding. Reduction or centralization of the pain with lumbar extension suggests a good prognosis for successful treatment by mechanical means.[27]

With any of the conditions that produce nerve root impingement, localization of hypesthesias to a specific dermatome or dermatomes identifies the nerve root or roots involved and rules out facet syndrome as the cause of the sciatica. Paresis and diminished or pathological reflexes are uncommon findings. Their presence indicates advanced disease and a poor prognosis for successful treatment by simple means.

With piriformis syndrome, sciatica is reproduced by increasing the tension in the muscle—by passive stretch or resisted action (Fig. 7–16). This test is both sensitive and quite specific, but not pathognomonic. For example, because the nerve is also stretched, these maneuvers can reproduce or exacerbate discogenic pain.

Tenderness over the course of the sciatic nerve in the buttock is a nonspecific finding. A rather more specific finding in piriformis syndrome is point tenderness lateral to the course of the nerve and posteromedial to the greater trochanter over the muscle and its tendon of insertion.

RADIOGRAPHIC EXAMINATION

If the clinical findings are consistent with piriformis syndrome, radiographic examination is not required. Otherwise, radiographic examination of the lumbosacral spine is indicated, although not necessarily on an acute basis.

Disc herniation may be evidenced by narrowing of a disc space. Spinal stenosis may be evidenced by osteophyte formation, particularly along the posterior margins of the vertebral bodies. Less commonly, spinal stenosis may be evidenced by a finding of spondylolisthesis.

OTHER DIAGNOSTIC TESTS

Although there are some false-negative studies, myelography, computed tomography, and magnetic resonance imaging are the most accurate diagnostic tests for disc herniation and spinal stenosis. Of these, magnetic resonance imaging has the advantages of being noninvasive and not involving radiation and is now our diagnostic procedure of choice. Neurogenic claudication can

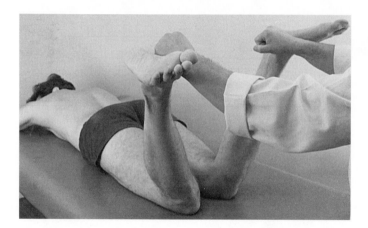

Figure 7–16. Tests for piriformis syndrome. The range of hip rotation is assessed as shown in Figure 7–3. With piriformis syndrome there is likely to be limitation of external rotation and pain at the limit of internal rotation of the hip. Then, with both hips internally rotated, the patient is asked to squeeze the feet together while the examiner holds them apart. The resisted action of the external rotators should reproduce sciatica attributable to piriformis syndrome.

be confirmed by studies of postexercise-evoked potentials. Corticosteroid/local anesthetic injection of a facet joint can be both diagnostic and therapeutic for facet syndrome.

Such tests would certainly be appropriate before surgical treatment of the conditions discussed. They have limited utility, however, in the primary care of the athlete with sciatica.

INITIAL TREATMENT

As discussed in part D, the acute pain is almost always self-limited. Time and relative rest are the most important aspects of successful treatment. Pharmacological, manipulative, and physical therapy are sometimes useful adjuncts.

Gentle manipulation, or preferably therapist-directed self-manipulation, can sometimes provide dramatic relief of symptoms associated with a bulging disc.[27] This is perhaps most evident with sciatic scoliosis.[25]

REFERRAL

In the acute setting, indications for referral to a back specialist are motor nerve deficits and pain that is constant and severe regardless of position. Subsequently, symptoms that persist for more than a few weeks despite appropriate treatment or activity modification, or both, are indications for referral.

The presence of sciatic scoliosis or demonstrable reduction or centralization of pain with lumbar extension is indication for referral to a therapist familiar with McKenzie's rehabilitation techniques.

REHABILITATION

As discussed in part D, symptoms that are clearly related to particular postures or motions are most likely to be amenable to rehabilitation.

In general, if examination reveals motion or strength deficits, then rehabilitation is directed at restoring those deficits. Abdominal strengthening is indicated when symptoms are associated with lumbar hyperextension, and paraspinous strengthening is indicated when they are associated with lumbar flexion.

Discogenic pain produced or exacerbated by lumbar flexion and relieved or centralized by lumbar extension is appropriately treated with McKenzie's rehabilitation exercises.[27] These include, sequentially, therapist-supervised self-correction of any lateral shift, progressive lumbar extension exercises, and flexion and rotation exercises.[25] Instruction in the maintenance of normal postural lumbar lordosis is also emphasized.[26]

Activity modification may be the only effective simple measure for treating neurogenic claudication. This is particularly relevant for the older fitness and recreational athlete with degenerative lumbar spinal stenosis who may be able to swim or bicycle without symptoms, even though unable to walk or run.

The definitive treatment of piriformis syndrome comprises appropriate

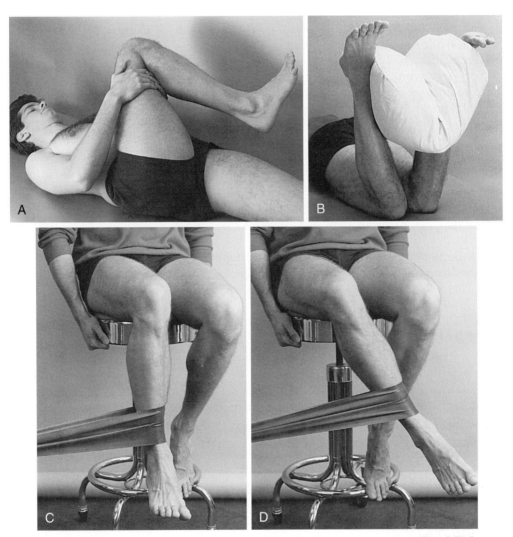

Figure 7–17. Stretching (A), isometric (B), and Theraband resistance exercises (C and D) for the piriformis (hip external rotator).

stretching and strengthening exercises (Fig. 7–17) and attention to mechanical factors such as avoiding forced turnout in ballet.

G. SCHEUERMANN'S DISEASE (BUTTERFLIER'S BACK)

Scheuermann's disease is an uncommon cause of back pain in skeletally immature athletes.[73] The essential lesion is a growth disturbance of the epiphyseal plates of the vertebral body anteriorly. As with spondylolysis, it appears that the cause may be developmental, traumatic, or both. To the extent that the condition is the result of injury, it appears that the mechanism of injury is repetitive flexion loading of the spine.

Classically, Scheuermann's disease involves the thoracic spine. The usual presentation is backache associated with thoracic kyphosis. The pain is typically provoked by flexion of the thoracic spine, such as occurs in swimming butterfly, hence the name "butterflier's back." Radiographic examination confirms the kyphosis and reveals the cause to be anterior wedging of the vertebral bodies. Schmorl's nodes, which are nodular erosions of the vertebral bodies, are common findings.

"Atypical" Scheuermann's disease may involve the lumbar vertebrae, apparently as a result of repetitive flexion loading of the lumbar spine. We have encountered the problem in gymnasts and figure skaters. The radiographic findings are similar to those of "typical" Scheuermann's.

The aim of treatment is prevention of permanent deformity. If there is involvement of three or more vertebrae, with kyphosis exceeding 30 degrees, treatment with a Milwaukee brace is probably indicated, and the patient should be referred for orthopedic evaluation. Whether or not bracing is required, extension stretching and strengthening exercises are indicated. Some athletes may be able to continue to train and compete while being treated with bracing, provided that the brace is worn at all other times, appropriate rehabilitation exercises are incorporated into the training program, and aggravating activities, e.g., swimming butterfly stroke, are avoided.[73] As with spondylolysis, all athletes with Scheuermann's disease should be followed radiographically until vertebral growth is completed.

REFERENCES

1. Addison R, Schulz A: Trunk strengths in patients seeking hospitalization for chronic low back disorders. Spine 5:539–544, 1980.
2. Albright JP et al: Non-fatal cervical spine injuries in interscholastic football. JAMA 236:1243–1245, 1976.
3. Albright JP et al: Head and neck injuries in college football: An eight year analysis. Am J Sports Med 13:147–152, 1985.
4. Blyth CS, Arnold DC: The forty-seventh annual survey of football fatalities: 1931–1978. Athletic Training 4:234–236, 1979.
5. Ciullo JV, Jackson DW: Pars interarticularis stress reaction, spondylolysis, and spondylolisthesis in gymnasts. Clin Sports Med 4:95–110, 1985.
6. Clancy WG: Brachial plexus and upper extremity peripheral nerve injuries. In Torg JS (ed): Athletic Injuries to the Head, Neck, and Face. Philadelphia, Lea & Febiger, 1982, pp 215–220.
7. Clancy WG et al: Upper trunk brachial plexus injuries in contact sports. Am J Sports Med 5:209–216, 1977.
8. Clarke KS: Calculated risk of sports fatalities. JAMA 197:894–896, 1966.
9. Clarke KS: Survey of spinal cord injuries in schools and college sports, 1973–1975. J Safety Res 9:140–146, 1977.
10. Clarke KS: An epidemiological view. In Torg JS (ed): Athletic Injuries to the Head, Neck, and Face. Philadelphia, Lea & Febiger, 1982, pp 15–26.
11. Clarke KS, Powell JW: Football helmets and neurotrauma—An epidemiologic overview of three seasons. Med Sci Sports 11:138–145, 1979.
12. Crouch L: Neck injuries: Prevention to avoid rehabilitation. Natl Strength Conditioning Assoc 1:29–31, 1979.
13. Ferguson et al: Low back pain in college football linemen. Am J Sports Med 2:63–69, 1974.
14. Garrick JG, Requa RK: Epidemiology of women's gymnastics injuries. Am J Sports Med 8:261–264, 1980.
15. Halpern AA, Bleck EE: Sit-up exercises: An electromyographic study. Clin Orthop 145:172–178, 1979.
16. Hoshina H: Spondylolysis in athletes. Physician Sportsmed 8:75–79, Sept 1980.
17. Jackson CP, Brown MD: Is there a role for exercise in the treatment of patients with low back pain? Clin Orthop 179:39–45, 1983.
18. Jackson CP, Brown MD: Analysis of current approaches and a practical guide to prescription of exercise. Clin Orthop 179:46–54, 1983.
19. Jackson DW: Low back pain in young athletes: Evaluation of stress reaction and discogenic problems. Am J Sports Med 7:364–366, 1979.

20. Jackson DW et al: Spondylolysis in the female gymnast. Clin Orthop 117:68–73, 1976.
21. Jackson DW et al: Stress reactions involving pars interarticularis in young athletes. Am J Sports Med 9:304–312, 1981.
22. Kirkaldy-Willis WH et al: Lumbar spinal stenosis. Clin Orthop 99:30–50, 1974.
23. Leffert RD: Thoracic outlet syndrome and the shoulder. Clin Sports Med 2:439–452, 1983.
24. McCoy GF et al: Injuries of the cervical spine in schoolboy rugby football. J Bone Joint Surg Br 66:500–503, 1984.
25. McKenzie RA: Manual correction of sciatic scoliosis. N Z Med J 76:194–199, 1972.
26. McKenzie RA: Prophylaxis in recurrent low back pain. N Z Med J 89:22–23, 1979.
27. McKenzie RA: The Lumbar Spine: Mechanical Diagnosis and Therapy. Waikan, NZ, Spinal Publications, 1981.
28. Maroon JC: "Burning hands" in football spinal cord injuries. JAMA 238:2049–2051, 1977.
29. Maroon JC: Catastrophic neck injuries from football in western Pennsylvania. Physician Sportsmed 9:83–86, Nov 1981.
30. Maroon JC et al: A system for preventing athletic neck injuries. Physician Sportsmed 5:77–79, Oct 1977.
31. Mennen U: Survey of spinal injuries from diving: A study of patients in Pretoria and Capetown. S Afr Med J 59:788–790, 1981.
32. Micheli LJ: Low back pain in the adolescent: Differential diagnosis. Am J Sports Med 7:362–364, 1979.
33. Mooney V, Robertson J: The facet syndrome. Clin Orthop 115:149–156, 1976.
34. Mueller FO, Blyth CS: Catastrophic head and neck injuries. Physician Sportsmed 7:71–74, Oct 1979.
35. Mueller FO, Blyth CS: Fatalities and catastrophic injuries in football. Physician Sportsmed 10:135–140, Oct 1982.
36. Nachemson AL: The lumbar spine: An orthopedic challenge. Spine 1:59–71, 1976.
37. Oh S: Cervical injury from skiing. Int J Sports Med 5:268–271, 1984.
38. Pearl AJ, Mayer PW: Neck motion in the high school football player. Am J Sports Med 7:231–233, 1979.
39. Rapp GF, Nicely PG: Trampoline injuries. Am J Sports Med 6:269–271, 1978.
40. Robertson W Jr et al: Upper trunk brachial plexopathy in football players. JAMA 241:1480–1482, 1979.
41. Rogers WA: Fractures and dislocations of the cervical spine. J Bone Joint Surg Am 39:341–376, 1957.
42. Roy SP: Intercollegiate wrestling injuries. Physician Sportsmed 7:83–94, Nov 1979.
43. Salter RB: Textbook of Disorders and Injuries of the Musculoskeletal System, 2nd ed. Baltimore, Williams & Wilkins, 1983.
44. Scher AT: Diving injuries to the spinal cord. S Afr Med J 59:603–605, 1981.
45. Scher AT: Vertex impact and cervical dislocation in rugby players. S Afr Med J 59:227–228, 1981.
46. Scher AT: "Crashing" the rugby scrum: Avoidable cause of cervical spinal injury. S Afr Med J 61:919–920, 1982.
47. Scher AT: Rugby injuries of the upper cervical spine: Case reports. S Afr Med J 64:456–458, 1983.
48. Schneider RC: Serious and fatal neurosurgical football injuries. Clin Neurosurg 12:226–236, 1965.
49. Schneider RC: Head and Neck Injuries in Football. Baltimore, Williams & Wilkins, 1973.
50. Shields CL Jr et al: Cervical cord injuries in sports. Physician Sportsmed 6:71–76, Sept 1978.
51. Snook GA: A survey of wrestling injuries. Am J Sports Med 8:450–453, 1980.
52. Sovio OM et al: Cervical spine injuries in rugby players. Can Med Assoc J 130:735–736, 1984.
53. Stanish W: Low back pain in middle-aged athletes. Am J Sports Med 7:367–369, 1979.
54. Stanitski CL: Low back pain in young athletes. Physician Sportsmed 10:77–91, Oct 1982.
55. Strukel RJ, Garrick JG: Thoracic outlet compression in athletes. Am J Sports Med 6:35–39, 1978.
56. Subcommittee on Advanced Trauma Life Support (ATLS) of the American College of Surgeons (ACS) Committee on Trauma: Advanced Trauma Life Support Course. Instructor Manual. Chicago, American College of Surgeons, 1984.
57. Subotnick SI: Limb length discrepancies of the lower extremity (the short leg syndrome). J Orthop Sports Phys Ther 3:11–16, 1981.
58. Tator CH, Edmonds VE: National survey of spinal injuries in hockey players. Can Med Assoc J 130:875–880, 1984.
59. Tator CH et al: Diving: Frequent and potentially preventable cause of spinal cord injury. Can Med Assoc J 124:1323–1324, 1981.
60. Tator CH et al: Spinal injuries due to hockey. Can J Neurol Sci 11:34–41, 1984.
61. Teitz CC: Sports medicine concerns in dance and gymnastics. Pediatr Clin North Am 29:1399–1421, 1982.
62. Teitz CC, Cook DM: Rehabilitation of neck and low back injuries. Clin Sports Med 4:455–476, 1985.
63. Thompson AJ, Morris IM: Neck injury with quadriplegia: Avoidable training hazard. Br J Sports Med 16:59–60, 1982.
64. Torg JS: Problems and prevention. *In* Torg JS (ed): Athletic Injuries to the Head, Neck, and Face. Philadelphia, Lea & Febiger, 1982, pp 3–13.

65. Torg JS, Das M: Trampoline-related quadriplegia: Review of the literature and reflections on the American Academy of Pediatrics' Position Statement. Pediatrics 74:804–812, 1984.
66. Torg JS et al: Collision with spring-loaded football tackling and blocking dummies. JAMA 236:1270–1271, 1976.
67. Torg JS et al: Severe and catastrophic neck injuries resulting from tackle football. J Am Coll Health Assoc 25:224–226, 1977.
68. Torg JS et al: National football head and neck injury registry: Report and conclusions, 1978. JAMA 241:1477–1479, 1979.
69. Torg JS et al: National football head and neck injury registry: Report on cervical quadriplegia, 1971–1975. Am J Sports Med 7:127–132, 1979.
70. Wales LR et al: Recommendations for evaluation of the acutely injured cervical spine: A clinical radiologic algorithm. Ann Emerg Med 9:422–428, 1980.
71. Williams CF et al: Essentiality of the lateral cervical spine radiograph. Ann Emerg Med 10:198–204, 1981.
72. Williams PC: Lesions of the lumbar spine. II: Chronic traumatic (postural) destruction of the lumbosacral intervertebral disc. J Bone Joint Surg 29:690–703, 1937.
73. Wilson FD, Lindseth RE: Adolescent "swimmer's back." Am J Sports Med 10:174–176, 1982.

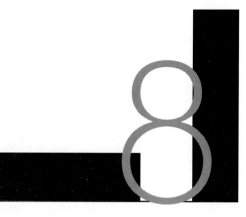

Pelvis, Hip, and Thigh Injuries

Conditions to Be Referred

- ◆ **Avulsion fractures (hamstrings, rectus femoris)**
- ◆ **Stress fracture of femoral neck**
- ◆ **Myositis ossificans (established)**
- ◆ **Degenerative joint disease (failure of conservative management)**

Triage

Indications for Referral

- ◆ **Acute**
  History
  Snap or pop with immediate loss of motion
  Examination
  Significant loss of motion (flexion or extension)
  X-ray films
  Avulsion fracture of pelvis
- ◆ **Gradual onset**
  History
  Thigh contusion with loss of knee motion
  Examination
  Swelling of anterior thigh with loss of knee flexion
  X-ray films
  Stress fracture of femoral neck

Indications for X-ray

- ◆ **Acute**
  History
  Painful snap or pop with abrupt flexion or extension
  Inability/unwillingness to bear weight
  Anterior thigh pain and loss of knee motion secondary to earlier contusion
  Examination
  Loss of flexion or extension
- ◆ **Gradual onset**
  History
  Hip pain with gelling or loss of motion (usually internal rotation and adduction), or both
  Examination
  Significant loss of motion
  Recurrent, activity-related proximal thigh pain

Nearly one fifth of all athletic injuries occur in the anatomical area between the iliac crest and the superior border of the patella.[7] Most of these injuries involve musculotendinous structures and, once precisely diagnosed, are managed like strains or overuse injuries anywhere else in the body. There are, however, three conditions unique to this anatomical region that present specific diagnostic or treatment problems—myositis ossificans, "hip pointer," and stress fractures of the femoral neck. These problems occur almost exclusively within the athletic environment. A fourth problem, degenerative joint disease, although not exclusive among athletes, is being seen with increasing frequency among the more active older population.

A. ACUTE HIP INJURIES

Acute hip pain in athletes is almost always the result of a strain or musculotendinous injury. In the skeletally immature athlete these injuries frequently are seen as avulsion fractures involving the iliac crest, anterior superior iliac spine (sartorius, tensor fasciae latae origin), anterior inferior iliac spine (rectus femoris origin), lesser trochanter, and ischial tuberosity (hamstring origin).[6, 10] Although more spectacular than many strains, the majority of these injuries can be managed similarly to musculotendinous injuries elsewhere in the body (see Chapter 2, part C). Acutely, operative management is indicated only when the avulsed fragment of bone is of appreciable size.

Hip fractures and dislocations sometimes occur during athletic participation—usually in collision sports or in activities involving high-speed falls such as skiing. In the vast majority of instances, the pain, disability, and deformity accompanying these injuries clearly set them apart from the much more common musculotendinous injuries discussed here.

HISTORY

MECHANISM OF INJURY. Like other strains, musculotendinous injuries around the hip are usually the result of an actively contracting muscle's encountering abrupt resistance: a misstep, an attempt at rapid acceleration, or abrupt stretching of a still-contracting muscle (as when a cheerleader improperly executes a split). Although most common in track and field activities, the injuries can be seen in any sport that involves running and rapid acceleration and deceleration. Adductor strains are particularly common in soccer, in which powerful muscular action may be abruptly opposed by the ball, the ground, or an opponent's foot.[20] Inadequate warm-up, fatigue, a cold environment, or inadequate rehabilitation of a previous injury are common predisposing factors.

SYMPTOMS. The injury occurs with a *pop or snap* (often audible). There is usually *sudden, severe, well-localized pain* as well as immediate *disability*. Occasionally the onset of pain is delayed; nonetheless, the athletes know they have sustained a significant injury. Ambulation may be impossible or, at the least, accompanied by a significant limp.

PHYSICAL EXAMINATION

The site of injury is *tender*. The area of tenderness enlarges with time, especially in the more severe strains. *Swelling*—the result of local hemorrhage—is variable and may not even be evident because the injured structures are buried deep in the other soft tissue surrounding the hip. Occasionally the hemorrhage is noted as an area of ecchymosis, often some distance removed from the site of injury. The locations of swelling or areas of ecchymosis are often not an accurate indicator of the site or severity of injury.

The involved muscle is usually *tense* and in *spasm*. The athlete is unlikely to tolerate either passive stretching or active contraction of the muscle. Pain and resistance to quadriceps stretching usually indicate an injury to the origin of the rectus femoris; pain and resistance to straight-leg raising usually mean an injury of the origin of one of the hamstrings. Muscle testing may be carried out as shown in Figures 8–5 and 7–16.

RADIOGRAPHIC EXAMINATION

Radiographic study is indicated for injuries resulting in immediate, significant disability. An anteroposterior view of the pelvis and a lateral view of the involved hip are usually adequate to visualize the avulsion fractures associated with these strains.

If radiographs are first obtained some weeks after the injury, the presence of new, immature bone at the site of the avulsion may lead to the erroneous diagnosis of a bony neoplasm. This possibility is usually ruled out by ascertaining a history of a specific incident of injury and visualizing the avulsed fragment of bone lying within the area of bony proliferation.

OTHER DIAGNOSTIC TESTS

Radionuclide bone scanning is sometimes of value in determining the completion of healing. Avulsion fractures of the ischial tuberosity are sometimes accompanied by new bone formation of a magnitude great enough to result in mechanical problems such as difficulty in sitting. It is our impression that vigorous activity during the phase of new bone formation increases the ultimate size of the bony mass. Being able to document the cessation of bone formation is therefore valuable in staging the rehabilitation program.

INITIAL TREATMENT

Although compression and icing are desirable, they are difficult to accomplish about the hip. It is more important to put the injured musculotendinous unit at rest. Because it is difficult to splint the hip, bed rest may be necessary in the more severe injuries. If the athlete can ambulate comfortably with the aid of crutches, this may provide adequate rest.

REFERRAL

Acutely, referral to an orthopedic surgeon is indicated for large avulsion fractures (i.e., greater than 2 to 3 cm). Referral is also indicated for symptomatic nonunion of fractures initially managed nonoperatively.

DEFINITIVE TREATMENT

Musculotendinous injuries around the hip are managed the same as strains anywhere in the body. Active, painless stretching and isometric exercises are started at 48 hours. The usual rehabilitative tasks are altered only in the presence of large avulsion fractures.

Strains, particularly those involving the hamstring muscles, have a bad reputation for becoming chronic and recurrent. After the acute injury it is readily apparent to the athlete that the muscle is abnormally tight. Thus even without medical advice, a stretching program is usually undertaken. In most cases the athlete has also embarked on a retraining program involving such activities as cycling or running. Examination of these athletes reveals normal flexibility but deficient strength.

It is usually impossible to run, cycle, or "play" an injured muscle back to normal strength and endurance. Specific efforts must be directed at the involved muscle. Thus in addition to stretching and the gradual resumption of athletic activity, the injured muscle should be subjected to daily efforts toward increasing strength and endurance. Once parity is achieved with the opposite, uninjured side, recurrent strains will become rare.

B. CONTUSIONS OF THE ILIAC CREST (HIP POINTER)

Even in the well-muscled athlete, the iliac crest is poorly protected and vulnerable to direct blows. A contusion in this region is called a *hip pointer*. Because the iliac crest serves as an anchor for both abdominal and hip muscles, injuries to this structure result in more global disability than the uninitiated might imagine. The medical importance of this condition lies in the fact that it may result in severe disability that can be mistaken for a potentially life-threatening ruptured viscus.

HISTORY

MECHANISM OF INJURY. The injury occurs as the result of a *direct blow* (usually from a football helmet) to the relatively unprotected iliac crest. It is seen most commonly in football but may occur in other contact sports such as wrestling, soccer, and lacrosse. Appropriately designed and properly worn hip pads can prevent or minimize the injury. Unfortunately, many football players view hip pads as an unnecessary encumbrance and modify them so that their effectiveness is nullified but they still pass the officials' inspection.

SYMPTOMS. The injury is usually instantly *disabling* and exceedingly *painful*. The trunk is flexed forward and toward the side of the injury. Because of the pain the athlete is often unable to take a deep breath or cough. Muscle spasm of the tensor fasciae latae and gluteus may make ambulation difficult.

PHYSICAL EXAMINATION

The iliac crest is exquisitely *tender*. *Swelling* may be limited to just the area overlying the iliac crest, or it may be more extensive, involving the oblique abdominal muscles as well as those muscles arising from the external surface of the ilium. The abdomen is often held *rigid*. Although rebound tenderness is absent, it is often difficult to test because of abdominal muscle spasm.

Within 24 to 48 hours the swelling becomes more diffuse, and an area of ecchymosis may become evident. The doubled-up posture may last for 3 or 4 days, and local tenderness may last for weeks.

RADIOGRAPHIC EXAMINATION

Careful scrutiny of films of the iliac crest may reveal evidence of a compression fracture. Rarely the entire iliac crest apophysis may be displaced. Radiographs may be helpful in ruling out a ruptured (hollow) viscus by the absence of air beneath the diaphragm.

OTHER DIAGNOSTIC TESTS

Other diagnostic tests are rarely necessary.

INITIAL TREATMENT

The application of ice provides (some) local analgesia and may assist in decreasing bleeding. A compression wrap is desirable but usually not well tolerated because of the tenderness. Analgesics, even narcotics, should be administered as necessary.

Some physicians inject the hematoma with local anesthetics (with epinephrine) and one of the cortisone preparations. We feel that the possibility of introducing bacteria into the hematoma overshadows the temporary analgesia gained by such a practice and thus do not inject these injuries. Oral administration of anti-inflammatory medications is started on the day of injury. The use of a 6- or 8-day corticosteroid "burst" often appreciably lessens the length of disability.

REFERRAL

If there is any evidence of intra-abdominal trauma or displaced fractures of the iliac crest, referral is indicated.

DEFINITIVE TREATMENT

The use of high-intensity galvanic stimulation may assist in decreasing swelling. Gentle abdominal muscle stretching is started as soon as the swelling has stabilized. Abdominal strengthening exercises are begun as soon as they can be done with reasonable comfort.

A protective pad should be worn with the return to athletic participation. The pad should be constructed in the form of an elongated doughnut; it should surround, but not overlie, the iliac crest.

C. ACUTE THIGH INJURIES

Acute injuries involving the thigh are diagnosed and managed in much the same fashion as those involving the hip. As with the hip, most of these injuries involve musculotendinous structures. Because grade III strains usually involve tendons or their junctions with bone or muscle, these injuries are more often seen near the hip. The less severe injuries, involving the muscle belly, are more commonly seen in the thigh.

The grading, assessment, and management of musculotendinous injuries are discussed in Chapter 2, part C. However, because strains of the thigh muscles are so common, some additional comments regarding the specific muscle groups are in order.

ADDUCTOR (GROIN) STRAINS

Adductor strains occur commonly in sports requiring quick direction changes (football and soccer) as well as in those in which the adductors are used for propulsion (figure skating and hockey). The more severe adductor strains virtually always occur at the muscles' attachment to the pelvis. The less severe but no less troublesome injuries occur more distally at the level of the muscle bellies.

Adductor strains merit special mention for two reasons: because rehabilitative strengthening is often ignored, and because postinjury stretching is usually inadequate.

The adductors are usually all but ignored in strength-training workouts, especially those employed by high school teams. Although weight-training machines designed for strengthening the adductors are available, they are seen far less commonly than those for the hamstrings and quadriceps. Thus the injured athlete is likely to have some difficulty in devising a restrengthening program after an adductor injury.

Endurance training of the adductors can be accomplished with some ease by utilizing the antigravity techniques popularized by aerobic dance programs (Fig. 8–1). Although the strengthening aspects of these exercises can be enhanced by draping weights or sandbags over the ankle, weights in excess of 5 or 10 lb may cause discomfort at the medial aspect of the knee.

Therabands or wall pulleys can be utilized in adductor strengthening as can isometric techniques (Fig. 8–2). By directing the resistance to the distal

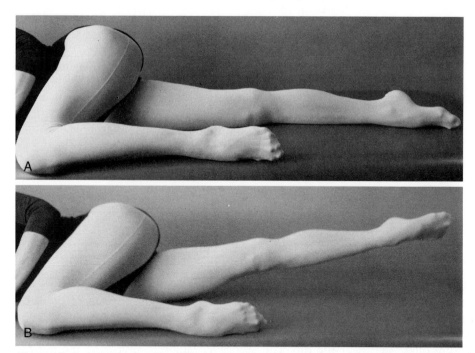

Figure 8–1. Side-lying, gravity-resisted adductor exercises. *A*, Start position. *B*, Lifted position.

aspect of the thigh, one spares the knee, and by undertaking the exercises in the upright position, one uses the muscle in its position of function.

Unlike strengthening, adductor stretching is commonly employed in most stretching and warm-up programs. Although the common straddle stretch seems adequate for preventive stretching (Fig. 8–3*A*), it falls short when used as a therapeutic stretch because the sitting position both flexes the hips and (slightly) relaxes the adductors. In this position the athlete may run out of hip motion before an adequate adductor stretch is accomplished. Thus we teach stretching with the hips in a neutral or even extended position (Fig. 8–3*B*).

Another inadequacy of the straddle stretch is that it is a simultaneous bilateral stretch. As a general rule, therapeutic stretching should be done unilaterally as it is easier to control and is unaffected by idiosyncrasies of the contralateral limb.

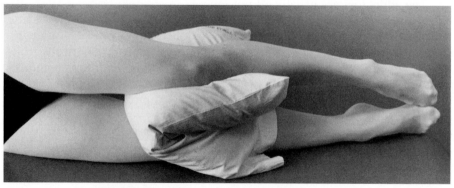

Figure 8–2. Isometric adductor-strengthening exercises.

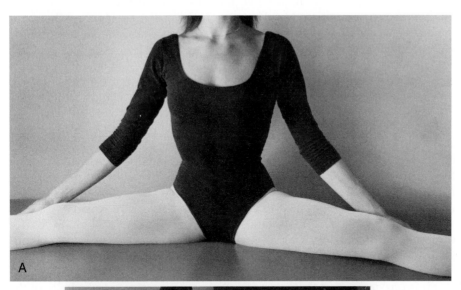

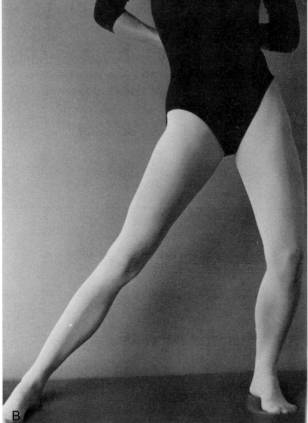

Figure 8–3. Adductor stretches. *A,* The straddle stretch is a common adductor-stretching exercise. *B,* The single-leg adductor stretch is an excellent therapeutic stretching exercise in a position of function. The stretch should be felt along the inner thigh and not at the knee.

QUADRICEPS/RECTUS FEMORIS STRAINS

The vast majority of strains involve muscles that cross two joints, and the quadriceps is no exception. Nearly every quadriceps strain involves the rectus femoris—that single component of the quadriceps that acts on both the hip and the knee.

Quadriceps (rectus femoris) strains merit special attention for two reasons: (1) They may result in complete ruptures of the muscle belly, and (2) they may produce a deformity out of proportion to their clinical significance.

Quadriceps strains frequently involve the rectus femoris at the level of the middle third of the thigh. Because the muscle overlies the remainder of the quadriceps and is subcutaneous, the presence of localized swelling or a defect is readily apparent. Integrity of the rectus femoris is tested by having the athlete flex the hip with the knee held in a 45-degree flexed position (see Fig. 8–5*B*). In this position the muscle should stand out on the anterior aspect of the thigh, and any localized swelling or defect is readily apparent.

In spite of the fact that these injuries may result in obvious loss of continuity of the muscle, they are managed as are other less visibly obvious strains. The preferred techniques for strengthening and stretching the rectus femoris are shown, respectively, in Figures 8–4 and 9–16.

It is our experience that even a complete rupture through the belly of the rectus femoris results in little or no functional disability. In a pragmatic sense this is fortunate because attempts at surgically repairing a midbelly tear of the rectus femoris are usually doomed to failure.

HAMSTRING STRAINS

Hamstring strains merit special mention because the axiom "once a strain, always a strain" is probably based on the experience with this injury. Hamstring strains or pulls have a deservedly bad reputation for recurrence and chronicity. We believe that this is because all athletes have been made aware of the importance of hamstring stretching and flexibility and, when faced with a hamstring injury, are acutely aware of the accompanying limitation of motion. Then they concentrate all their efforts on stretching and none on strengthening.

The hamstrings, like all other muscles, achieve normal functional flexibility only in the presence of normal strength. There is no better example of the adage "a weak muscle is a tight muscle" than the previously injured and inadequately rehabilitated hamstring muscle. The period of dysfunction following a hamstring strain results in profound weakness of this muscle group. Hamstring atrophy is not as visibly evident as, for example, quadriceps wasting is. In addition, the activities of daily living are little affected by hamstring weakness, as contrasted to the "giving way" and sense of instability that often accompany quadriceps weakness. Thus the athlete is not aware of the lack of strength but only the lack of flexibility.

The solution for the chronic hamstring pull is a comprehensive rehabilitation program utilizing both stretching and strengthening.

D. CHRONIC HIP PAIN

Pain in the hip or thigh, unassociated with acute trauma, is usually indicative of overuse injury. Such problems are most often seen in endeavors involving

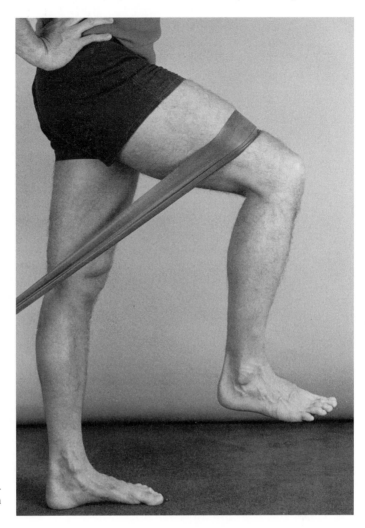

Figure 8–4. Hip flexor–strengthening exercises using a Theraband.

repetitious movements such as distance running, ballet dancing, gymnastics, or track and field events. The vast majority of the injuries are variations of tendinitis and, once precisely identified, can be managed in the manner described in Chapter 3.

The clinical significance of chronic "hip" pain in athletes is twofold: first, appropriate treatment of musculotendinous injury depends on the accuracy of the diagnosis, and second, musculotendinous injury must be differentiated from the much less common but more serious bone and joint problems, e.g., degenerative joint disease, slipped femoral capital epiphysis, and, especially in the athlete, femoral stress fracture—a truly serious injury requiring urgent and appropriate management.

HISTORY

MECHANISM OF INJURY. Overuse injuries in these anatomical regions are usually the result of repetitive, weight-bearing activities such as running and jumping. Typically they are early-season injuries resulting from activity changes that occur too abruptly for proper conditioning to take place. In the older athlete with degenerative joint disease the onset may be even more insidious and follow a seemingly benign change in activity such as an extra round of golf or set of tennis or merely more than accustomed walking during a vacation.

SYMPTOMS. The symptoms are those of activity-related pain. *Pain* and a sensation of *tightness* first occur after a workout and, with time, actually occur during the activity. The athlete usually does not seek medical care until the symptoms preclude normal workouts, or, in some cases, the activities of daily living. Frequently the athlete is unable to date the onset of the symptoms precisely.

With tendinitis, the location of the pain is consistent, although with time the painful area may enlarge. In the case of femoral stress fractures, the location of the pain is usually inconsistent, appearing, for example, in the adductor region one day and the buttock the next. Stress fractures of the inferior pubic ramus may also present as groin, buttock, or thigh pain.[17] The symptoms accompanying degenerative joint disease often present in the groin (adductor muscles) or buttock (hip extensors). True "hip pain," presenting anteriorly in the vicinity of the inguinal canal, is often absent in the patient with degenerative joint disease.

Athletes, quite appropriately, tend to be concerned about joint pain, but perhaps most are unaware of the true location of the hip joint and the referral pattern of hip joint pain. An athlete often says, for example, "It hurts right here in the [hip] joint," while pointing to the prominence of the greater trochanter. Pain from degenerative joint disease, arthritis, slipped femoral capital epiphysis, and the like is almost invariably perceived in the distribution of the femoral and obturator nerves, i.e., along the anteromedial aspect of the thigh, as far distally as the knee or among the muscles acting on the hip (adductors and extensors). Indeed, some athletes with hip joint disease present with activity-related *knee* pain. Conversely, lateral and posterior hip pain is seldom related to hip joint disease.

PHYSICAL EXAMINATION

The inflamed tendon is *tender* but rarely swollen. Stretching or resisted action of the involved muscle is painful (Fig. 8–5; see also Fig. 7–16).

Pain on motion, particularly internal rotation, limitation of motion, antalgic gait, and the like, is a nonspecific sign suggestive of hip joint disease. Crepitation, although rare, is rather more suggestive of degenerative joint disease. An antalgic gait with adduction and external rotation of the hip, a positive Trendelenburg sign (abductor weakness), and limitation of internal rotation and flexion of the hip are characteristic signs of slipped femoral capital epiphysis. This condition is classically, but not invariably, found in flabby, nonathletic, prepubescent males; females and thin athletic males are occasionally affected.

With femoral stress fractures there are no typical findings on examination.

RADIOGRAPHIC EXAMINATION

Radiographic study is indicated if the clinical findings are suggestive of or consistent with femoral stress fracture or hip joint disease, as opposed to musculotendinous injury.

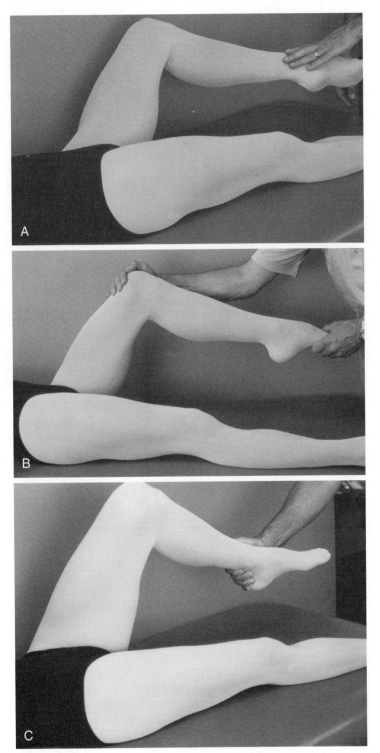

Figure 8–5. Specific muscle testing. *A,* Sartorius. The examiner applies downward pressure on the foot. *B,* Rectus femoris. The athlete is instructed to hold this position with her foot above the table. *C,* Medial hamstrings (semimembranosus and semitendinosus). With the leg internally rotated, the athlete attempts to resist extension of the knee by the examiner.

Illustration continued on following page

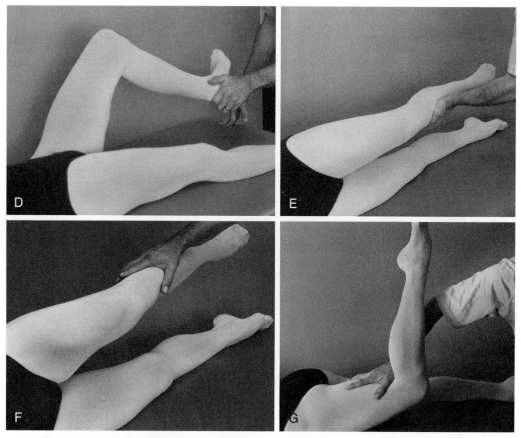

Figure 8–5 *Continued.* *D,* Lateral hamstrings (biceps femoris). With the leg externally rotated, the athlete attempts to resist extension of the knee by the examiner. *E,* Adductors. The athlete is told to press down against the examiner's hand. *F,* Abductors. The athlete is told not to let the examiner push the leg down. *G,* Gluteus maximus. The athlete is told to raise the thigh against the resistance of the examiner's hand.

Stress fractures of the femoral shaft may be evidenced by localized areas of periosteal new bone formation. Actual fracture lines are often not seen. Stress fractures of the femoral neck are more likely to be evidenced by small breaks in the superior cortex or condensations of the inferior cortex. Frequently the neck of the femur appears normal.

A slipped femoral capital epiphysis is best demonstrated in a lateral view of the hip.

Diminished joint space, femoral or acetabular osteophytes, and even subchondral cysts characterize degenerative joint disease. The magnitude of these changes is not always predictive of the clinical severity of the condition. We have observed aggressive skiers, golfers, and tennis players with total loss of the joint space but virtually no symptoms. Conversely, minimal radiographic changes may result in appreciable disability.

OTHER DIAGNOSTIC TESTS

As the clinical findings may be vague and radiographic examination may be (falsely) negative, radionuclide bone scanning should be undertaken with any suspicion of stress fracture.[2, 8, 11, 17, 19] In our experience, this test is exceedingly sensitive and "false negatives" almost nonexistent.

INITIAL TREATMENT

Both tendinitis and degenerative joint disease should be treated with relative rest, anti-inflammatory medications, and modalities such as icing, ultrasonography, and high-intensity galvanic stimulation. Although pain-producing activities should be halted, other activities such as cycling, swimming, and weight training should be continued to maintain as high a level of conditioning as possible.

REFERRAL

Athletes with the presumptive diagnosis of femoral stress fracture or slipped femoral capital epiphysis or with advanced degenerative joint disease that has failed to improve with rehabilitative efforts should be referred to an orthopedic surgeon.

DEFINITIVE TREATMENT

Treatment of overuse tendinitis involves alleviation of the symptoms and a rehabilitation program aimed at re-establishing strength, endurance, and flexibility of the involved muscle. Treatment of the athlete with one of these conditions is not complete until the cause has been identified in order that re-injury might be prevented in the future.

The treatment of choice for femoral neck stress fractures is often prophylactic internal fixation, as overt fracture with displacement may be accompanied by avascular necrosis of the femoral head. Similarly, slipped femoral capital epiphysis is usually best treated surgically.

Degenerative joint disease can often be satisfactorily managed by rehabilitation of the major muscle groups about the hip—and modification of activity, especially avoiding activities such as running that involve not only full weight bearing but also considerable joint motion (see Chapter 3, part D). Definitive treatment of advanced degenerative joint disease may require total joint arthroplasty. We are, however, continually surprised by the symptomatic improvement associated with strengthening of the musculature acting on the hip even in the face of rather spectacular radiographic changes.

E.   ILIOTIBIAL BAND SYNDROMES (ILIOTIBIAL BAND OR TRACT FRICTION SYNDROME, ILIOTIBIAL BAND TENDINITIS, TROCHANTERIC BURSITIS)

The term *iliotibial band or tract friction syndrome* or, more simply, *iliotibial band tendinitis* refers specifically to a syndrome of lateral knee pain related to irritation and inflammation of the distal portion of the iliotibial band at, or just distal to, the point at which it crosses the lateral femoral epicondyle. It is a well-recognized cause of knee pain in runners.[12–14, 16, 18, 21] In one reported series of more than 1000 distance runners, it accounted for some 5% of all cases of lower-limb musculoskeletal complaints.[21]

The condition is not unique to distance runners, however, nor is lateral knee pain the only manifestation of iliotibial band injury. Typical iliotibial band tendinitis has been reported in hammer throwers, racquet sports participants, and sprinters.[3, 5] We have found it to be a not infrequent cause of knee pain in aerobic dancers and cyclists. We have also found, as have others,[3, 4] that injury to the iliotibial band and related structures may be noted as lateral "hip" or lateral thigh pain, as well as lateral knee pain.

Because the mechanisms of injury, diagnostic approach, and treatment of all these syndromes are similar, we have chosen to discuss them collectively in this section.

ANATOMY

The iliotibial band or tract is a thickened band of the deep fasciae of the thigh extending from the tubercle of the iliac crest (about a handbreadth posterior to the anterior superior iliac spine) down the lateral aspect of the thigh to Gerdy's tubercle on the lateral tibial condyle. The tensor fasciae latae, arising from the anterior portion of the iliac crest and the anterior superior iliac spine, inserts obliquely from the front onto the iliotibial band. The upper part of the gluteus maximus and the superficial fibers of the lower part insert onto it obliquely from behind. The iliotibial band thus functions as the conjoint tendon of insertion for both muscles and permits them to act on the knee as well as the hip joint.

The iliotibial band and the aponeurosis of the gluteus maximus overlie the greater trochanter of the femur and are separated from it by the large trochanteric bursa. The distal iliotibial band moves over the lateral femoral epicondyle as the knee is flexed and extended. It is anterior to the epicondyle when the knee is fully extended and overlies it when the knee is flexed to about 30 degrees. A bursa also separates these two structures.

As demonstrated by electromyography, both the tensor fasciae latae and the upper part of the gluteus maximus are active when most of the body weight is supported on one leg.[1] Apparently the ability to modulate tension on the iliotibial band is an important mechanism for stabilizing the pelvis and thigh against adduction/varus-bending forces during such activities as walking, running, and landing jumps on one foot.

HISTORY

MECHANISMS OF INJURY. Iliotibial band tendinitis is characteristically a running-related overuse injury. *Training error*, especially an abrupt increase in distance, speed work, or hill running, seems to be the most common etiologic factor.

The pathomechanics are probably related to the previously noted anatomical relationships and function of the iliotibial band. It seems that either *excessive friction* among the distal iliotibial band, underlying bursa, and lateral femoral epicondyle or *excessive tension* on the iliotibial band during the stance phase of the running gait may result in tendinitis. A correlation has been noted with such variables as genu varum and increased prominence of the lateral epicondyle,[13, 21] limb-length discrepancy, crossover gait (in which the foot is brought toward the midline rather than straight ahead), overstriding, and excessive supination or pronation of the foot.[13] Running on a banked or very short track and consistently running on one side of a crowned road have also been implicated.[3, 14] In both cases it is the supinated foot side, or outside limb, that tends to be involved.

Similar mechanisms also seem to account for most cases of iliotibial band problems in sports such as walking, backpacking, and aerobic dancing. In cycling, however, the most common mechanism of injury seems to be *excessive internal rotation torque* at the knee, usually the result of improper cleat adjustment (see Chapter 3, part D and Fig. 3–2). Also in runners who pronate excessively, it is probably the associated internal rotation torque at the knee that causes increased tension on the iliotibial band.

In our experience, *quadriceps insufficiency* seems to predispose to iliotibial band tendinitis. When the hip is internally rotated, the iliotibial band mechanism can be recruited to assist with or to maintain extension of the knee. Some of our patients have even developed mild iliotibial band tendinitis as a complication of doing "quad setting" isometrics incorrectly and have had to be instructed specifically to avoid internal rotation of the hip while doing these exercises.

Trochanteric bursitis (see the discussion of olecranon bursitis in Chapter 5, part D, and of prepatellar bursitis in Chapter 9, part H) may be caused by repetitive pressure and friction, by mechanisms similar to those that cause typical iliotibial band tendinitis. *Direct blows*, such as commonly occur with sliding-out crashes in cycling or falls in figure skating, can produce acute, hemorrhagic bursitis.

Acute *strains* of the proximal part of the iliotibial band have also been reported in dancers and runners.[4]

SYMPTOMS. The hallmark symptom of typical iliotibial band tendinitis is activity-related *lateral knee pain*.

Less commonly, *lateral hip pain* is the presenting symptom of iliotibial band injury. As noted previously, the athlete often says, "It hurts right here in the joint," pointing to the prominence of the greater trochanter.

In either case, as with other overuse injuries, there are often a characteristic onset and progression of symptoms. A runner, for example, may at first have pain only after running. Subsequently the runner may start to have pain while running, and eventually the pain may become so constant and severe as to preclude further running and to interfere with activities of daily living.

With trochanteric bursitis, *swelling*, more than pain, may be the chief complaint.

PHYSICAL EXAMINATION

The hallmark signs are *point tenderness* and *pain with provocative testing*.

Characteristically, point tenderness is elicited over the distal iliotibial band, underlying bursa, and lateral femoral epicondyle. However, tenderness may be found anywhere in the course of the iliotibial band from its origin to its insertion.

Various provocative tests for iliotibial band tendinitis have been described.[12, 14, 18] In each case the band is placed under tension with the knee flexed to about 30 degrees. We have found the following to be a simple and reliable test (Fig. 8–6). The athlete lies on the uninjured side with the hip of the injured limb abducted and knee flexed to 30 degrees. Applying downward pressure on the leg results in an adduction force at the hip and a varus force at the knee, which the athlete is instructed to resist. With any of the iliotibial band syndromes, this usually reproduces the athlete's symptoms or enhances tenderness over the site of injury, or both. Often there is also demonstrable weakness of the hip abductors compared with the uninjured side.

Flexibility of the iliotibial band and tensor fasciae latae is best tested as follows (Fig. 8–7):[14, 15] The athlete lies on the uninjured side with that hip flexed slightly to eliminate any lumbar lordosis. The knee of the injured limb is flexed to 90 degrees, and the examiner holds the leg with one hand and stabilizes the pelvis with the other. The hip is then widely abducted, extended to bring the iliotibial band in line with the greater trochanter, and then adducted toward the table. Normally there is adduction to 15 or more degrees past horizontal. If there is any tightness of the iliotibial band and tensor fasciae latae, the hip remains passively abducted in direct proportion to the amount of tightening.

In our experience with iliotibial band syndromes, tightness of the gluteus maximus seems to be at least as common as tightness of the iliotibial band and tensor fasciae latae.

Flexibility testing of the gluteus maximus (hip external rotators) is carried out as shown in Figure 7–3.

With trochanteric bursitis there is a *discrete, fluctuant,* variably tender *mass overlying the greater trochanter.* It may be several centimeters in diameter.

RADIOGRAPHIC EXAMINATION

Radiographic study and other diagnostic tests are *not required.*

OTHER DIAGNOSTIC TESTS

Magnetic resonance imaging is employed with increasing frequency in an attempt to document changes associated with iliotibial band tendinitis at the

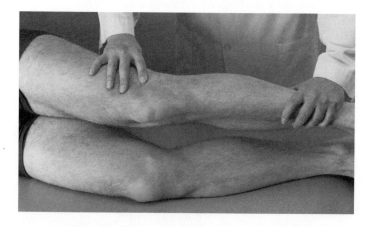

Figure 8–6. Provocation of pain with iliotibial band tendinitis. The examiner applies downward pressure on the limb with one hand and palpates the distal iliotibial band with the other.

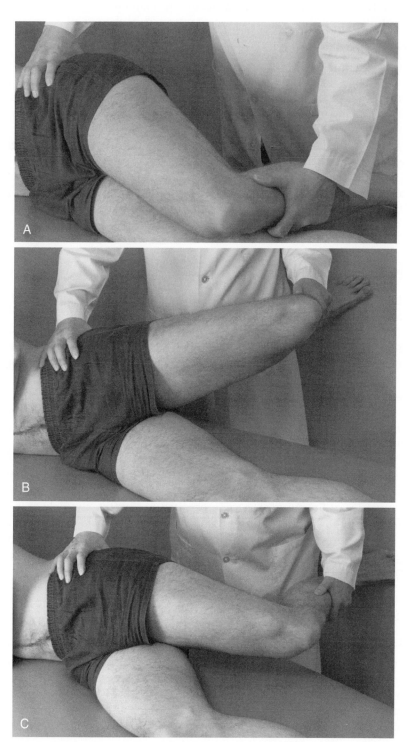

Figure 8–7. Technique of assessing flexibility of the iliotibial band. The examiner stabilizes the pelvis with one hand and controls the limb with the other. The hip is first abducted *(A)*, then extended *(B)*, and then adducted toward the table *(C)*.

knee. Although these studies are interesting, we have not found them particularly helpful in choosing or altering treatment regimens.

INITIAL TREATMENT

The treatment is symptomatic and anti-inflammatory. *Relative rest* is the most important aspect of treatment. Nonsteroidal anti-inflammatory medication, ice massage, and ice and electrogalvanic stimulation treatments are useful adjuncts.

Aspiration of the trochanteric bursa is indicated if the clinical findings are consistent with either acute hemorrhage or long-standing inflammation. The bursa is aspirated under sterile conditions, care being taken not to introduce the needle into the bursa through an area of skin abrasion (contamination) or infection. A snug compression wrap is then applied, using 4 × 4s and elastic tape.

REHABILITATION

Rehabilitation is aimed at restoring the flexibility of the iliotibial band and the strength and flexibility of the muscles acting on it.

Stretching the iliotibial band and tensor fasciae latae is most readily carried out as follows (Fig. 8–8): The athlete stands with knees straight and crosses the limb to be stretched behind the other, extending and adducting the hip as far as possible. The trunk is then flexed laterally as far as possible to the opposite side. Alternatively, the athlete lies on the side with the limb to be stretched on top, using the opposite leg, as shown, to assist in adducting the hip. Stretching the gluteus maximus is carried out as previously described for the piriformis and other external rotators of the hip (see Fig. 7–17A).

We routinely use a Theraband for strengthening the hip abductors. Standing on one leg with the Theraband looped around the other ankle, the athlete abducts the hip against resistance. This exercises the abductors on both sides, as the muscles of the support leg are recruited to stabilize the pelvis. Indeed, some patients may find it more difficult or even painful to have the "weak side" be the support leg. Strengthening the hip flexors is carried out as shown in Figure 8–4. Strengthening the external rotators is carried out as previously described for the piriformis (see Fig. 7–17B–D).

REFERRAL

Referral to an orthopedist is indicated if symptoms persist or recur despite appropriate treatment and rehabilitation or if there is persistent inflammation, recurrent fluid accumulation, or progressive enlargement of the trochanteric bursa despite appropriate initial treatment. Referral to a podiatrist may be indicated if excessive supination or pronation of the foot seems to be a causative factor (see later).

DEFINITIVE TREATMENT

In most cases, all that is required for definitive treatment of any of the iliotibial band syndromes is adequate initial treatment, complete rehabilita-

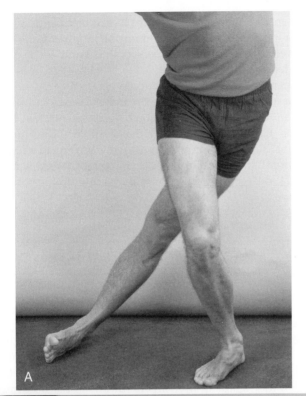

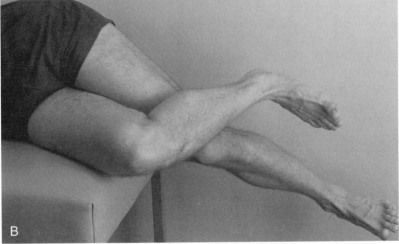

Figure 8–8. Stretching exercises for the (left) iliotibial band. *A,* Standing. *B,* Lying, using the opposite limb for assistance.

tion, correction of any biomechanical problems, and gradual resumption of activity with attention to avoiding training error.

Some authors routinely use a lateral or valgus heel wedge in the treatment of iliotibial band tendinitis,[14] apparently to reduce the varus stress at the knee. We do not subscribe to this recommendation, because, as discussed previously, iliotibial band problems may be associated with either pronation or supination of the foot. We suggest *trying* a valgus wedge only when there is clearly excessive supination. Sorting out this aspect of the problem may be deferred to a podiatrist.

Inflammation not responding to any of the previously described measures may sometimes be treated successfully with local corticosteroid injection. Some authors have reported operative treatment of iliotibial band tendinitis by release or division of the posterior fibers of the band with or without osteotomy of the lateral femoral epicondyle.[9, 12, 13] However, most authors, ourselves included, have not found surgery to be necessary.

Persistent trochanteric bursitis may be treated by repeat aspiration and corticosteroid injection. Under sterile conditions, fluid is aspirated, the needle is left in place, and a 1:1 mixture of betamethasone and 0.25% bupivacaine with epinephrine is instilled. A compression dressing is applied as previously described. The patient must understand that *continuous compression* is not only important, it is critical. Bursectomy is the only remaining option for definitive treatment.

F. MYOSITIS OSSIFICANS

With athletic injuries the anterior aspect of the thigh is the most common site for myositis ossificans—a condition in which heterotopic bone growth occurs within the quadriceps muscle. The medical importance of this condition lies in the fact that contusions (anywhere) are usually viewed as minor injuries by coaches and athletes and thus often treated too aggressively. Common with thigh contusions that result in myositis ossificans is the occurrence of a subsequent re-injury that, in this instance, may be due to vigorous massage or equally vigorous passive stretching in an effort to regain knee motion. It is our impression that appropriate management of the initial injury precludes the development of myositis ossificans in the vast majority of instances.

Myositis ossificans of the quadriceps is not only a season-ending condition but may preclude significant athletic activity for 4 to 6 months. Occasionally the mass of bone resulting from this condition is so large as to interfere with normal quadriceps function and thus to require surgical removal.

HISTORY

MECHANISM OF INJURY. The condition is a complication of a contusion resulting from a direct blow to the anterior (anteromedial or anterolateral) aspect of the thigh that usually occurs during active use of the quadriceps muscle. The contusion most often results when a running football player is struck in the thigh by a another player's helmet. In addition, the history usually reveals a second traumatic episode, such as abrupt flexion of the knee before regaining full knee motion, or vigorous massage or passive stretching before resumption of normal quadriceps function.

SYMPTOMS. The injury may be instantly disabling, giving rise to the assumption that the femur has been fractured. Just as frequently the injury, although painful, allows continued participation for a few minutes, becoming disabling only after the athlete has stood or sat for a few minutes, during which time the quadriceps goes into spasm, thereby limiting knee motion.

Swelling usually occurs rapidly and may be massive. (Based on circumference measurements, we have observed hematomas containing in excess of 1000 mL of blood.) Ecchymosis may or may not be evident at 24 to 48 hours.

Quadriceps function is impaired and knee flexion is limited by quadriceps spasm. Ambulation is painful to the point that weight bearing may be impossible.

Unfortunately the athlete is usually not seen at the time of injury but rather seeks medical assistance some 2 to 3 weeks later because of limited knee flexion, difficulty in running (or even walking), and the presence of a painful lump in the anterior thigh.

PHYSICAL EXAMINATION

The acutely injured athlete seeks a position in which the leg is supported with the *knee extended*. An attempt to lift the leg from the examining table, thus holding the knee extended against gravity, is usually impossible because of pain. Active or passive knee flexion is usually resisted and painful.

The thigh is *swollen* and diffusely *tender*, even fluctuant, to palpation. During the first few days after the injury, the area of swelling often extends distally. Although not present originally, a knee effusion may become evident at 4 or 5 days.

Measuring the range of painless knee flexion present 24 hours after the injury provides a rough estimation of the severity and perhaps the likelihood of development of myositis ossificans. With the athlete prone, the knee is gently, passively flexed by the examiner. If flexion is limited to less than 45 degrees, the contusion is considered serious, with a significant potential for the development of myositis ossificans. If flexion between 45 and 90 degrees is possible, treatment should be completed and athletic activity resumed in 4 to 6 weeks. With greater than 90 degrees of painless flexion, disability should last only 7 to 10 days.

The examination differs appreciably when the athlete is first seen 2 to 4 weeks after the initial injury. With the establishment of myositis ossificans the anterior aspect of the thigh is tender only to deep palpation. Swelling is woody, often in the form of a well-demarcated mass. There is usually significant quadriceps atrophy, causing the swollen area to appear overly prominent. There is a firm limitation to knee flexion—less painful than in the acute phase.

RADIOGRAPHIC EXAMINATION

Radiographs taken at the time of the acute injury give no clue to the likelihood of development of myositis ossificans. Evidence of bone formation within the quadriceps may be present as early as 3 weeks after injury. The initial appearance is usually fluffy calcification with indistinct margins lying in the soft tissue anterior to the femur. As the lesion matures it enlarges, with the margins becoming more clear-cut (Fig. 8–9).

OTHER DIAGNOSTIC TESTS

Radionuclide *bone scans* are routinely employed to assess the maturity of the lesion. The course of myositis ossificans is usually followed clinically and radiographically. When two radiographs taken 1 month apart show no change in the lesion, a bone scan is obtained. A negative, or cold, scan confirms that the lesion has matured.

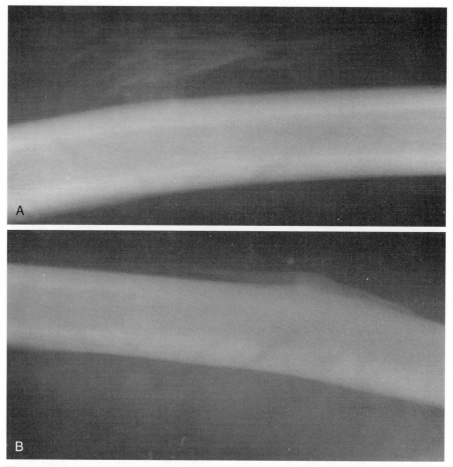

Figure 8–9. Radiographs of the thigh demonstrating myositis ossificans traumatica. *A,* Early, 3 weeks after injury. *B,* Late, 3 months after injury. Note greater density and increasing sharpness of the margins of the new bone with maturity.

We have also found that myositis ossificans may be clearly demonstrated on bone scan *before* there is any radiographic evidence of the lesion (Fig. 8–10). As with stress fractures, bone scan appears to be the more sensitive indicator of an active process. We recommend that a bone scan be obtained early to confirm the clinical diagnosis of myositis ossificans if initial radiographic examination fails to do so.

INITIAL TREATMENT

Immediate treatment of the contusion is aimed at halting the hemorrhage and preventing quadriceps spasm. This can be accomplished by flexing the knee to the limits of comfort and holding it in this flexed position for 24 to 48 hours. This can be accomplished by means of an anterior plaster splint extending from the hip to the ankle, held in place with an elastic wrap. Alternatively, a circumferential wrap can be used around the upper aspect of the thigh and distal area of the leg (Fig. 8–11). Commercially available hinged knee braces can also be used by "locking" the brace at the maximal flexion attainable by the athlete, preferably greater than 90 degrees.

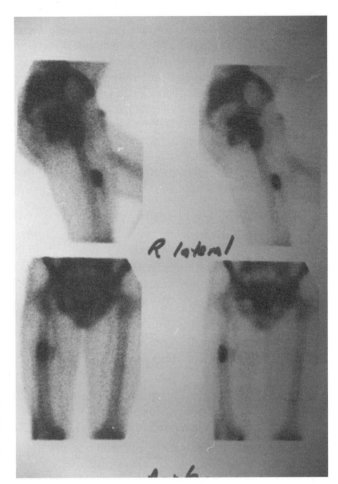

Figure 8–10. Radionuclide bone scan showing myositis ossificans in the thigh of a cyclist at less than 2 weeks after injury (a collision with an automobile with a direct blow to the anterior thigh). Radiographic examination at this time was negative.

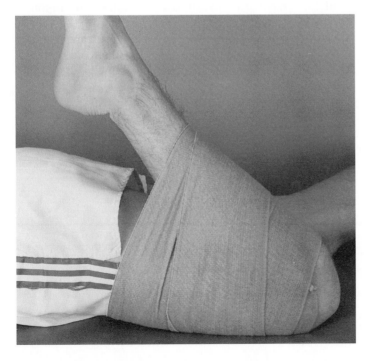

Figure 8–11. Method of maintaining knee flexion with circumferential elastic wrap.

If the knee cannot be comfortably flexed, pressure should be exerted over the site of injury. This is best accomplished by having the athlete forcibly hold an ice bag against the site of injury. The pressure should be maintained for at least 30 minutes and then replaced with a compression wrap employing a firm pad over the site of injury.

Regardless of the method of compression, the athlete should not bear any weight on the extremity, and the knee should be splinted in as much flexion as can be obtained. Splinting the knee allows the quadriceps to be rested and decreases the extravasation of blood within the muscle.

Anti-inflammatory medications are started at the time of injury. The use of a 6- or 8-day oral corticosteroid burst appears to have some merit.

REFERRAL

The presence of a mature, bony mass large enough to interfere with normal quadriceps function may require surgical removal. Such a procedure should not be undertaken until the radionuclide scan is "cold." In our experience, if left alone the mass usually shrinks and will not require removal.

DEFINITIVE TREATMENT

The treatment of the acute contusion after the period of pressure and immobilization is aimed at re-establishing quadriceps strength and flexibility in a *painless* manner. Active, painless knee flexion exercises are started at 48 hours, as are painless, isometric quadriceps exercises. As motion is obtained, isotonic lifting is begun, utilizing only the painless range of motion. We prefer to employ a splint or hinged brace limiting flexion for ambulation until 90 to 100 degrees of painless knee flexion are present. Allowing an athlete to ambulate unprotected with less than 90 degrees of knee flexion seems all too often to result in a fall that inevitably "overflexes" the knee—the re-injury that often results in myositis ossificans.

The treatment of radiographically confirmed myositis ossificans is aimed at maintaining as much quadriceps function as possible while avoiding irritation of the bony lesion. From the athlete's standpoint, this means the avoidance of *any and all painful activities*. Isometric quadriceps sets and active range-of-motion exercises are encouraged. A splint is used for all ambulation until there is evidence that the bony lesion has matured. A full rehabilitation program is instituted with radiographic and bone-scanning evidence that the lesion is no longer active.

REFERENCES

1. Basmajian JV, Deluca CJ: Muscles Alive: Their Functions Revealed by Electromyography, 5th ed. Baltimore, Williams & Wilkins, 1985.
2. Butler JE et al: Subtrochanteric stress fractures in runners. Am J Sports Med 10:228–232, 1982.
3. Ciullo JV, Jackson DW: Track and field. *In* Schneider RC, Kennedy JC, Plant ML (eds): Sports Injuries: Mechanisms, Prevention, and Treatment. Baltimore, Williams & Wilkins, 1985, pp 212–246.
4. Cyriax J: Textbook of Orthopedic Medicine. I: Diagnosis of Soft Tissue Lesions, 8th ed. London, Baillière Tindall, 1982.
5. Easterbrook M, Cameron J: Injuries in racquet sports. *In* Schneider RC, Kennedy JC, Plant

ML (eds): Sports Injuries: Mechanisms, Prevention, and Treatment. Baltimore, Williams & Wilkins, 1985, pp 553–571.

6. Fernbach SK, Wilkinson RH: Avulsion injuries of pelvis and proximal femur. AJR 137:581–584, 1981.
7. Garrick J, Requa R: Injuries in high school sports. Pediatrics 61:465, 1978.
8. Lombardo SJ, Benson DW: Stress fractures of the femur in runners. Am J Sports Med 10:219–227, 1982.
9. Lutter LD: The knee and running. Clin Sports Med 4:685–698, 1985.
10. Miller ML: Avulsion fractures of the anterior superior iliac spine in high school track. Athletic Training 17:57–59, 1982.
11. Noakes TD et al: Pelvic stress fractures in long distance runners. Am J Sports Med 13:120–123, 1985.
12. Noble CA: Treatment of iliotibial band friction syndrome. Br J Sports Med 13:51–54, 1979.
13. Noble CA: Iliotibial band friction syndrome in runners. Am J Sports Med 8:232–234, 1980.
14. Noble HB et al: Diagnosis and treatment of iliotibial band tightness in runners. Physician Sportsmed 10:67–74, April 1982.
15. Ober FR: The role of the iliotibial band and fascia lata as a factor in the causation of low back disabilities and sciatica. J Bone Joint Surg 18:105–110, 1936.
16. Orava S: Iliotibial tract friction syndrome in athletes—An uncommon exertion syndrome on the lateral side of the knee. Br J Sports Med 12:69–73, 1978.
17. Pavlov H et al: Stress fractures of pubic ramus. Report of 12 cases. J Bone Joint Surg Am 64:1020–1025, 1982.
18. Renne JW: Iliotibial band friction syndrome. J Bone Joint Surg Am 57:1110–1111, 1975.
19. Skinner HB, Cook SD: Fatigue failure stress of femoral neck: A case report. Am J Sports Med 10:245–247, 1982.
20. Smodlaka VN: Groin pain in soccer players. Physician Sportsmed 8:57–61, Aug 1980.
21. Sutker AN et al: Iliotibial band syndrome in distance runners. Physician Sportsmed 9:69–73, Oct 1981.

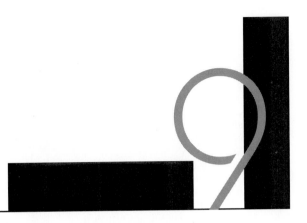

Knee Injuries

- **Grade III sprains**
  Medial collateral ligament
  Anterior cruciate ligament
  Posterior cruciate ligament
- **Torn meniscus with**
  Displaced fragment ("locked")—acute
  Recurrent impingement/locking—gradual onset
- **Osteochondritis dissecans**
- **Patellar dislocation (initial)**
- **Intra-articular fracture (tibial plateau, patella)**
- **Symptomatic loose body**
- **Intra-articular infection**
- **Infected prepatellar bursa**

T r i a g e

Indications for Referral

- **Acute**
  History
  Neurological symptoms distal to knee
  Inability to fully extend since instant of injury ("locked")
  Inability to bear weight
  "Instability"
  Immediate, significant effusion (hemarthrosis)
  Examination
  Tense effusion (hemarthrosis)
  Fat droplets in aspiration of blood
  Instability (any direction)
  Lack of extension due to anterior pain
  X-ray films (anteroposterior, lateral, notch view, and sunset view)
  Any fracture
- **Gradual onset**
  History
  Recurrent "locking"
  Tense effusion or localized swelling, local heat, redness, tenderness, and fever
  Loose body sensation
  Examination
  Palpable loose body
  X-ray films
  Loose bodies
  Osteochondritis dissecans (osteonecrosis)

Indications for X-ray Films

- **Acute**
  History
  Direct blow to knee
  Inability/unwillingness to bear weight
  Rapid onset of effusion (hemarthrosis)
  Fat droplets in bloody aspirate
  Examination
  Instability
  Bony tenderness (patella, femoral condyles, proximal fibula)
- **Gradual onset (include standing anteroposterior in 20 degrees of flexion—Rosenberg's view)**
  History
  Loose body sensation
  Recurrent locking
  Examination
  Palpable loose body
  Varus or valgus deformity compared to normal side

In sports the knee is subject to a wider variety and larger number of injuries than any other area of the body. Both acute and overuse injuries are common; together they account for about 15% of all sports injuries.[23] In clinical practice, knee problems are even more ubiquitous, accounting for nearly 50% of all sports-injury–related patient visits.[22]

The knee is a complex structure and subject to a variety of injuries, the diagnosis and treatment of which are often less than perfectly straightforward. In this chapter we discuss our recommended approach to the acutely injured athlete and to athletes with symptoms of impingement, instability, or chronic (anterior) pain. The acute and long-term manifestations of ligamentous and meniscal injuries, quadriceps mechanism insufficiency, and so on are thus considered in the contexts of their usual presentations. We also separately discuss medial collateral ligament sprains; anterior cruciate ligament sprains; posterior cruciate ligament sprains; lateral collateral ligament sprains and associated injuries; patellar dislocation; prepatellar bursitis; and popliteus tendinitis. Iliotibial band tendinitis, a common cause of lateral knee pain in runners, has already been discussed in the chapter on hip and thigh injuries (see Chapter 8, part E).

A. PROBLEM-ORIENTED APPROACH TO DIAGNOSIS AND TRIAGE

Knee problems in athletes characteristically present in one or more of the following ways:

Acute injury or the immediate sequelae of acute injury
Activity-related pain
Swelling
Locking
Functional instability (giving way)

This section gives an overview of our basic approach to these problems with emphasis on diagnostic and therapeutic pitfalls to avoid and when consultation/referral is appropriate. The discrete diagnostic entities mentioned are discussed in greater detail in subsequent sections.

ACUTE INJURY OR THE IMMEDIATE SEQUELAE OF ACUTE INJURY

"I hurt my knee in the game last night." "I twisted my knee skiing last month. I thought it would get better, but I still can't . . . ."
Of primary importance is the establishment of a precise diagnosis or, failing that, an appropriately inclusive differential diagnosis with a plan for further evaluation. When a precise diagnosis can be made, initial treatment, indications for referral, definitive treatment, and rehabilitative treatment generally follow. When a precise diagnosis cannot be determined from the data available, initial treatment and referral should be carried out as for the most serious *possible* injury. In most sports (nonvehicular) situations, the differential diagnosis of concern includes

Fractures of the distal femur, patella, and proximal tibia and fibula
Patellar dislocations and subluxations
Sprains (medial and lateral collateral and anterior and posterior cruciate
    ligament injuries)
Meniscal injuries
Strains (quadriceps, patellar, and hamstring musculotendinous injuries)
Contusions and hemorrhagic prepatellar bursitis

The diagnostic pitfall of greatest consequence is failure to recognize grade III ligamentous injuries, especially anterior cruciate ligament injury. The unwary examiner is liable to be trapped by over-reliance on the physical examination, which is frequently compromised in the acute setting by pain, swelling, muscle spasm, and guarding. It cannot be overemphasized that a careful history is the examiner's most important diagnostic tool. It should include

Circumstances and mechanism of injury
Immediacy, severity, and localization of pain
Associated noise or other sensation
Ability/willingness to bear weight
Localization, extent, and *rapidity* of swelling

Frank instability (perceived "giving way")
True locking

A noncontact, running/deceleration or mislanding-a-jump injury associated with a perceived "pop," perceived instability, and rapid swelling is an anterior cruciate ligament injury until proved otherwise. Similarly, a contact or noncontact injury associated with an "awesome" sound audible to the patient and others, perceived instability, perceived severe injury, and rapid swelling is a patellar dislocation until proved otherwise. A contact or noncontact injury with immediate inability to extend the knee is a locked meniscal tear or osteochondral loose body until proved otherwise. Positive physical and radiographic examinations may be confirmatory; however, negative examinations do not disconfirm the diagnoses. *An absence of proof does not constitute a proof of absence.*

Displaced fractures; intra-articular fractures; confirmed or suspected grade III sprains of the anterior or posterior cruciate ligaments; confirmed or suspected grade III strains of the quadriceps muscles or tendons, patellar tendon, or hamstring muscles or tendons; suspected acute meniscal tears; and any acute internal derangement associated with true locking are relatively common, unambiguous indications for orthopedic referral. Referral to an appropriate facility on an emergent basis is indicated for fractures or dislocations complicated by vascular impairment.

Nondisplaced transverse patellar fractures; nondisplaced or minimally displaced Salter I or II fractures; acute patellar dislocation or subluxation not associated with intra-articular fractures; and grade III collateral ligament injuries are possible indications for orthopedic referral.

Some primary care physicians may choose to manage some conditions themselves, e.g., patellar fractures (transverse, nondisplaced); patellar dislocations and subluxations (not associated with intra-articular fractures); and grade III medial collateral ligament injuries. The patellar injuries are best treated acutely by immobilization in extension; medial collateral ligament injuries, by bracing in 30 degrees of flexion.

As always, for acute injuries in which the precise diagnosis is uncertain after initial evaluation, consultation or referral is indicated.

ACTIVITY-RELATED PAIN (OVERUSE INJURY)

"My knee hurts a bit at the start of the run. Then it goes away. Then it really hurts afterward." "It hurts when I squat, go downstairs, and especially when I jump."

Knee overuse injuries are the bane of many endurance athletes and would-be endurance athletes. Virtually any major structure may be involved. Localization of pain and point tenderness provide a reasonable first triage of the differential diagnoses (see Fig. 9–2).

- Anterior knee pain
  Quadriceps mechanism dysfunction
  Patellofemoral mechanical dysfunction with excessive traction on medial soft tissues (medial peripatellar pain)
  Patellofemoral mechanical dysfunction with impingement of lateral soft tissues (lateral peripatellar pain)
  Patellofemoral mechanical dysfunction with chondromalacia patellae (retropatellar pain)
  Patellofemoral mechanical dysfunction with anterior fat pad impingement (infrapatellar pain)

Patellar tendinitis/tendinosis (infrapatellar pain)
Superficial and deep infrapatellar bursitis (infrapatellar pain)
Osgood-Schlatter disease (traction apophysitis of the anterior tibial tubercle; anteroinferior pain)
Quadriceps tendinitis (suprapatellar pain)
Pathological plica syndrome (medial or lateral peripatellar or suprapatellar pain)
Prepatellar bursitis
- Medial knee pain
    Medial meniscus tear
    Medial compartment arthrosis (degenerative joint disease)
    Hamstring tendinitis/anserine bursitis
    Chronic medial collateral ligament sprain
    Pathological plica syndrome
- Lateral knee pain
    Lateral meniscus tear
    Lateral compartment arthrosis (degenerative joint disease)
    Hamstring tendinitis
    Iliotibial band tendinitis
    Popliteus tendinitis
    Pathological plica syndrome
- Posterior knee pain
    Baker's cyst (suspect meniscal injury)
    Hamstring or gastrocnemius tendinitis/overuse strain, or both
    Fabella syndrome

Less severe, shorter-duration problems often respond to basic intervention comprising relative rest, anti-inflammatory measures, "home program" rehabilitation exercises, and gradual resumption of activity that avoids training error. As guidelines for treating and resuming activity, delayed soreness and overall trends are more important criteria than are the odd twinges of pain during activity.

The cause of most knee overuse injuries is multifactorial. Unless the patient has the luxury of avoiding the pain-provoking activity indefinitely, anti-inflammatory treatment alone will likely prove insufficient. As is true for all overuse injuries that do not resolve promptly and completely with basic intervention, *the essential diagnostic and therapeutic task is to identify and reverse as many of the causative factors as possible.*

Accordingly, follow-up with the physician is essential and should be scheduled every 3 weeks or so. Physical therapy referral is clearly appropriate if there has been no improvement by the first follow-up visit. Sports medicine/orthopedics consultation/referral is indicated for problems not demonstrably improving over time. Special diagnostic tests, e.g., biomechanical activity analysis or magnetic resonance imaging (MRI) examination of the knee, specialized treatment, e.g., prescription and dispensation of functional orthoses, or surgical intervention, e.g., lateral retinacular release for patellofemoral dysfunction, may be required.

SWELLING

"It swelled up right away after I hurt it." "I haven't noticed any swelling, but, yes, I have noticed I can't bend it as much as the other knee." "I've got this lump that seems to be getting bigger."

Soft tissue swelling about the knee may be associated with acute or overuse injuries or various arthritides. Characterization of the swelling as to location, diffuse versus discrete, intra-articular versus extra-articular, fluctuant versus nonfluctuant, rapidity of onset, and associated symptoms and signs provides the keys to sorting out the differential diagnosis. The examiner should differentiate

Knee joint effusion (hemorrhagic, synovial, inflammatory, septic)
Bursitis (prepatellar, deep and superficial infrapatellar, anserine)
Extra-articular hemorrhage, edema
Synovitis
Cysts
Tumors

"Swelling" about the knee may also be attributable to bony or cartilaginous enlargement. The differential diagnosis of "hard tissue swelling" includes

Osgood-Schlatter disease (traction apophysitis of the anterior tibial tubercle)
Benign exostoses (commonly of the distal femoral metaphysis)
Osteophytosis associated with degenerative joint disease
Tumors

Knee joint effusions are characterized by diffuse fluctuant swelling that tends to obscure the medial margin of the patella and often also distends the suprapatellar pouch (see Fig. 9–3).

Owing to the incompressibility of fluid, with acute knee effusions there is limitation of flexion proportionate to the size of the effusion. Indeed, with small effusions, patients may be aware only of some limitation of motion and not of frank swelling. In contrast, with chronic effusions, even large ones, there may be little or no abnormal limitation of motion, as the joint capsule becomes stretched over time.

Knee joint swelling that becomes obvious within an hour after the injury is indicative of intra-articular bleeding. Because acute hemarthrosis implies a high likelihood of significant structural injury, e.g., intra-articular fracture, cruciate ligament tear, or meniscus cartilage tear, the historical finding of rapid knee joint swelling should in itself be considered an indication for orthopedic referral.

Joint swelling that becomes obvious 12 or more hours after the injury is characteristic of synovial effusion. This is a typical presentation of meniscus cartilage tears. However, "water on the knee" is a nonspecific finding and is not in itself an indication for orthopedic referral.

Joint swelling associated with rubor, calor, and dolor is characteristic of septic or inflammatory arthritis. These findings constitute an indication for arthrocentesis with further treatment as indicated by synovial analysis. A diagnostic pitfall to avoid is mistaking a superficial infection, e.g., infected abrasion, cellulitis, or septic prepatellar bursitis, for a septic knee joint arthritis. A needle should not be introduced into the knee joint through an overlying extra-articular infection.

Bursitis is characterized by discretely demarcated, fluctuant swelling. A prepatellar "goose egg" is a classic presentation (see Fig. 9–4).

Prepatellar bursitis may be caused by direct trauma (acute, traumatic, hemorrhagic bursitis) or repetitive friction trauma (nonhemorrhagic bursitis). Because the overlying skin is liable to injury by either mechanism, either condition may be complicated by infection (septic bursitis). Aspiration is generally indicated. If the aspirate is nonpurulent and there are no other signs of infection, a corticosteroid may be instilled into the bursa. Adequate compression, however, is the most important aspect of preventing reaccumulation of blood/synovial fluid. For bursitis uncomplicated by infection, we recommend a continuous compression wrap for the first 48 hours following aspiration and continuous for the first week thereafter, except for showering.

Rapid onset of nonfluctuant, extra-articular swelling is commonly noted with medial collateral ligament sprains. Tenderness may be discretely localized to the origin (medial femoral epicondyle), insertion of the deep part (medial tibial plateau just distal to the joint line), or insertion of the superficial part (medial tibial metaphysis a handbreadth distal to the joint line). Swelling may be similarly discrete or somewhat more diffusely localized along the course of the ligament depending on the extent of injury and amount of bleeding.

With acute, traumatic patellar dislocation or subluxation, there may be both nonfluctuant, extra-articular swelling and a demonstrable joint effusion. The amount of swelling varies with the extent of structural injury (medial patellar retinaculum and patellofemoral articular surfaces) and the amount of bleeding. If present, extra-articular swelling and ecchymosis are usually diffusely localized over the medial aspect of the knee.

A complaint of aching popliteal pain may be attributable to a Baker or popliteal cyst. One might expect that a discrete, fluctuant mass in the popliteal space would be readily and reliably discernible by inspection and palpation, but in our experience, this has not proved to be the case. The principal clinical significance of a popliteal cyst is its probable association with an internal derangement of the knee, e.g., a meniscus cartilage tear, and both the cyst and the meniscal injury are best demonstrated on MRI examination of the knee.

Meniscal cysts localized to the joint line are more readily appreciated on physical examination. Their clinical significance also relates essentially to the underlying meniscal abnormality.

Synovitis associated with various arthritides may present as boggy, nonfluctuant joint line swelling and tenderness. There may or may not be an associated joint effusion.

In the skeletally immature, and particularly during the adolescent growth spurt, quadriceps mechanism overuse is commonly manifested as Osgood-Schlatter disease. Classically there is tenderness over the enlarging "bump" of the anterior tibial tubercle and pain localized to this site with quadriceps-intensive exercise, especially with eccentric action of the muscle, e.g., in landing jumps. For tenderness, horseshoe pads may afford some protection. Possible underlying causative factors, e.g., training error, flexibility, strength, and gait mechanics, should also be addressed. The mainstay of treatment, however, is relative rest. Osgood-Schlatter disease commonly tests the patience of the young athlete, the concerned parents, and the treating physician. Consultation for "second opinion/reassurance" purposes may be appropriate.

Benign exostoses represent another skeletal growth aberrancy. They are commonly located on the distal femoral metaphysis. Rarely, they may become large enough to cause muscular (quadriceps or hamstring) or neurovascular impairment, in which case referral for surgical excision is appropriate.

Lastly, regardless of the presenting circumstances, the examiner needs to keep in mind that bony or soft tissue swelling at the knee might represent a tumor. Swelling first noted after a sport-related injury is a not uncommon presentation of osteogenic sarcoma in young athletes.

LOCKING (AND PSEUDOLOCKING)

"My knee will sometimes lock up on me, and I can't straighten it. Then I have to take it and [manually] move it from side to side or something, and then I can usually straighten it again." "After I've been sitting for a while and then try to get up and start to walk, I can't straighten my knee out all the way. Then I have to tighten my quads and force it straight, and then it works OK again." "When my knee hurts, it gets real stiff, and I can hardly bend or straighten it."

Patients do not always use the term *locking* in a medically precise way. "My knee locks up on me" may imply abrupt onset of pain, limitation of motion, or functional instability. The examiner must first clarify that the patient is attempting to describe abnormal limitation of knee motion and then differentiate *true locking* (mechanical block of normal joint motion) from *gelling* or *joint stiffness* secondary to pain, swelling, or muscle spasm, or all of these.

True locking is characterized by an abrupt onset of inability to extend the knee completely. Subsequently, there may be equally abrupt unlocking, i.e., an abrupt return of normal knee motion. Less commonly, patients may present with their knees' having remained locked in flexion.

Mechanical blocking of knee extension may occur at the patellofemoral or tibiofemoral articulations and may be attributable to

Advanced chondromalacia
Delaminated articular cartilage flap
Meniscus cartilage tear
Osteochondral loose body
Remnant of torn anterior cruciate ligament

Episodes of true locking with active unlocking ("I tighten my quads and can then force the knee straight") are characteristic of patellofemoral chondromalacia, whereas episodes of true locking that require passive unlocking ("I have to manipulate the knee") represent internal derangement such as meniscal tear or loose body until proved otherwise.

A locked knee is an indication for prompt orthopedic referral and surgical intervention. The experienced clinician may attempt to unlock the knee manually as follows: The limb is supported as in Garrick's test for meniscal impingement such that the weight of the limb alone applies a gentle varus or valgus stress to the knee (see Fig. 9–10). The clinician then gently assists the patient's actively extending the knee. Forcible extension of the knee (which may actually be tolerated if the knee is anesthetized) and torsional maneuvers should be avoided. They risk extending a meniscus cartilage tear or amputating a bucket-handle meniscus tear.

A history of true locking episodes with passive unlocking is a clear indication for orthopedic referral, as is a history of true locking with a loose body sensation. In our experience, patients' perception of intra-articular loose bodies is virtually always accurate.

FUNCTIONAL INSTABILITY (GIVING WAY)

"My knee goes out on me" (in sports or activities of daily living [e.g., descending stairs or walking on uneven terrain], or both). "I can't cut on that leg" (in football

or soccer). "I can't cut, make a strong move to the hoop, or land a jump on that leg" (in basketball). "I can't turn on that leg" (in skiing).

Functional instability of the knee is not synonymous with ligamentous insufficiency or any specific structural abnormality. Rather, it implies only that the knee does not work reliably. The differential diagnosis of functional instability of the knee includes

Muscular or neuromuscular insufficiency
Internal derangement (meniscus cartilage tears, osteochondral loose bodies)
Uncompensated ligamentous insufficiency
Patellofemoral instability (dislocation or subluxation)

Although patients' perception of their knees' being functionally unstable is by definition accurate, their perception of the nature, severity, and cause of the instability is often inaccurate. "My knee dislocates" may describe moderate patellofemoral instability, whereas, "I sometimes feel something" may describe gross pivot shift instability associated with uncompensated anterior cruciate ligament insufficiency.

The most common cause of functional instability of the knee is muscular insufficiency, especially of the quadriceps. Common presenting complaints are backward buckling, giving-way episodes while standing, and pain, apprehension, or frank giving way while descending stairs. Causes of quadriceps mechanism insufficiency include

Disuse atrophy secondary to unrehabilitated prior injury
Reflexive pain or joint effusion inhibition of normal quadriceps function
Neuromuscular weakness secondary to L4 radiculopathy or femoral neuropathy
Exhaustive exercise (e.g., during the run after hard bicycling in a triathlon)

Another common cause of functional instability is episodic painful inhibition of normal quadriceps function secondary to an internal derangement such as a meniscus cartilage tear. A careful historian may note, "I get a jab of pain, and then the knee gives out," as opposed to, "The knee gives out, and then it hurts."

The least common, but most serious, cause of functional instability is uncompensated ligamentous laxity. There is not a perfect correlation between the extent of abnormal ligamentous laxity measurable or demonstrable on physical examination and the clinical problem of functional instability. Many individuals are able to use their quadriceps to compensate quite well for medial collateral ligament insufficiency. Similarly, some are able to use their quadriceps to compensate for posterior cruciate ligament insufficiency, and some are able to use their biceps femoris to compensate for anterior cruciate ligament insufficiency.

Individuals who are unable to compensate for their ligamentous laxity are liable to episodes of giving way with various activities. The more unpredictable the activity (e.g., going up in the air and not coming down as expected because someone has collided with you), the greater the risk of instability episodes. Because episodes of frank instability are neuromuscularly disconcerting, the individual often falls. There may or may not be associated pain or subsequent swelling.

Symptomatically, acute patellar dislocation or subluxation can be quite similar to acute anterior cruciate ligament tears. In either case, there may be a contact or noncontact mechanism of injury, immediate pain, associated joint noise, perceived instability, falling, an inability to continue the activity, and subsequent rapid and marked swelling. Similarly, recurrent patellofemoral instability episodes may be easily symptomatically confused with tibiofemoral (pivot shift) instability episodes secondary to anterior cruciate ligament insufficiency. Although certain historical and physical findings may favor one diagnosis over the other, the more serious possibility of ligamentous insufficiency should not be discounted until disproved. Especially in the setting of acute injury, *failure to elicit a positive Lachman test or pivot shift does not rule out anterior cruciate ligament injury/insufficiency.*

Treatment of functional instability basically entails identification and treatment of the underlying cause. Treatment of muscular insufficiency is rehabilitative, emphasizing combined strength/proprioception progressive resistance exercises. Similarly, the initial treatment of patellofemoral instability is rehabilitative.

Indications for orthopedic referral include

Functional instability secondary to proven or suspected internal derangement (e.g., meniscus cartilage tear with episodic impingement)
Functional instability secondary to proven or suspected ligamentous insufficiency
Proven or suspected acute grade III ligamentous injuries (potential functional instability)
Patellofemoral instability unresponsive to appropriate physical therapy

Treatment for functional instability secondary to ligamentous insufficiency may be either surgical or rehabilitative. The objective of specific rehabilitative treatment of anterior cruciate ligament insufficiency is reliable hamstring control of pivot shift instability. The rehabilitation comprises essentially motor skill learning with progressively more challenging functional tasks, as opposed to the more basic rehabilitation techniques appropriate for most other knee injuries. Accordingly, we recommend that whether surgical or nonsurgical treatment is elected, instability related to ligamentous insufficiency be managed and followed by a specialist.

B. ACUTE INJURY (INTERNAL DERANGEMENT)

Acute knee injuries in sports include contusions, sprains, strains, fractures, and dislocations. Some of these injuries, such as patellar tendon rupture, are clinically obvious. Others, such as anterior cruciate ligament tears, are likely to be misdiagnosed initially, perhaps as much as 90% of the time.[44]

Adding to the problem of diagnostic uncertainty is the fact that in many cases, even given the diagnosis, there is no consensus as to the preferred treatment. Take, for example, severe ligamentous injuries, the hallmark sign of which is instability. All of the following have been advocated in the literature: operative treatment even without instability, i.e., for grade II as well as grade III sprains; operative treatment for instability in any plane, i.e., for all grade III sprains; operative treatment only for instability combined with meniscal injury or for instability in two planes, e.g., for grade III sprains of both the anterior cruciate and medial collateral ligaments; and nonoperative treatment, even for two-plane instability.[13, 16, 24, 30, 33, 39–41, 45–47, 64]

In general, the importance of a given diagnostic test, such as examination under general anesthesia to rule out instability or MRI to rule out a posterior horn tear of the medial meniscus, depends on how the results of the test alter subsequent treatment. Our recommendations regarding the work-up of an acutely injured athlete obviously reflect our judgment as to the best way of treating the various injuries. Suffice it to say that we are not necessarily offended by the notion that a gifted athlete might sustain a significant knee injury and not even have an arthroscopy scar to show for it.

We cannot, however, neatly dichotomize all acute knee injuries as either definitely requiring or definitely not requiring operative intervention. Clearly, some injuries such as isolated grades I and II sprains of the medial collateral ligament can be satisfactorily treated nonoperatively.[13] Others such as displaced transverse fractures of the patella clearly ought to be treated operatively. Nevertheless, for many acute knee injuries, especially meniscal and grade III ligamentous injuries, the best treatment is and will remain a matter of clinical judgment, personal preference, and, therefore, controversy.

We recognize and appreciate the dilemma faced by the primary care physician, who must try to make logical and consistent treatment/referral decisions, despite the conflicting opinions of various authorities. We have attempted to get around this dilemma by underscoring the distinction between management by a surgeon and operative treatment. As a general rule, we suggest that an orthopedic surgeon be involved in the management of all cases in which the diagnosis or preferred treatment is uncertain, as well as those in which surgery is clearly required. Specific indications for referral therefore include (1) fractures, (2) grade III sprains, (3) grade III strains, and (4) mechanical disruption of normal knee motion.

Our recommended approach to the acutely injured athlete emphasizes those aspects of the history and physical and radiographic examinations that indicate severity of injury sufficient to merit orthopedic consultation. We only briefly review the use of special diagnostic tests and the definitive treatment of severe injuries. We discuss in greater detail the management of those injuries that can be appropriately treated by protection and rehabilitation alone.

HISTORY

Athletes are asked about the mechanism of injury, their symptoms, their perception of the severity of injury, the extent of any disability, especially any symptoms of instability, their postinjury course, and any prior injury to the knee.

When injury is the result of a high-speed, tumbling fall, the athlete's understanding of the mechanism of injury may be vague or inaccurate. Much of the time, however, the athlete can accurately describe just how the injury occurred, and in most cases, careful direct questioning permits the examiner to ascertain the critical details.

It is important first of all to determine whether a *definite, distinct injury* occurred. Not infrequently athletes present with acute or subacute pain and swelling of the knee following a bout of unaccustomed activity, as after hiking with a heavily loaded pack or playing consecutive games in a tournament. Physical examination may be consistent with internal derangement of the knee but may otherwise be nonspecific. In our experience, the athlete who does not remember a specific incident (having twisted the knee, felt it give out, felt a sharp pain, or felt something tear) is unlikely to have sustained a significant injury. A possible exception is the older athlete with a "degenerative" meniscal tear.

It is also important to characterize as precisely as possible the activity being pursued at the time of injury. Straight-ahead walking or running, for example, rarely produces significant injury other than recurrent patellar dislocation or dislodgment of an osteochondral fragment. However, if *deceleration or cutting* (turning) was involved, then injury to a meniscus or the anterior cruciate ligament must also be considered.

An *unanticipated move*, such as stepping in a hole or slipping on a wet surface, can result in injury to any of the dynamic (musculotendinous) or static (capsular, meniscal, ligamentous) stabilizers of the joint. Sudden, *eccentric loading* of the quadriceps mechanism, as may occur in attempting to prevent a backward fall, can produce sufficient tensile force to fracture the patella or rupture the patellar tendon. Awkwardly *mislanding a jump* is especially likely to cause anterior cruciate ligament injury. It is important to determine whether the injured knee was *bearing weight* at the time of injury. Keep in mind that weight bearing can occur while standing, kneeling, crawling, squatting, landing jumps, and the like. Midair, non–weight-bearing injuries, as may occur during jumping or diving, are for the most part limited to patellar dislocation or subluxation or other quadriceps mechanism injuries.

Contact, collision, or other externally applied force increases the risk of severe injury and increases the probability of certain specific injuries. A classic example is the "unhappy triad" of O'Donoghue, i.e., combined tears of the medial collateral ligament, anterior cruciate ligament, and medial meniscus, caused by a direct blow to the lateral aspect of the weight-bearing knee.[47]

Complete tears of the medial collateral ligament are almost always the result of externally applied force. The force may be either direct, as typically occurs in football when a player is tackled or illegally blocked, or indirect, as may occur when a skier falls and the bindings fail to release.

Sprains of the lateral collateral ligament are the result of direct trauma to the medial aspect of the knee. Such injuries typically occur in wrestling. They are uncommon in other sports, as the medial aspect of the knee is usually well protected by the other leg. Isolated sprains may occur, but usually there is associated injury to other structures, including the lateral capsule, iliotibial band, biceps femoris tendon, one or both cruciate ligaments, and often the peroneal nerve.

A direct force to the anterior aspect of the flexed knee may result in any of several typical "dashboard" injuries, depending on exactly where and how the force is applied. A blow to the anterior aspect of the proximal aspect of the tibia tends to cause *posterior cruciate ligament* injury, whereas a blow over the patella may produce acute hemorrhagic *prepatellar bursitis* or a *patellar fracture*.

In contrast to the injuries previously described, isolated tears of the menisci or anterior cruciate ligament are seldom the result of externally applied force. Rather, such injuries are usually the result of deceleration or rotational forces on the weight-bearing knee, as may occur in any running or jumping activity or in skiing.

Such very severe injuries as dislocation of the knee or structurally significant fractures are usually but not invariably the result of major trauma, as may occur in motor sports, rock climbing, motor vehicle/pedestrian, or motor vehicle/cyclist accidents. Notable exceptions are the noncontact fractures of the patella (see earlier) and tibia (Fig. 9–1).

Pain is to a greater or lesser extent a feature of all significant injuries.

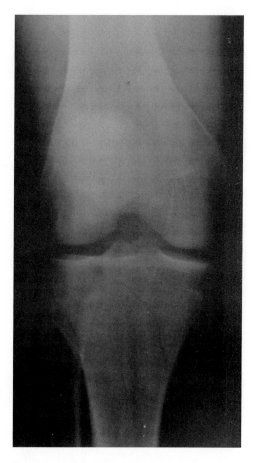

Figure 9–1. Anteroposterior radiograph of the knee of a football lineman who sustained a noncontact, deceleration injury while running with the ball. Although the mechanism of injury was suggestive of anterior cruciate or meniscal injury, physical examination revealed marked swelling and ecchymosis, tenderness over the proximal aspect of the tibia, and an inability to bear weight. Radiographic examination confirmed a comminuted, intra-articular (Y-condylar) fracture.

However, the extent of pain and the *perceived severity of injury* can be misleading. An athlete who has sustained a grade II sprain of the medial collateral ligament is likely to have quite a bit of pain and to be reluctant to continue playing. The athlete may even be hesitant to bear weight on the injured limb. The athlete who has dislocated the patella will likely be absolutely convinced that something terrible has happened to the knee and be unwilling even to move the knee, much less to bear weight. Conversely, the athlete with a grade III sprain of the medial collateral ligament is likely to have had some immediate but not persistent pain and may very well attempt to continue playing unless or until he or she perceives some sensation of instability.

For a while after injury, *pain and tenderness* may be *well localized* to the injured structure or structures. Thus the torn medial collateral ligament hurts on the medial aspect of the knee; the patellar dislocation hurts over the adductor tubercle and medial retinaculum (the site of soft tissue injury); and meniscus tears hurt over the respective (medial or lateral) joint lines. Anterior cruciate ligament tears are characteristically perceived as pain on either side of the patellar tendon at the front of the tibial plateau (Fig. 9–2) or at the posterolateral corner of the knee.

A snapping, popping, ripping, or tearing sensation at the time of injury is generally indicative of severe injury but is not, as a rule, diagnostically specific. A notable exception is the characteristic, awesome sound of patellar dislocation, which has been likened by one of our patients to that of pulling apart a chicken drumstick and thigh. An injury that is *audible to someone other*

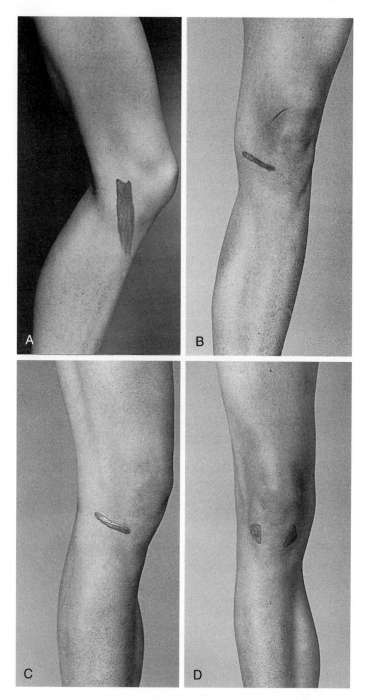

Figure 9–2. Anatomical location of pain and tenderness in various knee disorders. *A,* Medial collateral ligament sprain (mark denotes the most common site). *B,* Medial meniscus injury. *C,* Lateral meniscus injury. *D,* Anterior cruciate ligament sprain.

than the person injured is almost invariably a patellar dislocation. A snap or pop during a deceleration or cutting maneuver implies anterior cruciate or meniscal injury until proved otherwise.

A history of locking must be pursued and clarified. The limitation of motion caused by pain, swelling, or muscle spasm must be differentiated from true locking, which is caused by mechanical impingement of an osteochondral loose body or a torn fragment of meniscus. Some limitation of both flexion and extension is common after injury. Athletes are particularly likely to notice this after the injured knee has been held in one position for a while.

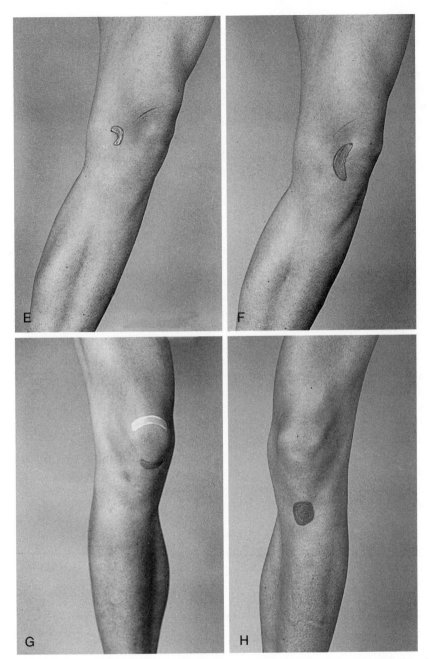

Figure 9–2 *Continued. E*, Patellar dislocation (mark denotes frequent point of maximal tenderness. *F*, Patellofemoral dysfunction (mark denotes more common site). *G*, Jumper's knee (lower mark denotes more common site). *H*, Osgood-Schlatter disease.

They may then find that as they attempt to move the knee, they can gradually gain some motion. They may refer to this phenomenon as *locking* (and *unlocking*), although better terms are *gelling* or, simply, *stiffness*. In contrast, true locking occurs abruptly and definitely blocks further motion, almost always extension. When this occurs the knee must usually be "unlocked" (twisted or manipulated) until motion is regained, usually as abruptly as it was lost. Further history will reveal whether the athlete ever feels something loose moving around inside the knee. A positive response implies osteochondral loose body until proved otherwise.

A history of having had a *full range of knee motion* at some time after the knee was injured can be diagnostically important. Usually by the time the athlete seeks medical attention, there is at least some limitation of motion secondary to pain, swelling, and muscle spasm, whereas there may or may not have been any limitation of motion just after injury. Pain permitting, most athletes "try the knee" shortly after it has been injured. Such trials usually involve attempts at full extension and flexion. It is important to ask whether the knee was able to be completely straightened at any time after the injury. Knowing that full extension was possible practically precludes the possibility of a dislocated, locked, bucket-handle meniscus tear.

Any symptom suggestive of *instability* must be heeded. Typically athletes who have sustained an anterior cruciate ligament tear say that the knee "went out," causing them to fall. Athletes with a torn medial collateral ligament may very perceptively observe that the knee bends the wrong way. Alternatively, athletes may simply admit that the knee does not feel right, feels loose, will not support them, or that they do not trust it. The presence of any such symptoms in association with acute injury implies *severe ligamentous injury* until proved otherwise.

Disability may be the result of pain, swelling, or muscle spasm, as well as significant structural injury. Immediate and marked disability such as an inability to bear weight or to move the knee is generally indicative of severe injury. However, an absence of disability does not by any means rule out severe injury. An important case in point is the grade III sprain of the medial collateral ligament, the only major symptom of which may be instability (see earlier).

Similarly, the extent of *swelling* and the rapidity with which it occurred may or may not correlate with the severity of injury. A rapid onset of tense, painful hemarthrosis suggests an intra-articular fracture or a patellar dislocation. Moderate hemarthrosis occurring over 12 to 24 hours is characteristic of a torn anterior cruciate ligament. However, even a minor sprain or contusion, treated initially by immersion in a hot tub, may present as a markedly swollen, painful knee, whereas appropriate immediate treatment of a severe injury with ice and compression minimizes the amount of swelling that occurs.

Finally, the *past history* may be contributory. Patellar subluxations and dislocations tend to be recurrent. Prior anterior cruciate ligament tears may predispose to meniscal injuries. More generally, any incompletely rehabilitated prior injury may render the knee vulnerable to recurrent, and often more severe, injury.

PHYSICAL EXAMINATION

INSPECTION AND PALPATION. This begins with simple observation of the athlete and the position of the injured limb. Deformity, marked swelling and ecchymosis, an inability to move the knee or to bear weight, and so on are all indicative of severe injury.

Assessment of the neurovascular status of the limb is particularly important if any deformity or marked swelling is present. The popliteal nerve and vessels are especially liable to injury with posterior dislocation of the knee or supracondylar fractures of the femur. The peroneal nerve is vulnerable to injury with any trauma to the lateral aspect of the knee.

The hallmark, though diagnostically nonspecific, sign of acute knee injury is *joint effusion or hemarthrosis*. This must be differentiated from other soft tissue swelling, especially traumatic prepatellar and infrapatellar bursitis.

Normally, with the knee extended, the contour of the patella is well defined by the recesses above and on either side of it. If the knee joint is distended by blood or synovial fluid, inspection will reveal obliteration of these hollow spaces. This is particularly evident on the medial side (Fig. 9–3*A*). Squeezing the suprapatellar pouch with one hand and palpating medially with the other demonstrates fluctuation, confirming that the swelling actually represents fluid within the joint (Fig. 9–3*B*). Alternatively, the presence of fluid within the joint can be demonstrated by ballottement of the patella. If fluid is present, compression above and on both sides of the patella will float the patella away from the femur. Sharply pushing downward on it with the other hand will cause it to strike the femur with a palpable tap. Demonstration of a fluid wave by "milking" the fluid away from the medial

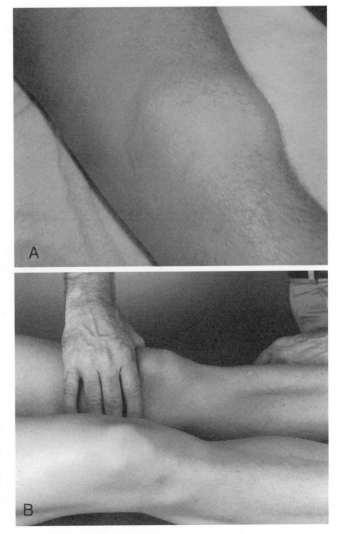

Figure 9–3. *A*, Large effusion resulting in obliteration of the hollow spaces normally found on each side of the patella. *B*, Compressing the suprapatellar pouch moves joint fluid beneath the patella. Then, alternately compressing medially and laterally may reveal fluid moving from side to side.

recess and then watching it refill is a less reliable sign of joint effusion. Too little or too much fluid yields a false-negative result.

With prepatellar bursitis, or housemaid's knee, there is a sharply demarcated, fluctuant goose egg directly overlying the patella (Fig. 9–4) appearing much more prominent when the knee is flexed. Similarly, with (superficial) infrapatellar bursitis, or clergyman's knee, there is a discrete, fluctuant mass overlying the patellar tendon.

Physical examination continues with systematic inspection and palpation of possibly injured structures. An appreciation of the surface anatomy of the knee is essential.

Major landmarks anteriorly are the femoral condylar ridges, tibial plateau, patella, patellar tendon, anterior tibial tubercle, vastus medialis obliquus, and adductor tubercle. With patellar tendon strain or tendinitis, tenderness is often localized to the central, proximal portion of the patellar tendon. The medial patellar retinaculum, which is torn with patellar dislocation, lies between the patella and the adductor tubercle. The pes anserinus, formed by the tendons of sartorius, gracilis, and semitendinosus, and beneath it the anserine bursa, overlies the medial tibial condyle. The Q angle is that formed by the intersection of the line of the femur and that of the patellar tendon.

Major landmarks medially are the medial femoral epicondyle, the tibial plateau, and the tendons of the semitendinosus and, just deep to it, semimembranosus. The superficial part of the medial collateral ligament extends a handbreadth below the joint line. Particularly with a twisting mechanism of injury, as may occur in skiing, the site of injury is likely to be the distal attachment of the ligament, and hence the importance of palpating the entire length of the structure is evident (see Fig. 9–2*A*).

Major landmarks laterally are the lateral femoral epicondyle, the head of the fibula, Gerdy's tubercle (onto which the iliotibial band inserts), the iliotibial band, the tendon of the biceps femoris, and the lateral collateral ligament. The popliteus tendon is most accessible to palpation in the interval between the lateral collateral ligament, the iliotibial band, and the biceps tendon. The peroneal nerve is quite superficial and therefore vulnerable to injury, as it crosses the neck of the fibula just distal to the insertion of the biceps tendon.

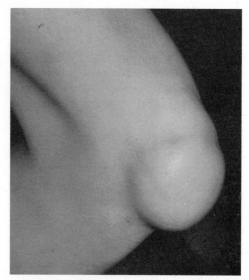

Figure 9–4. Distended prepatellar bursa.

Point tenderness, swelling, and ecchymosis may initially be well localized to the injured structure or structures. For a few hours after injury, discrete swelling may be apparent, e.g., over a sprained ligament or strained tendon. Ecchymosis usually takes longer to become apparent and may be a sign of either contusion or tearing. Thus, for example, with a medial collateral ligament sprain, there may be bruising laterally where the knee was struck and medially where the ligament was torn. Indeed, ecchymosis localized to the medial or anteromedial aspect of the knee implies severe medial collateral ligament injury or patellar dislocation until proved otherwise. However, these well-localized, and thus highly specific, signs tend to become obscured over time, as swelling and tenderness become more diffuse and gravity and compressive dressings cause ecchymosis to spread subcutaneously.

The *range of motion* of the acutely injured knee may or may not be diagnostically significant. With *true locking* there is a definite end point, as further motion, usually extension, is abruptly blocked. Such limitation of motion implies a torn meniscus or osteochondral loose body until proved otherwise. Conversely, a full, pain-free range of motion after injury effectively rules out significant meniscal injury. Usually, however, by the time the athlete is examined, there is some limitation of both flexion and extension, due to effusion and hamstring muscle spasm, respectively. Such limitation of motion without a definite end point has no diagnostic significance.

If there are such signs of severe injury as point tenderness over bone (especially in the skeletally immature), marked swelling and ecchymosis, and inability to move the knee or to bear weight, then further examination of the injured knee is deferred until indicated radiographic examination has been carried out. Otherwise, physical examination continues with specific testing for ligamentous, musculotendinous, and meniscal injury.

TESTS FOR LIGAMENTOUS INSTABILITY. Testing the knee for instability is perhaps the most critical part of the examination. The decision to primarily repair a torn ligament is an urgent one. Results are compromised if repairs are delayed for more than a few days.

As with other aspects of the history and physical examination, positive findings are generally true positives, whereas negative findings may or may not be true negatives. Even with severe ligamentous injury, if there is any muscle spasm or guarding, the knee may falsely appear to be completely stable. Examination, which may be technically easy immediately after injury, becomes increasingly more difficult as pain, swelling, and muscle spasm increase over time.

A careful explanation of what is intended and a *gentle* approach are essential. Attempts to overpower a contracted muscle will cause more spasm, to say nothing of pain and distrust. Examination of the uninjured knee first provides a basis for comparison and helps prepare the athlete for examination of the injured knee.

The examiner's main task is to determine whether there is any *abnormal joint motion* and whether there is a *definite end point* of motion. Abnormal motion and the absence of a definite end point are the hallmark signs of grade III injury. A firm, definite end point, as opposed to a soft, indefinite one, differentiates grades I and II sprains from grade III sprains.

With grade II sprains there may or may not be any demonstrable abnormal motion. Also, especially with acute grade II sprains of the medial collateral ligament, and more so than with grade III sprains, ligament testing is likely to cause some pain localized to the injured structure.

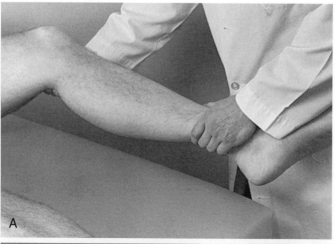

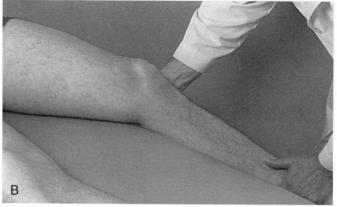

Figure 9–5. Technique of testing the medial collateral ligament. The thigh is supported and the knee is flexed to 20 or 30 degrees. Gentle valgus stress is applied by moving the leg laterally. *A,* Thigh supported by the examiner. *B,* Thigh supported by the examining table (often necessary with a large patient or a small examiner).

Medial/lateral instability is first tested with the knee extended as much as possible, and then with the knee in 20 to 30 degrees of flexion (Fig. 9–5). The examination is facilitated by having the athlete completely recline. The injured limb must be painlessly and securely supported to permit relaxation of the quadriceps and hamstring muscles. The examiner may hold the distal area of the thigh with one hand and the leg with the other, or allow the thigh to rest on the examination table, or hold the knee with two hands and the leg between the arm and the torso. Then, gentle valgus stress is applied. Rapid, jerky, or forceful manipulation precludes reliable examination. The examiner notes any abnormal motion, any pain produced, and the presence or absence of a definite end point. With the knee fully extended, any instability, i.e., abnormal motion compared with the uninjured side, implies severe capsular/ligamentous injury and is a clear indication for referral.

If flexion of the knee to 90 degrees is tolerated, anterior instability is assessed with the traditional *anterior drawer* test (Fig. 9–6). Although this test has recently fallen into disfavor because of the relatively high likelihood of "false negatives," the test is easier to perform than the Lachman test. If positive, the test establishes the diagnosis of a significant injury to the anterior cruciate ligament and eliminates the necessity of trying to perform the more difficult Lachman test. The knee in neutral rotation is flexed to 90 degrees. The examiner stabilizes the foot by sitting on it and confirms relaxation of the hamstring muscles by palpation. The examiner then gently pulls on the posterior aspect of the leg in an attempt to displace the tibia anteriorly on the

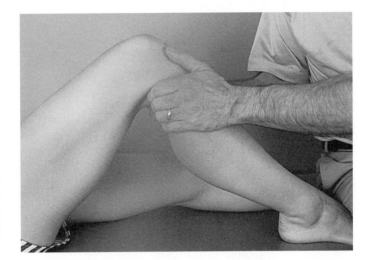

Figure 9–6. Anterior drawer test. The knee is flexed to 90 degrees, the foot stabilized beneath the examiner, and the tibia gently pulled forward. Note the examiner's fingers against the medial and lateral hamstring tendons to ensure relaxation.

femur. Any abnormal motion and the presence or absence of a definite end point are noted. The test is repeated with the knee externally and internally rotated. A positive test, in which there is abnormal motion without a definite end point, usually implies injury to the anterior cruciate ligament and to a meniscus or another of the secondary support structures. A negative test, in which there is no abnormal motion, does *not* rule out a torn anterior cruciate ligament.

Anterior instability is best assessed with the *Lachman test* (Fig. 9–7). As described by Torg and coworkers,

> The test is performed with the patient lying supine on the examining table with the involved extremity to the side of the examiner. With the involved extremity in slight external rotation and the knee held between full extension and 15 degrees of flexion, the femur is stabilized with one hand and firm pressure is applied to the posterior aspect of the proximal tibia, lifting it forward in an attempt to translate it anteriorly. The position of the examiner's hands is important in performing the test properly. One hand should firmly stabilize the femur, while the other grips the proximal tibia so that the thumb lies on the anteromedial joint margin. When an anteriorly directed force is applied by the palm and four fingers, anterior translation of the tibia in relationship to the femur can

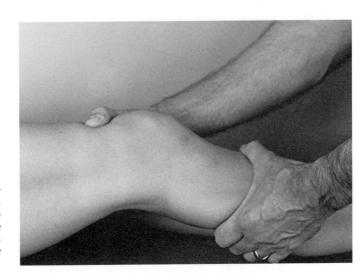

Figure 9–7. Lachman test for anterior cruciate ligament instability. The examiner stabilizes the thigh with one hand and with the other attempts to move the tibia gently forward from beneath the femoral condyles.

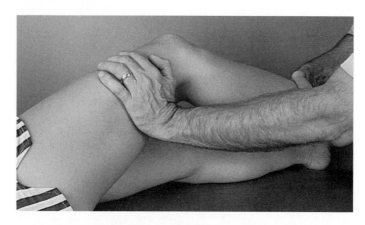

Figure 9–8. Pivot shift test for anterolateral rotatory instability (see text for description).

be palpated by the thumb. Anterior translation of the tibia associated with a soft or mushy end point indicates a positive test.[64]

The test is well tolerated by the acutely injured athlete, and it is the most sensitive and reproducible clinical test for anterior cruciate ligament instability.[14, 21, 31, 36, 41, 53, 64] It is probably the only reliable clinical test for diagnosing isolated acute anterior cruciate ligament sprains.

The *pivot shift test* is still another test for anterior instability or, more precisely, anterolateral rotatory instability (Fig. 9–8). The basis for the test is the fact that with anterior cruciate ligament deficiency, the lateral tibial plateau may abruptly subluxate anteriorly as the knee is extended or abruptly relocate as the knee is flexed.[18–20, 37, 57, 58] The test is described by Galway and associates as follows:

> *The leg is picked up at the ankle with one of the examiner's hands, and if the patient is holding the leg in extension, the knee is flexed by placing the heel of the other hand behind the fibula over the lateral head of the gastrocnemius. The patient must be completely relaxed. As the knee is extended, the tibia is supported on the lateral side with a slight valgus strain [sic] applied to it. The femur falls backward as the knee approaches extension, and the tibial plateau subluxes forward. This subluxation can be slightly increased by subtly rotating the tibia with the hand that is cradling the foot and ankle. A strong valgus force is placed on the knee by the upper hand. This prevents easy reduction as the tibia is flexed on the femur. At approximately 30 degrees of flexion, and occasionally more, the [anteriorly] displaced tibial plateau will suddenly reduce in a dramatic fashion. At this point, the patient [with recurrent instability episodes] will indicate that subluxation has occurred.*[19, 20]

The pivot shift test is a reasonably sensitive and specific test when the knee is examined under anesthesia.[31, 41] It is, however, not likely to be well tolerated or appreciated by the awake, acutely injured patient. In the primary care setting, its use is probably best limited to the work-up of chronic functional instability. It is discussed here mainly for the sake of completeness.

Posterior instability is assessed with the *posterior sag* and *posterior drawer* tests (Fig. 9–9). These tests are usually performed in conjunction with the anterior drawer test. The posterior sag test is performed as follows: With both of the patient's knees flexed to 90 degrees and viewed from the side, the anterior contours of both legs are compared. With posterior cruciate ligament tears the tibia tends to sag backward beneath the femur, and the prominence of the anterior tibial tubercle is lost. The posterior drawer test is performed

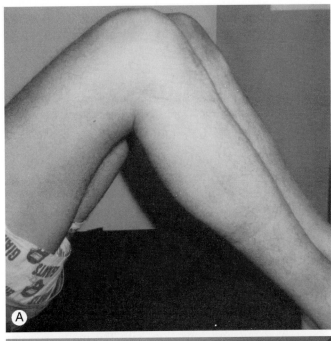

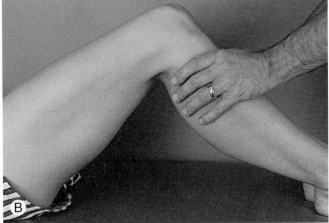

Figure 9–9. Tests for posterior cruciate ligament instability. *A*, Posterior sag test. This downhill skier sustained a hyperextension injury to the right knee. Note, on the right, the loss of the usual prominence of the anterior tibial tubercle and the "flat" profile of the patella, patellar tendon, and tibia. *B*, Posterior drawer test (see text for description).

identically to the anterior drawer test except that the examiner gently pushes on the anterior aspect of the leg in an attempt to displace the tibia posteriorly on the femur. The examiner must not confuse reduction of a "sagging," posteriorly subluxated tibia with a positive anterior drawer test. If either the posterior sag or posterior drawer test is positive, the examiner has an important obligation to rule out associated injury to the popliteal vessels and nerve.

TESTS FOR MENISCAL INJURY. As a rule, the need to know about acute meniscal injuries is less urgent than with acute ligamentous injuries. Many, perhaps most, torn menisci cause no further symptoms, degenerative joint disease, or other problems once the effects of the acute injury have subsided.[7, 12]

A notable exception is the injury, typically a bucket-handle tear of the medial meniscus, that is mechanically disrupting to normal knee function.

The locked knee merits prompt referral. Delay makes definitive treatment technically more difficult and needlessly prolongs the athlete's pain and downtime. Thus the first task with respect to acute meniscal injury is to determine the presence or absence of true locking (see earlier).

Another exception is combined meniscal and anterior cruciate ligament injury. Tears of the medial meniscus, especially, seem to increase the risk of chronic functional instability in the anterior-cruciate–deficient knee. A second diagnostic priority, therefore, is to confirm or rule out anterior cruciate ligament injury, as discussed earlier.

None of the tests that specifically attempt to reproduce the symptoms of meniscal impingement are likely to be very well tolerated by the acutely injured athlete. These tests have their greatest value in the work-up of recurrent impingement symptoms (see part I).

The simple *impingement test* that we describe here, which requires only 90 degrees of knee flexion, is the best tolerated of the group (Fig. 9–10). With the athlete supine and relaxed, the knee is flexed to 90 degrees. The athlete is then asked to let the knee flop to the inside, which opens the medial aspect of the joint. A fingertip is then pressed into the opened joint space, and the hip is abducted and the knee extended. Normally with this maneuver, the fingertip is painlessly pushed out of the joint by the intact meniscus. Pain or a catching sensation with the maneuver implies a medial meniscus lesion. The lateral meniscus is tested similarly, except that the athlete is asked to let the knee flop to the outside (the "figure-four position"), and the fingertip is pressed into the opened lateral joint space. This must be done gently, as it is possible to painfully displace even a normal lateral meniscus. The knee is then simply extended, and any pain or catching sensation is noted.

McMurray's test requires full flexion of the knee. We do not generally use or recommend it in the setting of acute injury but describe it here for the sake of completeness. The knee is gently but fully flexed, externally rotated, and then extended. One hand is used to control the leg and the other to palpate the medial joint line and to apply a slight varus stress to the knee. Pain and an audible or palpable click with this maneuver imply a lesion of the medial meniscus. The lateral meniscus is tested similarly, except that the knee is internally rotated, the lateral joint line is palpated, and slight valgus stress is applied.

Apley's grind test involves flexion to 90 degrees, rotation, and forcible compression of the tibia against the femur. In our opinion, it seems as likely to cause as to detect meniscal injury, and we do not recommend it in any setting. The same applies to "duck walking" and other unnecessarily draconian tests.

OTHER TESTS. The *patellar apprehension test* involves manual lateral displacement of the patella with the knee slightly flexed. A positive test, i.e., provocation of apprehension, might imply dislocation or subluxation of the patella; however, the test is usually impossible to perform in acute injury.

The diagnosis of acute musculotendinous injury by inspection, palpation, and specific muscle testing is rather straightforward. With complete rupture of the patellar tendon or transverse fracture of the patella, there may be a visible or palpable defect, or both, in the injured structure.

RADIOGRAPHIC EXAMINATION

Radiographic examination is indicated if there are any signs of severe injury, such as point tenderness over bone (especially in the skeletally immature),

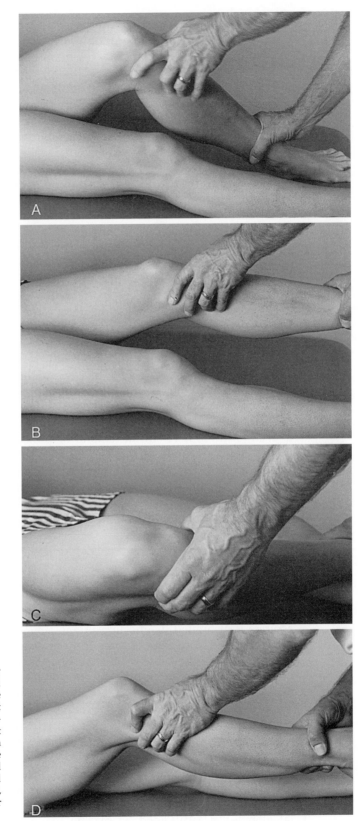

Figure 9–10. Simple tests for impingement of the medial and lateral menisci, respectively (see text for description). *A,* The joint is opened medially and a fingertip pressed into the opened joint space. *B,* The joint is closed with the finger pressing firmly on the meniscus. *C,* The joint is opened laterally and a fingertip pressed into the opened joint space. *D,* The joint is closed with the finger pressing firmly on the meniscus.

marked swelling and ecchymosis, and an inability to move the knee or to bear weight. Then anteroposterior and lateral views should be obtained "as is," without any manipulation of the injured knee.

"Decision rules" for the use of radiography in the acutely injured knee are being promulgated.[60] Any of the following is an indication for obtaining x-rays films on an acutely injured knee: (1) an age of 55 years or older, (2) tenderness at the head of the fibula, (3) isolated tenderness of the patella, (4) an inability to flex to 90 degrees, and (5) an inability to bear weight (for four steps) both immediately and in the emergency department.

If the clinical findings permit the diagnosis of isolated grade I or II sprains or strains, then radiographic examination is not required. Otherwise, standard anteroposterior and lateral views should be obtained to rule out intra-articular fractures, avulsion fractures at the attachments of tendons and ligaments, and the like. If the athlete can comfortably flex the knee, we also recommend "notch" and "sunrise" views to visualize the intercondylar notch area, the posterior aspects of the femoral condyles, and the patellofemoral joint. We do not routinely order or recommend oblique views, which are of little value except in localizing loose bodies or osteochondral fractures.

We believe that valgus stress views are seldom, if ever, indicated, especially in the primary care setting. In the skeletally mature individual with a medial collateral ligament sprain, even if it were possible exactly to document the physical examination radiographically, it is unnecessary to do so. Given the difficulty of stressing both knees and obtaining precisely comparable views, a few millimeters or degrees of difference in medial "opening" of the knee should hardly constitute a rationale for specific treatment. In the skeletally immature, an apparent medial collateral ligament injury may in fact be a fracture through the distal femoral or proximal tibial growth plate. Stress views, which essentially involve reproducing the injury, may indeed confirm the diagnosis, whereas standard views might not. However, unnecessary or repeated manipulation of the fracture may cause additional injury to the growth plate and is generally contraindicated. A decision to obtain stress views, rather than simply to treat the possible growth plate injury as such, is best left to an orthopedist.

OTHER DIAGNOSTIC TESTS

ARTHROCENTESIS. Arthrocentesis for the purpose of analyzing the joint aspirate is of limited diagnostic value in acute injury. Synovial fluid analysis is essential only to rule out septic or inflammatory arthritis, not a usual consideration in the acutely injured athlete. The presence of hemarthrosis, as opposed to simple synovial fluid effusion, can usually be surmised by the rapidity with which the swelling occurred. More importantly, the presence or absence of blood in the aspirate is not necessarily indicative of the severity of injury, and it is certainly not diagnostically specific.[11, 28] Bleeding into the joint is indeed characteristic of anterior cruciate ligament tears and patellar dislocation. It may also occur, however, with peripheral meniscal tears, capsular tears, osteochondral fractures, and simple contusion with synovial bleeding. Fat globules in the aspirate are characteristic of intra-articular fractures but may also (rarely) occur with synovial or fat pad injury. The presence of fat globules is ascertained by placing the aspirate in an emesis basin and putting it aside for a few minutes, allowing the globules to rise to the surface. The presence of fat globules is in itself an indication for referral and is the least expensive and (perhaps) most accurate screening test for an intra-articular fracture. Conversely, such severe injuries as complete tears of the medial collateral ligament may result in little or no effusion/hemarthrosis, as the joint capsule may be completely torn, allowing the joint fluid to leak into the soft tissues.

A possible indication for arthrocentesis may be to permit better examination of the acutely injured knee. Decompression of a large, tense, painful effusion and instillation of some local anesthetic should permit a greater range of motion and facilitate testing for ligamentous instability.

Asepsis and adequate local anesthesia are essential. A needle can usually be safely and easily inserted into the joint at a point 4 cm proximal to the joint line and 1 cm medial to the patella. Either a large-gauge needle or a plastic intravenous catheter may be used. The latter may be less traumatic to the articular cartilage. During introduction of the needle the suprapatellar pouch should be compressed in order to displace as much fluid as possible immediately beneath the aspiration site.

The pain relief provided by arthrocentesis is likely to be only temporary. The use of a longer-acting local anesthetic, e.g., 5 mL of 0.25% bupivacaine (Marcaine), helps. However, when the joint is aspirated, particularly during the first 24 hours after injury, the tamponade effect of the accumulated fluid is lost and the effusion/hemarthrosis tends to recur. Rest, ice, compression, and elevation, especially compression (Fig. 9–11), are essential after aspiration (see Initial Treatment).

Before attempting aspiration, it is especially important to have differentiated joint effusion from prepatellar bursitis (see Figs. 9–3 and 9–4). Acute, traumatic prepatellar bursitis is frequently septic and associated with an abrasion, cellulitis, or the like, whereas acute, traumatic knee effusions, unless associated with penetrating trauma, are almost always sterile. Unfortunately, we have seen cases of septic arthritis after ill-advised aspiration attempts in which a needle was inserted through an infected area into the knee joint.

MAGNETIC RESONANCE IMAGING. MRI undoubtedly provides more information than any other special noninvasive diagnostic test. The issue is, however, not how much information is *available* but how much is *needed*. We believe that *any* diagnostic test is valuable—or necessary—only when it provides information necessary or helpful in the treatment of the condition being studied. When the primary care practitioner manages acute knee injuries there are few indications for the use of this expensive procedure. The decision to refer can nearly always be based on the history and physical examination, leaving the decision to obtain an MRI in the hands of the treating orthopedic surgeon. For those conditions chosen to be treated by the primary care physician, information provided by an MRI will rarely influence management decisions.

ARTHROSCOPY AND EXAMINATION WITH ANESTHESIA. Arthroscopic examination is undoubtedly the single most accurate means of diagnosing an internal derangement of the knee. However, it is best considered complementary to, rather than a substitute for, careful clinical evaluation, standard radiographic examination, and so on. As with MRI, its greatest diagnostic value is in regard to meniscal lesions. Even in this regard, however, it is not perfectly diagnostic.[29, 61] It rarely produces false-positive results, but lesions, particularly of the posterior horn, are sometimes missed. The procedure is also expensive and not without potential complications.

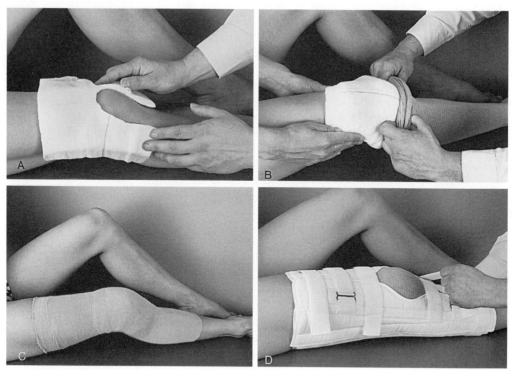

Figure 9–11. Application of a compression wrap and knee immobilizer. *A,* ABds or a horseshoe-shaped felt pad is placed just above and on each side of the patella. *B* and *C,* An elastic wrap or, preferably, elasticized stockinette (Tubi-Grip) is applied over the padding. The wrap should extend from below the calf to midthigh. *D,* A knee immobilizer is applied over the compression wrap. It may be necessary to bend the posterior stays or put some padding behind the knee so that the knee can be held in a position of comfort, i.e., 20 to 30 degrees of flexion.

Obviously the decision to examine the knee arthroscopically or under anesthesia rests mainly with the orthopedic surgeon. In our opinion, these, like other surgical procedures, should be undertaken selectively. In acute injury, we consider *mechanical disruption of normal knee function* to be the only *absolute indication for arthroscopy.*

INITIAL TREATMENT

As a rule, *knee dislocations and displaced fractures* should be padded and splinted "as is." In principle, such injuries should be reduced as quickly, gently, and safely as possible, particularly if there is any associated neurovascular impairment. However, because of the risk of causing further injury, reduction is best left to an orthopedist. Primary care is essentially aimed at preventing further injury.

A possible exception is the posterior dislocation of the knee complicated by occlusion of the popliteal artery. In this case, if no orthopedist is available, reduction may be attempted to restore arterial blood flow. This is achieved by applying gentle in-line traction on the leg and then lifting the proximal aspect of the tibia forward. It is important to assess and document the neurovascular status of the limb after any such attempt.

In most cases, *patellar dislocations* are spontaneously reduced at the time of injury as the athlete falls and the knee is extended. Occasionally, however, the patella remains laterally dislocated. In this case, reduction is achieved by extending the knee and then, if necessary, applying gentle, medially directed pressure.

After any severe injury, the knee must be protected. In most cases, this means using a *knee immobilizer*. The immobilizer should have stiff medial, lateral, and posterior stays. The posterior stays should be bent, or padding should be added, to allow the knee to be held in 20 to 30 degrees of flexion, the usual position of comfort (see Fig. 9–11).

Rest, ice, compression, and elevation are part of the initial treatment of all knee injuries. Rest may at first imply using both crutches and a knee immobilizer for ambulation. Non–weight-bearing crutch ambulation is advanced to partial weight-bearing ambulation with heel-to-toe gait as tolerated. Ice implies application of crushed ice for 20 minutes at least once every 4 waking hours. It can be applied over a compression wrap. Ice treatment is continued until the swelling stabilizes. As most knee immobilizers do not provide adequate compression, compression implies the application of a *compression wrap*. This consists of padding in the shape of an inverted horseshoe around the patella, held in place by a snug elastic wrap (see Fig. 9–11). Elevation implies keeping the injured knee at or above waist level at all times when the athlete is not actively using it, i.e., for ambulation. Both compression and elevation are continued until all swelling is resolved.

DECISION POINT: REFERRAL

Referral to an appropriate facility on an *emergent* basis is indicated for fractures or dislocations complicated by neurovascular impairment.

Orthopedic referral on an *urgent* basis is generally indicated for the definitive treatment of penetrating wounds of the knee, open or structurally significant fractures, grade III sprains, and mechanical disruption of normal knee function. Orthopedic referral is also indicated if the physical examination reveals any ligamentous instability, if radiographic examination reveals an avulsion fracture of either the femoral condyle or the anterior or lateral tibial plateau, or if the mechanism of injury or the symptoms are suggestive of severe ligamentous injury and this cannot be ruled out by physical examination.

This does not imply that all grade III sprains necessarily require acute operative intervention.[16, 24, 33, 39, 40, 45, 46, 64] Indeed, our present practice is to operate only if there is an associated meniscal injury resulting in a locked knee or if there is a bony avulsion of the distal attachment of the anterior cruciate ligament. Nevertheless, we believe that any severe ligamentous injury at least merits orthopedic evaluation to define the full extent of injury and to permit timely definitive treatment if necessary.

REHABILITATION

Rehabilitation begins with the initial treatment of the acute injury and continues until the athlete is fully recovered. Specific measures are used to achieve the following specific objectives: the prevention of swelling, the resolution of swelling, the restoration of motion, the restoration of strength, and the maintenance of fitness. Concomitantly there is gradual progression of functional use of the knee, during which time it must be appropriately protected from further injury. Decisions relating to the initiation and discontinuation of specific measures and to the progression of functional use of the knee are rather straightforward. They are depicted graphically in Figure 9–12 and further discussed later. There is some overlap as new exercises are added to, rather than substituted for, previous ones. Thus the time required for completion of the exercises increases as the athlete progresses through the program. Usually this does not pose any problem, for athletes are usually eager to do more and realize that as they are able to do more they are getting better.

The basic rehabilitation program described is generally applicable to almost all knee injuries and constitutes the definitive treatment for many. There are, however, some important injury-specific considerations.

As at the shoulder, the specifics of rehabilitation are largely determined by the presence and direction of any instability. Thus, for example, with anterior cruciate ligament deficiency, as dynamic control of the anterior instability is desired, hamstring as well as quadriceps strengthening is emphasized.

PREVENTION OF SWELLING. Measures to prevent swelling were discussed previously under Initial Treatment.

REDUCTION OF SWELLING. Measures to reduce swelling include relative rest, compression, elevation, ice, and electrogalvanic stimulation, contrast baths with active range-of-motion exercises, and anti-inflammatory medications. Those measures not already begun can be started as soon as the swelling

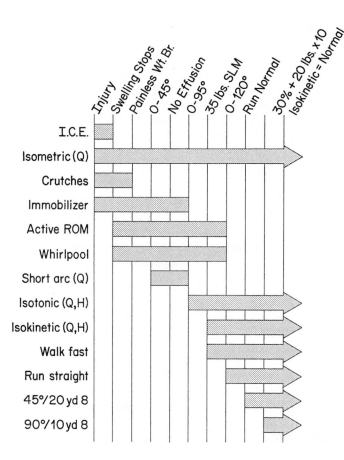

Figure 9–12. Basic knee rehabilitation program. Either knee extensions and hamstring curls or leg presses can be used for isotonic exercises. I.C.E., ice, compression, elevation; ROM, range of motion; Wt. Br., weight-bearing; SLM, single-lift maximum.

has stabilized, usually within 2 or 3 days after the injury. It is important to emphasize that active range-of-motion exercises be done during the warm phase of the contrast baths. These measures are continued until the swelling has resolved.

RESTORATION OF MOTION. Measures to restore motion are begun as soon as the swelling has stabilized. The knee is taken out of the immobilizer at least three or four times a day so that active range-of-motion exercises can be done. Initially the injured limb can be supported by the opposite limb when the patient is seated, by the table or bed when lying down, or by the buoyancy of water when in a whirlpool (Fig. 9–13). The knee is flexed to a point just short of discomfort, held in that position for 10 seconds, then extended as far as comfort allows, and again held for 10 seconds. This is repeated at least five times.

As a rule, range-of-motion exercises are continued until the full range of motion has been achieved (Figs. 9–14 and 9–15; see also Fig. 7–9). With anterior cruciate ligament sprains, however, no attempt is made to regain the terminal last few degrees of extension. This is because the ligament is under maximal tension as the knee is fully extended.

MAINTENANCE AND RESTORATION OF STRENGTH. Measures to maintain and restore strength are begun as soon as tolerated, usually when the athlete is first seen. Initially, isometric quad-setting exercises are used (Fig. 9–16).

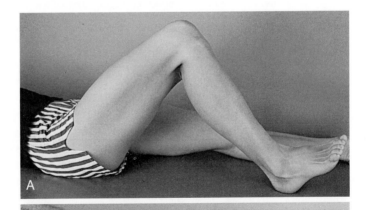

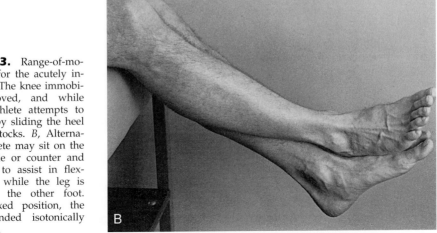

Figure 9–13. Range-of-motion exercises for the acutely injured knee. *A*, The knee immobilizer is removed, and while supine, the athlete attempts to flex the knee by sliding the heel up to the buttocks. *B*, Alternatively, the athlete may sit on the edge of a table or counter and allow gravity to assist in flexing the knee, while the leg is supported by the other foot. From the flexed position, the knee is extended isotonically against gravity.

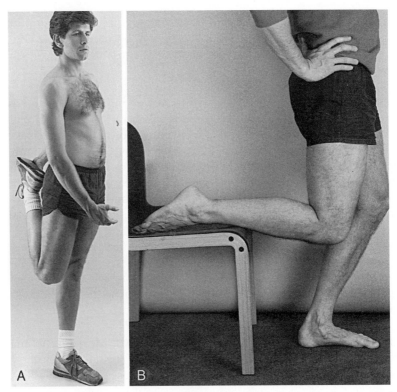

Figure 9–14. Quadriceps-stretching exercises. *A,* The foot is held with the opposite hand to prevent "cheating" by abducting the hip. The athlete is told to emphasize extending the hip rather than flexing the knee. The stretch should be felt in the anterior aspect of the thigh, not the knee. *B,* The chair stretch is used when the knee cannot be flexed far enough to allow grasping of the foot.

They may be done in or out of the immobilizer and are generally much more effective than straight-leg–raising exercises. Attention is directed to obtaining a good, strong contraction of the vastus medialis obliquus (VMO). The contractions are consecutively held for 6 to 10 seconds and released for 2 to 3 seconds. Two or three good (maximal) contractions at any one time are sufficient. These are repeated as often as the athlete thinks about it, at least twice every waking hour.

The athlete may find it more comfortable to do the isometrics with the knee slightly flexed rather than fully extended. This is permissible as long as the athlete can still maintain a good contraction of the VMO. It also usually allows the hamstrings as well as the quadriceps to be set. With anterior cruciate ligament injury, only flexed-knee quad sets should be done.

Occasionally, particularly with patellar dislocation, the athlete has difficulty doing the quad sets. If the athlete is still unable to obtain a good contraction of the VMO at 1 week after injury, we recommend the use of an electrical muscle stimulator (EMS) unit. A two-channel unit permits contraction of both the main bulk of the quadriceps and the VMO (Fig. 9–17). We prescribe the unit to be leased by athletes, which enables them to use it at home for the desired 2 hours a day.

Subsequently, usually as soon as swelling has stabilized, isotonic exercises are added and advanced as tolerated (Fig. 9–18). It is essential that all such exercises be performed within a pain-free range of motion and that there be

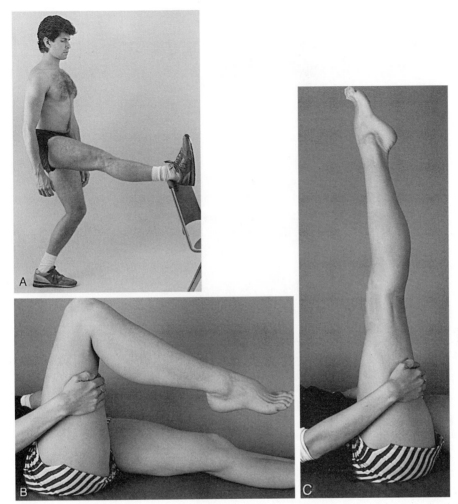

Figure 9–15. Hamstring-stretching exercises. *A*, Passive stretching. *B* and *C*, Active hamstring stretch using the quadriceps (resting and stretched positions, respectively). (Hamstring stretching is generally to be avoided with anterior cruciate ligament deficiency.)

no delayed pain or swelling. Leg presses are often better tolerated than knee extensions.

As with motion exercises, there are also certain injury-specific limitations. With vigorous, resisted contraction of the quadriceps, athletes tend to do a Lachman test on themselves.[52] Thus with anterior cruciate ligament injury, knee extensions should be done only within a limited arc of motion, i.e., from 90 degrees to 30 degrees of knee flexion, although single-leg leg presses can be done through a 90-degree to 0-degree arc of motion. Alternatively, shallow squats or leg presses may be done. Also, when doing hamstring curls, the athlete must protect the knee from being inadvertently snapped into full extension. With patellofemoral instability or pain, a patellar-supporting neoprene sleeve should be worn[38] (Fig. 9–19).

When the athlete is easily able to handle three sets of 20 repetitions of the strongest Theraband exercises, weight-lifting or isokinetic exercises can be started. Specific strengthening exercises are continued until desired injury- and sport-specific goals have been achieved.

It has been shown, in a prospective, blind study of high school football

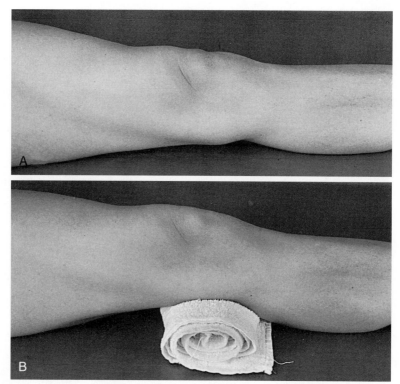

Figure 9–16. Isometric quadriceps exercises—quad sets. The vastus medialis obliquus may be palpated with the fingertips to ascertain a firm contraction. *A,* Knee extended. *B,* Knee slightly flexed. The athlete may be instructed to press the back of the knee into a rolled-up towel as shown.

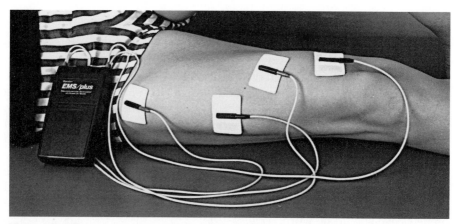

Figure 9–17. Two-channel electrical muscle stimulator unit applied so that both the bulk of the quadriceps (upper electrodes) and the vastus medialis obliquus (VMO) (lower electrodes) are stimulated. (A single-channel unit can be used for VMO-strengthening only.)

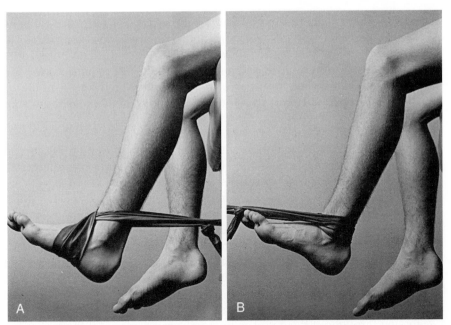

Figure 9–18. Theraband exercises for the quadriceps *(A)* and hamstrings *(B)*. (With anterior cruciate ligament injury, the quadriceps exercises are done only within an arc of 90 degrees to 30 degrees of knee flexion.)

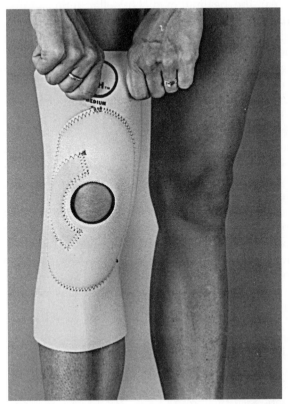

Figure 9–19. Patella-supporting neoprene sleeve. The C-shaped lateral pad stabilizes the patella.

players, that isokinetically measured right-to-left or quadriceps-to-hamstrings muscle imbalance of 10% or more does not predispose the athlete to knee injury.[25] As a practical matter, however, some reasonable end points of rehabilitation are required. On a single-leg maximal knee extension, for example, athletes should be able to lift at least 85% of the weight they can lift with the other leg. For contact and collision sports, the single-leg maximum should be at least 35% of body weight.

AMBULATION. Ambulation without crutches is permitted as soon as painless weight bearing is possible. However, the knee must be adequately protected as ambulation progresses (see Fig. 9–12).

Ambulation without a knee immobilizer is permitted when a good quad set can be demonstrated, little or no swelling (effusion) remains, and the knee can be nearly fully extended and flexed to more than 90 degrees without pain. At first, however, the patient should use crutches when going without the immobilizer. Completely unaided ambulation is not permitted until the athlete can also demonstrate a normal heel-to-toe gait and can lift at least 25 lb on a single-leg knee extension. Subsequently, increasing amounts of time without the immobilizer are permitted, starting in the morning and progressing throughout the day. The immobilizer is replaced if the athlete becomes fatigued or starts to limp.

Failure to heed these criteria risks re-injury, particularly in the case of patellar dislocation, in which a fall with forcible hyperflexion of the knee is likely to tear the healing medial patellar retinaculum. Also, allowing the athlete to limp risks secondary overuse problems, e.g., recurrent effusions, hamstring and Achilles tendinitis, low-back pain, and the like.

In the case of patellar dislocation or subluxation, when the immobilizer is no longer required a patellar-supporting neoprene sleeve is used (see Fig. 9–19). It is worn for all ambulation until there is no pain or apprehension with normal activities of daily living. Thereafter it is worn for all athletic activities for a minimum of 6 months after injury. Some athletes will continue to use it indefinitely.

Subsequently, ambulation is progressed by increasing first the cadence, then the length of the stride. A walk-jog-run program can be started when the athlete is able to walk briskly for at least ½ mile (see Chapter 2, part A). By this time the athlete is usually also able to cycle for ½ hour or longer. A reasonable predictor of the athlete's ability to start running is his or her ability to hop up and down on the injured side. It is usually apparent to the athlete that, if unable to do this, he or she is not yet ready to run.

We let the athlete start doing sprints, starts and stops, 20-yd figure of eights, and 45-degree cuts when a full (desired) pain-free range of motion and 85% strength have been achieved. This is advanced, as tolerated, to jumps, 10-yd figure of eights, and 90-degree cuts.

MAINTENANCE OF FITNESS. Measures to maintain fitness while the athlete's injury precludes the usual training regimen are begun as soon as tolerated. Strength of the uninvolved limbs can be maintained with appropriate weight training. Endurance fitness can be maintained or even improved with swimming or stationary cycling. As a rule, level I cycling can be started well before the athlete is able to run, or even to walk (see Chapter 1). With anterior cruciate injury especially, the athlete is instructed to "spin" in lower gears, rather than "push" against heavier resistance. The athlete is advanced to levels II and III as tolerated.

RETURN TO SPORTS PARTICIPATION

Ideally, return to sports participation is simply the final step in the sequence of rehabilitation. In our experience, sport-specific functional drills, e.g., figure-of-eight running, are the best predictors of the athlete's ability to resume the sport without undue risk of re-injury.

For the athlete whose sport makes lesser demands on the knee, a return to the sport can occur before completion of the full rehabilitation program discussed previously. However, for the athlete whose sport does place great demands on the knee, e.g., football, basketball, tennis, downhill skiing, completion of the entire program is strongly recommended.

With any substantial injury the physician should resist letting the athlete return to play prematurely. The risks and consequences of re-injury or further injury are too great. At best, it would only invite overuse problems and poor performance.

With grade III sprains of the anterior cruciate ligament and residual functional instability, use of one of the custom-made "derotational" braces may be required. With patellar dislocations and subluxations, a patellar-supporting neoprene sleeve is used for at least 6 months after injury, or longer if patellofemoral instability persists. In both cases, however, these appliances should be used in addition to, rather than as substitutes for, adequate rehabilitation.

In most cases of knee injuries in sports such as football, fixation of the foot on the ground is a necessary element in the mechanism of injury. Cleat penetration, and thus foot fixation, is enhanced by the lower number and greater length of cleats found on conventional football shoes. It has been shown that the risk of injury can be decreased by using multicleated, molded-sole, soccer-style shoes.[63]

C. MEDIAL COLLATERAL LIGAMENT SPRAINS

Medial collateral ligament sprains are among the most common knee injuries in sports. The medial collateral ligament can be injured alone or in combination with other structures. Combination injuries such as the unhappy triad of O'Donoghue (medial collateral ligament and anterior cruciate ligament sprains with a torn medial meniscus) are familiar to most physicians dealing with athletes. Other mixed injuries such as those involving a medial collateral ligament sprain and patellar dislocation are less familiar but may be no less common. Although some authorities suggest that the medial collateral ligament is never injured in a purely isolated fashion, the majority of the injuries can be managed as though they involve only this structure.

HISTORY

MECHANISM OF INJURY. The majority of medial collateral ligament sprains are the result of an outside force directed at the lateral aspect of the knee. This mechanism is best exemplified by the clipping injury in football—the sport most commonly associated with medial collateral ligament sprains.

Skiing is the only activity producing a significant number of medial collateral ligament sprains in which a blow to the lateral area of the knee is not involved. In this instance the ligament is injured by the valgus force produced by catching an inside edge and literally skiing away from the trapped foot.

The medial collateral ligament is also liable to overuse injury, a notable example of which is breaststroker's knee.[32, 34, 35, 54, 62]

SYMPTOMS. Pain in the medial aspect of the knee is the most common symptom. The pain is usually sharp and may be transient or lasting. In grade III sprains the pain often disappears within a minute, whereas the less severe injuries usually remain painful for longer periods. The absence of lasting discomfort accompanying grade III sprains often leads both the athlete and the examiner to underestimate the severity of the injury.

The pain may be located anywhere in the course of the ligament. It should be remembered that the medial collateral ligament extends from the adductor tubercle on the femur to well below the knee on the medial aspect of the tibia (see Fig. 9–2A).

Athletes with grade III sprains are often more impressed with *instability* than they are with discomfort. Indeed it is not uncommon for a football player or skier to attempt to continue participating, stopping only because the knee feels loose, it will not support the athlete, or it bends the wrong way. Complaints or comments suggesting *laxity* or *instability* should never go unheeded. In our experience, patients describing medial instability are rarely wrong.

Patients with grade II sprains may also note the presence of instability but are generally more impressed with the pain that accompanies any opening of the medial aspect of the knee. *Swelling* may be present in varied degrees. In the first 24 hours it is usually well localized over that portion of the ligament that was damaged. Swelling is a lesser symptom in these injuries.

PHYSICAL EXAMINATION

The most important aspect of the physical examination is *stability testing*. Stability testing should reveal the presence of abnormal motion and the existence or absence of an end point (see part B and Fig. 9–5).

The results of stability tests are valid only if the athlete is able to relax the quadriceps and hamstrings. "Attacking" the knee results in apprehension, pain, and reflex tightening of the muscles. Actively contracting the quadriceps and hamstring can make even the most grossly unstable knee "tight" during testing.

Tenderness may be present anywhere throughout the course of the ligament (see Fig. 9–2A). Maximal tenderness is usually located over the proximal 1 to 2 in. of the ligament—the most frequent site of injury.

Swelling is usually well localized at the site of maximal tenderness. After 24 hours a modest effusion may be present with grade I or II sprains. Large effusions are rarely seen even with the more severe injuries, as the capsule is often torn, allowing any collected fluid to leak into the soft tissues.

Motion is usually limited in both extension and flexion. Initially, motion is restricted by pain and muscle spasm; later, by soft tissue swelling or the presence of an effusion.

RADIOGRAPHIC EXAMINATION

In grade I or II sprains, radiographic study is unnecessary. Because subluxation of the knee occurred in the production of a grade III sprain, radiographs in both anteroposterior and lateral planes should be obtained to rule out intra-articular fractures or bony avulsions at the proximal attachment of the ligament.

We believe that valgus stress views are seldom, if ever, indicated, especially in the primary care setting. In the skeletally mature individual with a medial collateral ligament sprain, even were it exactly possible to document the physical examination, it is unnecessary to do so. In the skeletally immature, apparent medial collateral ligament injuries may in fact be fractures through the distal femoral or proximal tibial growth plates. These possible growth plate injuries can simply be treated as such or referred to an orthopedist who may or may not choose to obtain stress films to confirm the diagnosis (see part B for further discussion).

OTHER DIAGNOSTIC TESTS

Occasionally pain, swelling, and muscle spasm preclude the performance of accurate stability tests during the physical examination; thus an examination under anesthesia may be indicated. Usually this can be accomplished by injecting a few milliliters of local anesthetic into the area of maximal pain and tenderness 5 to 10 minutes before performing the stability test. (The injection should be done with the same sterile precautions used when aspirating the knee.)

INITIAL TREATMENT

Initial treatment should include application of *ice, focal compression, elevation, and avoidance of pain-producing activities. If the athlete is unable to ambulate comfortably—or demonstrates evidence of a painless grade III sprain—the knee should be placed in a knee immobilizer.* Since most immobilizers will not provide adequate compression, a compression wrap should be used also (see part B and Fig. 9–11).

Crutches may be necessary if weight bearing in the immobilizer produces pain.

It is our practice to start the administration of nonsteroidal anti-inflammatory medications as soon after injury as possible. Occasionally, in the case of an exceptionally painful grade I sprain, we prescribe a short course of oral corticosteroids. We use prednisone 15 mg four times a day for 2 days, 10 mg four times a day for 2 days, 10 mg twice a day for 2 days, and 5 mg twice a day for 2 days. We use this regimen only if we are sure there is no ligamentous laxity and the patient is compliant and can be trusted to carry out the rehabilitation program even if the knee becomes comfortable.

REFERRAL

All patients with *grade III sprains, coexisting injuries* (e.g., patellar dislocation, anterior cruciate ligament sprain, or meniscal injury), or *any attendant fracture* should be referred to an orthopedic surgeon.

DEFINITIVE TREATMENT

The treatment of the more severe medial collateral ligament injuries seems in a constant state of flux. Four decades ago all grade II and III medial collateral ligament sprains were treated nonsurgically with cast immobilization. O'Donoghue popularized the early surgical repair of grade III sprains, retaining a period of rigid (postoperative) immobilization.[47] Somewhat later, grade II sprains began to be managed by the earlier institution of rehabilitative efforts and shorter periods of immobilization until, at the present, these injuries are never rigidly immobilized.[13] The successes resulting from this treatment of incomplete ligament tears and mounting evidence that ligaments heal stronger and faster when not rigidly immobilized led to the practice of allowing early motion after surgical repairs and, most recently, the nonsurgical, aggressive rehabilitative approach to even grade III sprains.[16, 46]

Regardless of the severity of the sprain, management essentially consists of protecting the ligament until normal strength and motion have returned (see part B). The compression wrap and knee immobilizer are left in place, and icing (20 minutes every 2 to 4 hours) is continued until swelling has stabilized. Isometric quadriceps contractions, with the knee partially flexed, are started at the time of the first examination.

On the second or third postinjury day the immobilizer is removed three or four times to allow active range-of-motion exercises (see Fig. 9–13). Resisted (isotonic) exercises are also instituted through the comfortable range of motion. The resistance can be provided by a knee extension bench, Theraband, or surgical tubing. Three sets of 10 repetitions are done during each session (see Fig. 9–18).

As an alternative to the immobilizer, an adjustable, hinged knee brace can be used. Our practice is to adjust the hinge to allow slightly less than the painless range of motion. For example, if the knee can be flexed painlessly to 70 degrees, we would set the brace to stop at 50 degrees. Initially the brace can be locked at 10 degrees and thus serve as an immobilizer.

The knee brace or immobilizer is removed when pain-free motion is present between 5 and 100 degrees and the athlete is able to walk with a minimal or no limp. Allowing the patient unsupported ambulation in the face of a severe bent-knee limp invites recurrent effusions, calf pain and tightness, and low-back and hip discomfort—all conditions likely to severely compromise rehabilitation efforts.

The use of compression is continued until all swelling has disappeared. Usually the focal compression wrap can be replaced by a Tubi-Grip or neoprene sleeve when the immobilizer is discarded. Athletes may even continue to wear the sleeve after they return to participation.

Measures to maintain fitness while the athlete's injury precludes the usual training regimen are begun as soon as tolerated. The strength of the uninvolved limbs can be maintained with appropriate weight training. Endurance fitness can be maintained or even improved with swimming or stationary cycling. As a rule, level I cycling can be started well before the athlete is able to run, or even to walk (see Chapter 3, part D).

D. ANTERIOR CRUCIATE LIGAMENT SPRAINS

Sprains of the anterior cruciate ligament are surrounded by more controversy than any other sports injury. The injury is often exceedingly difficult to diagnose, and once diagnosed, there is some controversy regarding appropriate management. Our recommendation is that the primary care physician be thoroughly acquainted with the history and mechanism or mechanisms associated with this injury in order that a tentative diagnosis can be made and the athlete referred to an orthopedic surgeon.

Part of the confusion surrounding this injury stems from the fact that up until 20 years ago the most common test used to estimate the integrity of the anterior cruciate ligament—the drawer test—was grossly inaccurate.[64] This, coupled with the fact that the mechanism of injury is often reported as seemingly benign, led to gross underestimation of the frequency of occurrence and importance of the problem. Thus it is only within the past 2 decades or so that specific treatment regimens have been employed. In the majority of instances, the long-term efficacy of these many regimens still remains unknown.

HISTORY

MECHANISM OF INJURY. Although anterior cruciate ligament sprains have been reported as occurring in virtually every athletic activity, the largest numbers are sustained in the running/jumping sports. The injury is frequently seen in football, basketball, soccer, and gymnastics. The major exception to the running/jumping mechanism is skiing—a frequent cause of anterior cruciate ligament sprains.[4] There is increasingly compelling evidence that women and girls participating in sports such as basketball, soccer, gymnastics, and volleyball are significantly more likely to sustain anterior cruciate ligament injuries than their male counterparts.[2]

Among running activities the injury is usually reported as being the result of a cutting or turning maneuver or the result of abrupt deceleration. In jumping activities the injury is the result of "mislanding" or alighting in an awkward position. In skiing the history is usually of a twisting fall. Isolated sprains of the anterior cruciate ligament are almost never the result of contact or collision. Indeed, the mechanism often sounds so benign as to lull the examiner into dismissing the injury as a minor one. In virtually every reported study dealing with the management of chronic, recurrent injuries of the anterior cruciate ligament, the diagnosis was missed by the original treating physician—in as many as 90% of the instances in some reports.[44]

SYMPTOMS. The most important and consistent symptoms are a pop or snap and the knee abruptly "going out." Nearly always the athlete subsequently falls to the ground or floor.

Pain may be severe and lasting, minimal and transient, or anything in between. The pain is usually described as being located deep in the knee, but it may be at any specific location, most often anteriorly or laterally. The initial burst of pain is usually sharp. It may then become dull and aching or may disappear entirely.

Swelling, in the form of effusion or hemarthrosis, is usually present but may require 24 hours to become evident.

With attempts at weight bearing or ambulation or both, the athlete often describes a sense of ill-defined *instability.* This is frequently verbalized as the knee "not feeling right."

PHYSICAL EXAMINATION

The most significant, and perhaps only important, aspect of the physical examination is *stability testing* of the anterior cruciate ligament. The most discriminating and accurate test for the presence of anterior instability due to an anterior cruciate ligament sprain is the *Lachman test*.[64] Although this test is simply a drawer test performed with the knee flexed at 20 to 30 degrees rather than 90 degrees, it may be difficult to master. As with the classic drawer test, the hamstrings must be completely relaxed lest they hold the tibia posteriorly. The weight of the knee is supported by the examiner's upper hand beneath the distal aspect of the femur or by the examining table if the examination is performed with the leg off the side of the table (see Fig. 9–7). The lower hand then grasps and supports the upper leg while attempting to move the tibia *gently* forward from beneath the femoral condyles.

As with the drawer test, both the distance of abnormal anterior excursion and the presence and firmness of the end point are important in determining the presence and severity of the anterior cruciate ligament injury with the Lachman test. From the vantage point of the primary care physician, the Lachman test should be considered "positive" when, compared with the uninjured side, there is any perceptibly increased anterior excursion of the tibia or there is no definite end point.

The uninjured knee is examined first to allay the fears of the athlete as well as establish how much "normal instability" is present. The amount of anterior excursion is noted, as are the presence and sharpness of the end point. As with the evaluation of injuries of the medial collateral ligament the presence of a firm end point is as important as the amount of abnormal excursion. The test is then repeated on the injured knee.

Traditionally the *drawer test* was used to evaluate anterior and posterior stability of the knee (see Fig. 9–6). The athlete lies recumbent with the knees flexed at 90 degrees. This position is maintained by the examiner's sitting on the patient's feet, thus allowing the hamstring muscles to relax. The tibial tuberosities should be equally prominent. If one side is less prominent or flatter, it may be an indication of posterior instability (see Fig. 9–9). The upper area of the calf is then grasped by the examiner's hands and the upper aspect of the tibia gently pulled and pushed forward and backward. This maneuver should be performed *gently*.

A "positive" anterior drawer test—that is, abnormal forward excursion of the tibia with or without a firm end point—is indicative of a sprain of the anterior cruciate ligament. A "negative" drawer test means nothing! There is abundant evidence documenting the coexistence of grade II or III anterior cruciate ligament sprains and a negative drawer test. The anterior drawer test is of value mainly if it is positive.

Swelling in the form of an effusion/hemarthrosis is usually present if some hours have elapsed since the injury. A significant (i.e., ≥40 mL) effusion present within 24 hours of the injury is nearly always grossly bloody; thus aspiration should not be necessary to determine the character of the fluid.

Tenderness may be present anywhere about the knee. In our experience it is most commonly around the anterior portion of the tibial plateau, palpated on either side of the patellar tendon. Joint-line tenderness seems more common on the lateral side. Tenderness of the anterolateral tibial plateau, especially if accompanied by localized swelling, may indicate the presence of an avulsion fracture with the fracture fragment attached to the lateral capsule.

The *range of motion* is limited at the extremes. Nearly without exception the athlete is unable or unwilling to allow the knee to extend the last 10 to 20 degrees or flex beyond 90 degrees. The lack of extension may be so striking as to suggest that the knee is locked. Although meniscal tears commonly occur in conjunction with anterior cruciate ligament sprains, the lack of extension is usually not due to a fragment of meniscus caught in the anterior aspect of the joint.

RADIOGRAPHIC EXAMINATION

Anteroposterior and lateral radiographs should be obtained if a significant sprain of the anterior cruciate ligament is suspected. Fractures are uncommon but when present are not easily found on physical examination. Avulsion fractures of the lateral tibial plateau or tibial attachment of the anterior cruciate ligament are the most common.

MRI often allows visualization of the anterior cruciate ligament. We believe, however, that the Lachman test offers a much more accurate appraisal of the functional status of the knee and therefore do not routinely order MRI examinations.

OTHER DIAGNOSTIC TESTS

The most accurate appraisal of the status of the anterior cruciate ligament is obtained by arthroscopy. This technique not only allows visualization of tears, but an intact although lengthened ligament can also be identified by performing a Lachman test while viewing the ligament.

Arthroscopy is of value if the exact status of the ligament (i.e., completely or partially torn) is to determine the treatment regimen or if one seeks meniscal tears amenable to surgical repair. Suffice to say the role of arthroscopy in anterior cruciate ligament injuries is by no means uniformly formulated and should be left to the discretion of the orthopedic surgeon to whom the athlete is referred.

MRI can provide valuable insight into the status of both the cruciate ligaments and the menisci, although such insight may be of little value in structuring a program of initial management. The test is, however, expensive and, in our experience, less accurate than arthroscopy.

INITIAL TREATMENT

Initial treatment should include *rest,* the application of *ice, compression,* and *elevation,* with the knee comfortably flexed at about 20 degrees in a knee immobilizer. The athlete should be non–weight bearing with crutches.

REFERRAL

As noted previously, any of the following should raise the index of suspicion for anterior cruciate ligament injury: a deceleration, cutting, or jumping injury associated with a snap or pop; the knee's going out, causing the athlete to fall; the abrupt onset of the knee's feeling unstable; or the occurrence of significant swelling within the first 24 hours after injury. Orthopedic referral is indicated if the physical examination reveals any anterior laxity, if radiographic examination demonstrates a fracture of the anterior tibial plateau, or if the mechanism of injury or the symptoms are suggestive of a torn anterior cruciate ligament that cannot be ruled out by physical examination.

REHABILITATION

In several important respects, rehabilitation differs from that which is appropriate for other knee injuries (see part B). For example, aggressive hamstring stretching is avoided. Isometric quad sets are done with the knee slightly flexed rather than fully extended, and isometric quadriceps exercises are never undertaken in full extension against resistance. Isotonic and isokinetic quadriceps exercises, e.g., knee extensions, are limited to an arc of 90 degrees to 30 degrees of knee flexion and are never done at low speeds (<120 degrees per second). In cycling or using an exercycle, the athlete is instructed to spin in lower gears, rather than push against heavier resistance. Most importantly, the hamstrings are progressively strengthened through isometric, isotonic, isokinetic, and functional exercises.

DEFINITIVE TREATMENT

As evidenced by the number of procedures described for repair or reconstruction of the torn anterior cruciate ligament, the best way of treating this injury is yet to be determined. Indeed, there may not be a single best way of treating all such injuries and hence our recommendation that the athlete with an anterior cruciate–deficient knee be referred for orthopedic evaluation and treatment.

It seems clear, however, that primary repair of the anterior cruciate ligament with an intrasubstance tear is not effective and, at the time of this writing, all synthetic cruciate ligament substitutes have been doomed to failure. Thus if operative treatment is considered, the options are essentially limited to choosing a reconstructive procedure and deciding when to do it.

Proponents of primary reconstruction argue that restoration of mechanical stability is necessary to prevent progressive deterioration, recurrent instability episodes, meniscal tears, degenerative joint disease, and so on. However, mechanical stability does not necessarily imply normal function, particularly at such a complex joint as the knee. A fused knee, for example, is completely stable but not very functional. Daniel, in reporting the most comprehensive study of the consequences of anterior cruciate ligament sprains, notes that even those knees successfully reconstructed are no less likely to develop degenerative changes than those successfully treated nonoperatively.[9]

In our experience, about one third of patients with anterior cruciate ligament deficiency seem to do well with rehabilitation alone. Another third are unable to return to sports such as football, soccer, basketball, tennis, and downhill skiing without the use of a "derotational" brace of some sort, but they have little difficulty with other athletic, occupational, and daily activities. The remaining third are unable to resume their former level of activity, even with a brace and despite diligent rehabilitation. Some of these, however, may find a lesser level of activity acceptable.

Thus, we do not believe that a torn anterior cruciate ligament necessarily means the beginning of the end for the athlete's knee. Associated tears of the medial collateral ligament or medial meniscus do seem to imply a poor prognosis.[17] However, with isolated anterior cruciate ligament injuries, we are still unable to predict exactly who will do well and who will not.

Retrospectively, however, it has been shown which athletes with anterior cruciate–deficient knees have done well without operative intervention.[9, 65] By and large, those who have been able to return to athletics, who do not have functional instability, and who do not have long-term problems appear to be those who have learned to use their hamstring muscles automatically to compensate for their ligamentous deficiency. Such variable features as the severity of ligamentous laxity, pivot shift instability, and strength on isokinetic muscle testing do not correlate with long-term results.

Accordingly, our present approach to the athlete with an anterior cruciate injury emphasizes rehabilitation (see earlier). Newer rehabilitation techniques, such as teaching hamstring control of pivot shift instability, as is being done by Albright and coworkers,[1] seem to offer at least as much promise as do newer surgical techniques.

Our present practice is to operate on the acutely injured knee only if there is an associated meniscal injury resulting in a locked knee. In that case we do an arthroscopic examination and partial meniscectomy or meniscal repair as indicated. In a younger athlete, particularly one involved in "anterior cruciate ligament–intensive" activities such as basketball, soccer, volleyball, and gymnastics, who has intact menisci, we actively consider primary anterior cruciate ligament reconstruction once full motion has been regained and reactive synovitis has disappeared.

E. POSTERIOR CRUCIATE LIGAMENT SPRAINS

Posterior cruciate ligament sprains are relatively uncommon in sports. As is true with any ligament about the knee, the posterior cruciate ligament can be injured singly or in combination with other structures, although some authors suggest that the posterior cruciate ligament cannot be injured except in combination with other structures. Although this may be true in the strictest anatomical sense, from a practical clinical standpoint, injuries do occur in which there is no obvious evidence of involvement of structures other than the posterior cruciate ligament.

Most discussions of posterior cruciate ligament injuries center around complete tears (grade III sprains) of the ligament. Doubtless, as is true with any other ligament, grades I and II sprains far outnumber the more severe injuries. We suspect that the majority of these lesser sprains are diagnosed as hyperextension injuries and are thus never considered as posterior cruciate ligament sprains.

Because the role of the posterior cruciate ligament is somewhat controversial, the management of the more severe posterior cruciate ligament sprains is also less than well defined. Our philosophy of management is that surgical repair of (grade III) sprains is indicated only when nearly complete success of healing can be anticipated—a circumstance that exists only when an avulsion fracture of the tibial attachment has occurred. We manage the remainder of the injuries, regardless of their severity, with an aggressive rehabilitative approach. Our recommendations for referral, however, reflect our respect for the controversies surrounding the treatment of this injury.[8, 49, 51, 56]

HISTORY

MECHANISM OF INJURY. *Hyperextension* of the knee appears to be the most common mechanism of injury. This can be the result of a direct blow to the front of the knee or a misstep while running or jumping. In the former circumstance, the injury is seen in activities such as football, soccer, or other contact/collision sports; in the latter, it can be seen in any activity.

The injury can also result from a blow directed to the front of the upper part of the tibia with the knee flexed at 90 degrees, driving the tibia posteriorly beneath the femoral condyles. Although this mechanism is more often the result of striking the dashboard of an automobile, it is occasionally seen in athletic activities.

SYMPTOMS. With the more severe posterior cruciate ligament injuries, a pop or snap is usually heard or felt. Sprains of a less severe nature are usually accompanied by a sense of *stretching* in the posterior aspect of the knee.

Pain is posterior, often initially severe, but of variable duration. Because of concomitant posterior capsule and gastrocnemius stretching, attempts to extend the knee the last 20 degrees usually produce posterior pain. The knee *extension is limited.* Posterior knee pain may be the most consistent single symptom associated with injuries of the posterior cruciate ligament.

With grade III sprains, *effusion/hemarthrosis* usually occurs rapidly to a degree that the athlete is aware of *swelling.*

Although the more perceptive athlete may recognize a sense of *instability,* it is usually ill defined and unappreciated by most.

PHYSICAL EXAMINATION

An accurate assessment of *posterior instability* is the most important aspect of the physical examination. The *posterior sag and drawer tests* are performed with the patient supine with the hips flexed and the knees flexed to 90 degrees (see Fig. 9–9). The quadriceps must be allowed to relax. The examiner then views the profile of the front of the knees. The tibial tuberosities should be equally prominent. A flattening of the anterior contour of the knee indicates that the tibia has displaced posteriorly—impossible with an intact posterior cruciate ligament. This *sag sign* can also be demonstrated with both hips and knees flexed to 90 degrees and the athlete's feet held in the air by the examiner.

The drawer test is performed by grasping the upper part of the tibia and gently pushing and pulling the tibia backward and forward (see Fig. 9–9B). The amount of abnormal posterior excursion and the presence (or absence) of an end point are noted. Abnormal excursion and the absence of an end point indicate a grade III sprain; abnormal excursion with a firm end point suggests a grade II sprain.

It is essential that the examiner appreciate the position of the tibia before actually performing the test. If the tibia has sagged backward before the actual performance of the test, no additional posterior excursion will be possible, but the knee will displace forward to an abnormal degree, giving the impression of abnormal *anterior* instability. Actually what appears to be anterior instability is merely the tibia returning to its normal position.

Swelling and tenderness in the popliteal space (posterior aspect of the knee) and *effusion* are usually present with the more severe injuries.

Loss of motion, particularly extension, is nearly always present secondary to protective spasm of the gastrocnemius and hamstring muscles. Relaxation of these muscles reveals *abnormal hyperextension* in most grade II and III sprains.

RADIOGRAPHIC EXAMINATION

Radiographic study is indicated in the presence of demonstrable posterior instability, with a history of rapidly developing effusion/hemarthrosis, or with the presence of fat in the joint aspirate (which may be indicative of an intra-articular fracture). The region of the intercondylar eminence and posterior tibia must be carefully examined for evidence of an avulsion fracture.

OTHER DIAGNOSTIC TESTS

Although they are often unnecessary, if other diagnostic tests are required, MRI is probably the diagnostic procedure of choice owing to the difficulty of visualizing the posterior cruciate ligament through standard arthroscopic portals.

INITIAL TREATMENT

Initial treatment includes the application of *ice, focal compression*, and the use of a *knee immobilizer* bent to allow the knee to be stabilized in a position of comfort (see part B and Fig. 9–11). If painless ambulation is impossible, crutches should be used.

REFERRAL

Referral is indicated in the presence of measurable posterior instability or with radiographic evidence of fracture.

DEFINITIVE TREATMENT

Definitive treatment is focused on the re-establishment of normal or supranormal quadriceps strength. Contraction of the quadriceps muscle tends to displace the tibia anteriorly, i.e., reverse the posterior drawer sign. Conversely, hamstring muscle contraction displaces the tibia posteriorly. Thus the aim of the rehabilitation program is establishing quadriceps strength/function adequate to overpower the action of the hamstrings. In our experience this is usually possible and allows the return to most sports activities without surgical repair or reconstruction of the ligament.

Isometric quadriceps contractions are begun at the time of injury and continued throughout the entire rehabilitation program. Isotonic quadriceps exercises are instituted as soon as any painless range of motion is present. Single-leg maximal quadriceps strength goals should approach 30% to 40% of body weight regardless of the sport to which the athlete wishes to return. Hamstring strength is allowed to return spontaneously without specific exercises. Hamstring stretching is important and should be actively pursued, but hyperextension of the knee should be avoided.

With these exceptions, the standard knee rehabilitation programs should be followed (see part B).

F. LATERAL COLLATERAL LIGAMENT SPRAINS AND ASSOCIATED INJURIES

Among the four major ligaments of the knee, the lateral collateral ligament is the least important from the standpoint of stabilization. The biceps femoris, iliotibial band, and perhaps even the popliteal muscle all provide more of a stabilizing effect than the lateral collateral ligament. Injuries that truly compromise lateral stability of the knee often involve all these structures as well as the peroneal nerve, and thus they are very serious, with the potential of permanent disability.

Isolated sprains of the lateral collateral ligament are uncommon in most sports. Wrestling seems the only athletic activity in which isolated lateral collateral ligament injuries occur with any appreciable frequency, although the injury can be seen in an anecdotal fashion in any activity.

HISTORY

MECHANISM OF INJURY. Most isolated injuries of the lateral collateral ligament occur as a result of a blow directed at the medial side of the knee. This is a rare occurrence in most activities because the medial aspect of the knee is protected by the other leg. In wrestling, however, the opponent is often between the participant's legs and thus able to deliver the appropriate force to the medial surface of the knee. As a rule, isolated lateral collateral ligament injuries occur with the knee partially flexed; if the knee were fully extended a medially applied force would injure the other supporting structures as well.

Injuries of the lateral collateral ligament occasionally occur as the result of transmitted force such as a varus (adduction) thrust of the knee resulting from stepping into a hole or alighting off-balance from a jump.

SYMPTOMS. The athlete usually feels or hears a pop. The injury is accompanied by lateral *pain* that is usually initially sharp. The pain may last or disappear temporarily. *Instability* may be subtle and not impressive to the athlete. Swelling is usually neither immediate nor impressive.

PHYSICAL EXAMINATION

Swelling and tenderness are usually well localized over the ligament. Occasionally the tenderness is localized to the region of the head of the fibula—a possible indication of the presence of an avulsion fracture.

The most important part of the physical examination is determining the *integrity of the ligament*. This can be done by direct palpation. The patient lies supine, flexes the knee to 90 degrees, and places the lateral aspect of the ankle on the upper surface of the contralateral tibia. In this position the ligament can be palpated as a discrete, pencil-like structure running between the lateral femoral condyle and the head of the fibula. If the ligament is not palpable in this position one must assume it is torn.

RADIOGRAPHIC EXAMINATION

With evidence of a grade III sprain or well-localized tenderness over the head of the fibula, radiographs should be obtained in the anteroposterior and lateral planes. The head of the fibula should be carefully examined for any evidence of an avulsion fracture.

OTHER DIAGNOSTIC TESTS

Other diagnostic tests are not required.

INITIAL TREATMENT

Like the treatment provided for any acute soft tissue injury, initial treatment includes the application of *ice, focal compression,* and *rest* in the form of a *knee immobilizer* (see part B and Fig. 9–11). *Crutches* may be necessary for comfortable ambulation.

REFERRAL

Referral is indicated with grade III sprains, injuries suspected of involving other lateral supporting structures, or any evidence of peroneal nerve injury. Isolated grade III sprains of the lateral collateral ligament rarely merit surgical repair.

DEFINITIVE TREATMENT

Grade I and II sprains are treated with activity modification to relieve pain and an aggressive muscle-strengthening program emphasizing the quadriceps and lateral hamstrings (biceps femoris). Because full active extension of the knee often places painful tension on the ligament, isometric quadriceps exercise must often be undertaken in the bent-knee position.

The general guidelines for rehabilitation of the knee are followed throughout.

G. PATELLAR DISLOCATION

Dislocation of the patella is not one of the first conditions to come to mind when one considers acute athletic injuries involving the knee. Rather, the diagnosis of patellar dislocation produces visions of overweight, poorly muscled women with genu valgum (knock knees). Although these conditions are frequently associated with this injury, patellar dislocation is a real and frequently occurring injury in the athletic world.

Patellar dislocations are frequently associated with a number of biomechanical variations, including femoral anteversion, external tibial torsion, and genu valgum. In athletics the most frequent association may be with inadequate quadriceps strength, especially as it concerns the vastus medialis portion of that muscle. Frequently that strength deficiency is the result of inadequate rehabilitation of the quadriceps after a previous knee injury. Thus in some instances patellar dislocations may be almost unique among acute knee injuries in that they may be preventable.

HISTORY

MECHANISM OF INJURY. The mechanism of injury involves *external rotation of the leg, active contraction of the quadriceps, and extension of the knee.*

Patellar dislocations are self-induced injuries. These injuries are rarely the result of externally applied force but rather are the result of the "normal" action of the quadriceps. Extending the knee by contracting the quadriceps normally results in lateral displacement of the patella. This displacement is controlled and minimized by the buttress formed by the anterior aspect of the lateral femoral condyle, the counteracting pull of the vastus medialis, and the tethering effect of the medial retinaculum and patellofemoral ligaments.

When the tibia is externally rotated—as with cutting to the left off the planted right foot—the distal attachment of the quadriceps is moved farther laterally, increasing the tendency for the patella to displace in the same direction. As the knee extends, the lateral femoral condyle becomes less prominent, diminishing its effectiveness as a buttress. Although the injury usually occurs during weight bearing, dislocation can occur in midair, as in diving or gymnastics.

SYMPTOMS. The symptoms associated with the original dislocation of the patella are among the most spectacular seen with any knee injury. The athlete describes a tearing or ripping noise/sensation likened by one patient to the sound accompanying the disjointing of a chicken leg. The sound is often heard by other players—an important diagnostic point, as most knee injuries are heard only by the injured athlete. The more perceptive observers also describe something slipping out of place. Although the dislocation spontaneously reduces with the extension of the knee that nearly always occurs when the athlete falls to the ground, most are unaware that the reduction has occurred.

Swelling occurs rapidly because of the formation of a large hemarthrosis. The knee can become obviously swollen within minutes and often continues to swell until the overlying skin becomes taut and shiny. An area of ecchymosis is often noted in the area of the medial retinaculum.

The athlete is usually instantly *disabled*—unwilling or unable to move the knee, much less bear weight.

The symptoms are usually directly proportional to the excursion of the patella and inversely related to the frequency with which previous episodes have occurred. If the dislocation is but one in a series of many, or if the abnormal excursion is limited to only a few millimeters, all the associated symptoms may be lessened in magnitude but will nonetheless follow the same pattern.

PHYSICAL EXAMINATION

In the acute injury, one is faced with a *grossly swollen, tender, painful, extended knee*. Efforts to flex the knee are resisted by quadriceps spasm. Tenderness is most apparent over the medial retinaculum, with the point of maximal tenderness located at the superior aspect of the adductor tubercle (see Fig. 9–2E). The pain and swelling make it difficult to assess the integrity of the ligaments—important because the dislocation may occur in conjunction with sprains of the medial collateral ligament or anterior cruciate ligament, or both.

Often the presence of hemarthrosis is most apparent over the tear that has occurred in the medial retinaculum, giving the appearance of an elongated bulge adjacent to the medial side of the patella.

RADIOGRAPHIC EXAMINATION

Any injury resulting in the rapid production of massive swelling should be radiographed to rule out the presence of intra-articular fractures. A failure of spontaneous reduction of the dislocated patella is often the result of an intra-articular fracture of the articular surface of the patella or lateral femoral condyle. The examination should include anteroposterior, lateral, sunset, and notch views.

OTHER DIAGNOSTIC TESTS

Aspiration of the knee and examination of the aspirate for the presence of fat may be indicated to rule out the presence of an intra-articular fracture. Either computed tomography or MRI may be helpful in documenting the presence of intra-articular fractures or loose fracture fragments.

INITIAL TREATMENT

Application of *ice, focal compression, immobilization, rest, and elevation* are indicated. Even a well-applied compression wrap may fail to thwart the swelling. Any signs of painful constriction should prompt loosening of the wrap and immobilizer (see part B and Fig. 9–11).

Aspiration may be necessary for the relief of pain (see part B). If possible, it should be avoided for at least 24 hours lest hemarthrosis recur. Adequate compression after aspiration is imperative regardless of when the aspiration is carried out.

REFERRAL

Our practice is to operate on initial patellar dislocations *only* in the presence of a significant intra-articular fracture. Thus, we suggest referral under those circumstances. Referral is also indicated for dislocations that continue to recur in spite of rehabilitative efforts and the use of a sleeve.

DEFINITIVE TREATMENT

Treatment of patellar dislocations is aimed at re-establishing quadriceps (vastus medialis) strength while protecting the knee against subsequent dislocations.

Isometric quadriceps exercises are begun as soon as possible (see part B and Fig. 9–16). It is often difficult and painful for the athlete to produce a contraction that involves the vastus medialis. If a substantial quadriceps contraction is not present at 1 week, we begin the use of an EMS unit. A two-channel unit allows contraction of both the main bulk of the quadriceps and the vastus medialis (see Fig. 9–17). We prescribe the unit to be leased by the patient so that it might be used for up to 2 hours a day.

Active range-of-motion exercises are started at 1 week. The athlete removes the splint and, while supine, attempts to flex the knee by drawing the heel to the buttock (see Fig. 9–13A). If this fails to result in knee flexion, the athlete sits on the edge of a table or counter, allowing gravity to assist knee flexion while partially supporting the leg with the other foot (see Fig. 9–13B). From the flexed position the knee is extended isotonically against gravity.

A hinged knee brace can be substituted for the knee immobilizer at 1 week. The hinge is set to allow full extension but to block flexion just short of what can be comfortably accomplished (e.g., painless, active knee flexion of 60 degrees; hinge set to block flexion beyond 50 degrees.) The knee immobilizer or hinged brace is used for ambulation until 100 degrees of painless flexion is present, there is no effusion, the single-leg maximum for the quadriceps is at least 25 lb, and a normal heel-to-toe gait is possible. Patients are allowed to practice without the splint but with the aid of crutches. If unsupported and unprotected weight bearing is allowed before achievement of these goals, the athlete inevitably falls, hyperflexing the knee and tearing the (healing) medial retinaculum.

Patients are allowed increasing amounts of time without the immobilizer or brace, starting in the morning and progressing throughout the day. The device is replaced when fatigue or a limp becomes apparent. The immobilizer or brace is replaced with a neoprene sleeve with a lateral pad (see Fig. 9–19). The sleeve is worn during all ambulation until normal, painless activities of daily living are possible. Thereafter it is worn during all athletic activities for a minimum of 6 months. Many athletes choose to continue using the sleeve indefinitely.

H. PREPATELLAR BURSITIS

Falls on the anterior aspect of the knee often result in injury to the prepatellar bursa. Hemorrhage into the bursa results in inflammation of its walls and subsequent production of fluid. Repeated trauma to the fluid-filled, tense bursal sac leads to enlargement and occasionally rupture. Even though prepatellar bursitis does not involve the knee joint per se, the joint may enlarge to a point at which knee function is compromised. More commonly the patient appears for treatment because the condition is a tender, painful, unsightly annoyance.

This condition achieves true *clinical significance* under two circumstances: (1) when the bursa becomes infected as the result of an adjacent break in the skin or (2) when the fluid-filled bursa is mistaken for the presence of an effusion.

HISTORY

MECHANISM OF INJURY. Located between the skin and subcutaneous surface of the patella, the prepatellar bursa is vulnerable to any direct trauma to the anterior aspect of the knee. This trauma can be acute, as with a *direct blow* to the knee, or chronic, as seen with recurrent episodes of local pressure and *friction* (housemaid's knee).

The initial episode is usually a fall on the anterior aspect of the flexed knee. The problem occurs most often in wrestling, but it is also seen in other contact sports such as football.[43] Although the rate of occurrence may be diminished by the use of knee pads, these devices—in their current state of design—obviously do not offer complete protection.

As the condition becomes chronic, episodes of bursal swelling occur with progressively less trauma. With each episode the bursa enlarges.

Abrasions (turf burns, road rash, and the like), *lacerations, and puncture wounds* (including those rendered by needle and syringe) can result in septic bursitis. Turf burns about the knee are commonly seen in football and indoor soccer, both of which are frequently played on synthetic turf. These abrasions are often ignored, become secondarily infected, and thus pose a threat to the underlying inflamed bursa.

SYMPTOMS. The primary complaint is of a *discrete, swollen mass* on the anterior aspect of the knee. After the initial episode of trauma, the swelling may occur rapidly, within minutes, or more slowly, over a 24-hour period. *Pain*, although usually not severe enough to be debilitating, is proportional to the rapidity with which the swelling occurs and to the size attained. Usually athletes seek care because they fear that the injury has involved the knee joint.

Between acute episodes the athlete often notes the presence of subcutaneous masses or irregularities on the anterior aspect of the knee. Although these represent only the swollen, folded walls of the collapsed bursa, they are often perceived as loose bodies within the knee.

PHYSICAL EXAMINATION

During acute episodes the bursa is noted as a swollen, variably tender mass usually overlying the patella. Unlike the situation in effusion of the knee or subcutaneous hematoma, the margins of the mass are well defined (see Fig. 9–4). Pressure on one side of the mass brings into sharp contrast the confines of the opposite side. Partial flexion of the knee renders the outlines of the bursa even more distinct. Even if the bursa is decompressed, its thickened outlines are usually readily palpable.

The mass may transilluminate, especially in chronic cases when the sac is filled with clear fluid rather than blood. Knee motion should be normal except in the occasional instance in which the bursa is so large as to limit flexion.

There may also be signs of infection—erythema, calor, touch-me-not tenderness, purulent exudate, cellulitis, lymphangitis, lymphadenopathy. Usually these are found in association with some disruption of the integument, as an abrasion or laceration.

RADIOGRAPHIC EXAMINATION

Radiographic study is not necessary.

OTHER DIAGNOSTIC TESTS

Other diagnostic tests are not required unless there are symptoms or signs of infection, in which case aspiration of the bursa, with Gram's stain, culture, and sensitivity studies of the aspirate, is indicated.

INITIAL TREATMENT

Aspiration can be both diagnostic and therapeutic and is indicated if the clinical findings are consistent with acute hemorrhage, infection, or long-standing inflammation. The bursa is aspirated under sterile conditions, care being taken not to introduce the needle into the bursa through an area of skin abrasion (contamination) or infection. The needle (18 gauge) should enter the skin 2 or 3 cm from the wall of the bursa lest a fistula develop. Unless there is evidence of infection, the knee is then placed in a focal compression wrap and a knee immobilizer. The immobilizer is worn for 3 to 5 days, and the compression wrap is worn for at least 2 weeks. During the first 48 hours, the compression wrap should not be removed even for the application of ice.

If there is evidence of infection, additional treatment comprises the use of warm soaks four times a day, repeated aspirations as necessary, and the administration of specific antibiotics. Pending the results of the culture and sensitivity tests, we usually begin antibiotic therapy with cephalexin 500 mg four times a day.

REFERRAL

If infection does not respond promptly to treatment or if there is persistent inflammation, recurrent fluid accumulation, progressive enlargement of the bursa, and so on, despite appropriate initial treatment, referral is indicated.

DEFINITIVE TREATMENT

Treatment beyond that described previously, or referral, is necessary only with recurrent accumulations of fluid within the bursa. In these instances the fluid should be aspirated under sterile precautions. After the aspiration the needle should be left in place and used to inject one of the cortisone preparations. We use 1 mL of betamethasone mixed with 3 mL of 0.25% bupivacaine with epinephrine. The knee is then placed in a compression wrap and an immobilizer for a minimum of 1 week. The wrap and immobilizer are worn *at all times*, even during showering.

Knee pads are subsequently worn during athletic activities, especially those entailing a high risk of falling on the knees. A knee sleeve with double-thickness neoprene anteriorly is often easier to keep in place than the traditional knee pads and can be used as added protection worn beneath the standard knee pad provided with a football uniform.

I. IMPINGEMENT SYNDROMES

Impingement syndromes are due to prevention of the normal motion of the knee by a mechanical block. The block can occur in either the patellofemoral or tibiofemoral portion of the joint. The various causes of impingement include loose bodies, a fold of synovium (plica), or meniscal fragments—the last being by far the most common.

Because of the lack of precision with which many describe their complaints, true impingement must be differentiated from pseudoimpingement. What is often described as "catching" may actually be a momentary episode of instability due to weakness (see part K).

Impingement (or locking) may be momentary or prolonged. Prolonged, true locking, as might be seen with a displaced bucket-handle tear of the medial meniscus, is an uncommon condition. More often, painful, momentary impingement results in hamstring muscle spasm with a resultant inability to extend the knee.

The ability to recognize the presence of true impingement is particularly important, as this diagnosis usually carries with it the necessity for surgical intervention. The athlete with recurrent episodes of impingement is at risk not only of sustaining other injuries as a result of impingement-caused falls, but also of sustaining irreparable damage to the joint surfaces.

HISTORY

MECHANISM OF INJURY. The initial impingement episode associated with the acute tearing of a meniscus is usually obvious and easily recalled by the athlete. Acute meniscal tears are almost always the result of a combination of rotation (twisting) and *weight bearing*. A cutting maneuver in running sports (Fig. 9–20) is often the cause of a medial meniscus tear. Lateral meniscus injuries are more likely to occur while the knee is acutely flexed as in a squatting position—common in wrestlers (Fig. 9–21).

With advancing age the menisci become less resilient and more easily damaged. Thus the episode heralding the onset of a symptomatic meniscal tear in a 40-year-old tennis player may appear inappropriately benign.

Once a meniscus is torn, subsequent impingement episodes may occur in the absence of weight bearing. Sitting in the lotus position or merely

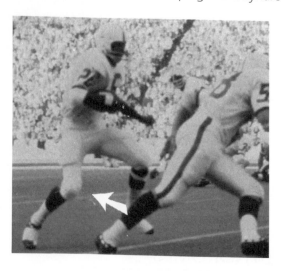

Figure 9–20. Medial meniscus injury is often associated with cutting maneuvers in football (right knee of ball carrier, arrow).

crossing the knees (Fig. 9–22) may be enough to displace the meniscus. Often getting out of a car results in impingement.

Impingement resulting from the presence of a loose body is much less predictable than that seen with meniscal injuries. Loose bodies can become momentarily trapped during virtually any activity but usually not in a reproducible manner. These episodes can occur during straight-ahead walking or merely arising from a chair. The hallmarks of loose-body impingement are the *absence of an obviously traumatic onset and the nonpredictability of recurrences.*

Impingement resulting from the presence of a thickened fold of synovium (plica) is usually very predictable.[5, 26, 42, 50] The symptoms occur at a certain point in the range of motion, usually between 30 and 60 degrees of flexion. Thus a cyclist will complain of pain at two distinct points on the pedal cycle, once on the downstroke as the knee is extended and again on the upstroke as the knee is flexed. The onset of symptoms is usually insidious, and the symptoms at first are easily confused with typical patellofemoral pain. In our experience, in sports other than cycling, the "pathological plica" is a rare condition and tends to be overdiagnosed.

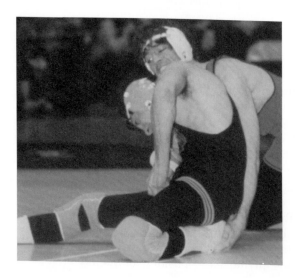

Figure 9–21. Weight bearing, rotation, and hyperflexion (left knee of wrestler in foreground) are often associated with injury to the lateral meniscus.

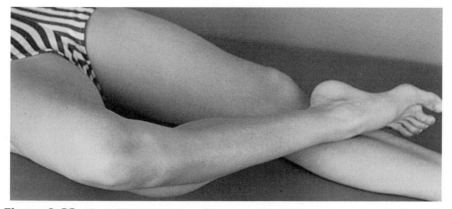

Figure 9–22. The half-lotus position often prompts impingement symptoms in the athlete with a torn medial meniscus.

SYMPTOMS. *Sudden, sharp pain* is the characteristic symptom of most forms of impingement. The pain may be the predictable consequence of the assumption of a particular posture or position of the knee, as seen with meniscus injuries, or it may be unpredictable, as in the case of loose bodies.

True locking—prolonged impingement—is distinguished by the necessity for *unlocking*. The athlete usually describes the knee as becoming abruptly and painfully locked and incapable of being fully extended. Manipulation—pulling, twisting, or jiggling—results in equally abrupt resumption of normal motion. A loss of flexion is almost never the result of true locking.

The location of the impingement within the knee may or may not be precisely described. Our experience is that if the patients are able to point to the site of the impingement, they are usually correct in its localization. The converse is not true. For example, inability of the athlete to localize the site of catching to the medial aspect of the knee does not rule out the possibility of a medial meniscus tear.

The description of "something floating" in the knee is almost always an accurate appraisal of the situation. This complaint should be assumed to indicate the presence of a loose body until proved otherwise. Often the athlete has learned to trap the loose body beneath the medial or lateral retinaculum and is thus able to demonstrate its presence to the examiner.

Impingement episodes may or may not be followed by continued pain or the presence of an effusion. Neither symptom is of particular value in establishing a definitive diagnosis.

PHYSICAL EXAMINATION

The most reliable finding on physical examination is *reproduction of the impingement episode* (see part B). In view of the fact that these episodes are often quite painful, it seems to us a bit draconian to force such an episode on an athlete when, in the majority of instances, the athlete is fully capable of describing it in very precise and colorful terms. Thus we do not routinely employ the various provocative tests (McMurray-type tests). These tests are designed to place the knee in a position that encourages the torn portion of the meniscus to become trapped between the articular surfaces of the tibia and femur. Aside from the fact that one is occasionally unable to subsequently unlock the joint, the tests often require that the knee be fully flexed—a position strenuously avoided by most patients with meniscal disorder.

We employ a more gentle impingement test that we believe is more discerning than the traditional provocative maneuvers. With the patient relaxed, the knee is flexed to 90 degrees. The thigh is then adducted (see Fig. 9–10) to open the medial aspect of the joint. A fingertip is then pressed into the open joint space while the thigh is abducted and the knee extended. Normally the fingertip is painlessly pushed out of the joint by the intact meniscus. If the maneuver is painful or accompanied by the catching sensation, the test is positive, indicating a medial meniscus lesion.

Integrity of the lateral meniscus is tested in a similar fashion but in the opposite direction. The lateral impingement can also be accomplished by placing the patient in the figure-four position (see Fig. 9–22) and then pushing the finger into the opened lateral joint space. The knee is merely extended from this position to close the joint. Pressure on the meniscus should be gentle, as it is possible to painfully displace even a normal lateral meniscus.

Tenderness over the respective joint line may be indicative of meniscal lesions. Tenderness of the medial retinaculum during flexion and extension of the knee might suggest the presence of a pathological plica. Tenderness of the weight-bearing portion of the medial femoral condyle is often found in the presence of osteochondrosis dissecans—the most frequent source of osteochondral loose bodies—or osteonecrosis in the older female patient.

RADIOGRAPHIC EXAMINATION

Standard radiographs should be obtained in the presence of clinical evidence of impingement. The notch view is particularly important, as it allows viewing of the contour of the posterior portion of the femoral condyles—the site of the majority of osteochondrosis dissecans lesions.

OTHER DIAGNOSTIC TESTS

Arthrotomograms are frequently helpful in determining the status of osteochondrosis dissecans lesions, particularly regarding the integrity of the overlying articular cartilage.

MRI may be very helpful in identifying both meniscal tears and osteochondrosis dissecans lesions. In our experience, however, displaced meniscal tears are frequently missed. Thus positive studies are of value but negative exams should be viewed with caution.

Arthroscopy now plays the major role in the diagnosis and treatment of impingement problems. The availability of arthroscopy, however, should not preclude the use of MRI, as this technique can often be used in a complementary fashion. In the absence of a truly locked knee, we now frequently employ MRI in an attempt to identify obvious meniscal tears. If none is found, or if such tears are located far at the periphery of the meniscus, we often institute a vigorous rehabilitation program, observing closely for recurrent effusions, pain, or evidence of impingement.

Although arthroscopy is the gold standard of diagnostic tests, it is more invasive and appreciably more expensive than the other diagnostic techniques. We reserve arthroscopy for cases in which the findings, whether abnormal or normal, will result in substantial alterations in treatment regimens.

INITIAL TREATMENT

If the knee is truly locked, it should be placed in an immobilizer that is bent to allow the knee to be rested in a position of comfort. Gentle manipulation can be attempted in the presence of true locking.

REFERRAL

The diagnosis of true impingement is an indication for referral to an orthopedic surgeon. If the knee is locked, referral should be undertaken with some urgency, as prolonging the time until operative intervention leads to chronic synovitis, substantial strength loss, and needless prolongation of the rehabilitation period.

DEFINITIVE TREATMENT

Definitive treatment usually calls for removal of the torn portion of the meniscus or the loose body if a definite pattern of impingement has been established. A single apparent impingement episode at the time of acute injury is not in itself an indication for arthroscopy. General knee rehabilitation is carried out postoperatively in a fashion similar to that following an acute injury.

J.   CHRONIC ANTERIOR KNEE PAIN

Chronic knee pain among athletes usually stems from either extensor mechanism problems or degenerative joint disease. Occasionally the pain accompanying an acute injury such as a grade I or II sprain of the medial collateral ligament lasts longer than anticipated, but usually, if properly managed, the discomfort associated with acute injuries is self-limited and disappears in a few weeks.

This discussion centers on three conditions: patellofemoral dysfunction, patellar tendinitis, and Osgood-Schlatter disease. The first of these conditions is most prevalent and variously referred to as *chondromalacia patellae, patellar subluxation, runner's knee, patellar compression syndrome,* or *quadriceps insufficiency syndrome.* The other two are actually forms of patellar tendinitis—Osgood-Schlatter disease occurring at the distal insertion of the tendon of the skeletally immature athlete. Even though there may be subtle differences among these conditions, they can be grouped together because their presentation and management are similar in the vast majority of instances.

To understand these conditions one must recall the anatomy of the extensor mechanism, particularly that of the vastus medialis (see Fig. 9–24). The vastus medialis is the smallest of the four components of the quadriceps, but because of its direction of pull, it is the most important from the standpoint of positioning and stabilizing the patella. Vastus medialis atrophy seems common to all these problems. Whether it is a cause or a result of the symptoms is unknown, and perhaps not important, as vastus medialis re-strengthening is usually associated with successful treatment of any of the conditions.

Osgood-Schlatter disease is probably inappropriately described as a disease. It is, rather, an overuse problem involving the insertion of a tendon into a growth center or traction apophysis.

HISTORY

MECHANISM OF INJURY. All these conditions are overuse syndromes (see Chapter 3), and, as such, their onset is gradual and usually associated with a change in activity or the athletic environment. Patellofemoral dysfunction is most often the result of involvement in a new activity (beginning aerobic dance classes or the start of soccer season), while patellar tendinitis seems more frequently associated with repetitious activities. Patellofemoral dysfunction is seen in virtually any sport but most often in running, dance forms, gymnastics, and figure skating. Patellar tendinitis was first described in high jumpers (hence the term *jumper's knee*) but is nearly endemic in basketball players. Patellofemoral dysfunction occurs more frequently in females; patellar tendinitis and Osgood-Schlatter disease, in males.

Any of the mechanisms of injury found associated with patellofemoral dysfunction or patellar tendinitis may also be found in Osgood-Schlatter disease. In addition, Osgood-Schlatter disease often occurs during or shortly after a growth spurt. By definition, Osgood-Schlatter disease occurs only in the skeletally immature, although the residually prominent tibial tuberosity may be associated with symptoms years after epiphyseal closure.

Patellofemoral dysfunction is often noted as the residual of an acute knee injury, usually the result of a return to athletic activity before adequate quadriceps restrengthening. Conversely, any of these conditions can result from inappropriate quadriceps rehabilitative or strengthening exercises. The most common example is attempting to perform heavily weighted isotonic quadriceps exercises or knee extensions before the development of a vastus medialis adequate to stabilize the patella.

The environment appears to play a role in all three conditions. Running or jumping on hard surfaces, such as cement floors or synthetic turf, is viewed as being associated with all three conditions although definitive evidence of a relationship between playing surfaces and knee complaints is lacking. Ascending or descending hills or stairs often prompts the symptoms of patellofemoral dysfunction. Osgood-Schlatter disease is often seen in gifted young athletes. The condition is not the result of possession of well-developed musculoskeletal skills, but rather of the fact that athletes possessing these skills are in high demand and thus often spend more time at risk than their less-talented peers.

Abnormal, or at least idiosyncratic, biomechanics also predisposes to these conditions.[6, 55] For example, the distance runner with "malicious mal-alignment" (i.e., femoral anteversion, external tibial torsion, and pronation), the ballet dancer who forces turnout, or the cyclist whose cleat positions do not correlate with his or her tibial torsion are all candidates for patellofemoral dysfunction.

Any of the conditions can have a sudden onset. Although uncommon, when this occurs it is usually the result of a strenuous jumping effort, ill-timed kicking, or sudden deceleration.

SYMPTOMS. The primary symptom for any of the problems is *pain* in the anterior aspect of the knee. In patellofemoral dysfunction, the pain usually overlies the medial retinaculum (see Fig. 9–2F) but may be lateral, retropatellar, or diffuse. Regardless of its location, the pain is rarely well localized. When asked to localize the pain, the athlete usually rubs the index and long fingers up and down along the medial border of the patella (Fig. 9–23). The pain with patellar tendinitis is well localized, most often at the inferior pole of the patella or, less frequently, at the superior border of the patella (see Fig. 9–2G). Osgood-Schlatter disease is characterized by pain over the tibial tuberosity (see Fig. 9–2H). The location of the pain in both patellar tendinitis and Osgood-Schlatter disease can be specifically pointed to with a fingertip.

The pain of Osgood-Schlatter disease and patellar tendinitis is exacerbated by activities involving running and jumping. Patellofemoral dysfunction usually worsens with the ascending or descending of hills or stairs, squatting or semisquatting maneuvers, weight bearing on a semiflexed knee (plié in ballet), and especially after sitting for long periods with the knee flexed—the *theater symptom*. Squatting is also often painful in Osgood-Schlatter disease.

After being seated for long periods, athletes with patellofemoral dysfunction often complain of their knees "locking." This is not true locking, but rather *gelling* or stiffness resulting in difficulty straightening the knee. The knee extends gradually, rather than abruptly, as would occur with true locking.

Giving way (of the weakness variety) may accompany any of these problems but is most common with patellofemoral dysfunction.

Swelling is reported to a variable degree. In both patellar tendinitis and Osgood-Schlatter disease, it is well localized at the area of maximal tenderness, but it is most evident in the latter. In the former the swelling appears diffuse, usually representing an *effusion*.

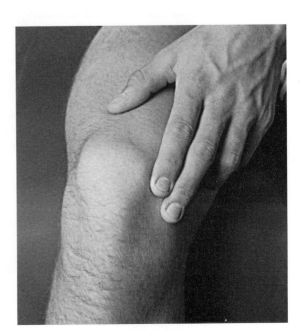

Figure 9–23. The site of pain with patellofemoral dysfunction is often demonstrated by rubbing the fingers up and down over the medial retinaculum.

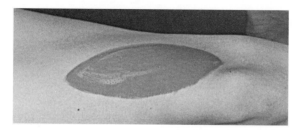

Figure 9–24. Vastus medialis obliquus of the right quadriceps.

The pain associated with any of these problems is increased with activities and decreased with rest.

PHYSICAL EXAMINATION

Vastus medialis weakness is nearly always evident in patellofemoral dysfunction. This may present as a loss of bulk (when compared with the opposite side), noted when the quadriceps is isometrically contracted with the knee fully extended (Fig. 9–24). Palpation of the contracting vastus medialis usually reveals it to be soft and lacking in tone compared with the opposite side.

Tenderness in patellar tendinitis is well localized and often deep in the tendon. The tender area is sought by tipping the inferior or superior aspect of the patella forward and then palpating deep into the fibers at their bony attachment (Fig. 9–25). Tenderness in patellofemoral dysfunction may be found over the medial or lateral retinaculum or on the undersurface of the patella—an area palpable only with the quadriceps well relaxed and the knee fully extended. Tenderness in Osgood-Schlatter disease is well localized over the distal 1 in. of the patellar tendon and the tibial tuberosity.

An *effusion* may be present in patellofemoral dysfunction. Localized swelling, often accompanied by redness and an increase in local temperature,

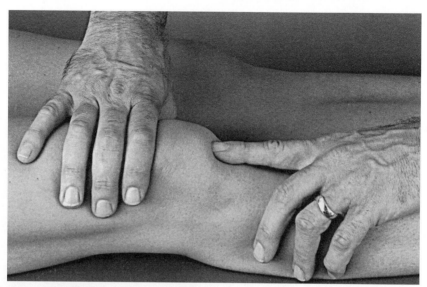

Figure 9–25. Palpation for point of maximal tenderness in jumper's knee. The athlete is told to relax the quadriceps. The superior border of the patella is gently pushed inferiorly and posteriorly while the index finger of the opposite hand palpates deep in the tendon at its attachment to the inferior pole of the patella.

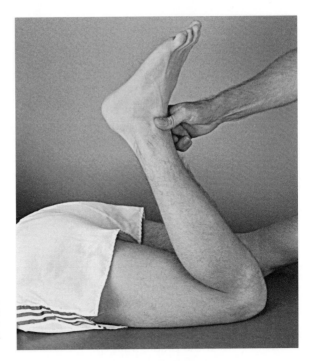

Figure 9–26. Passively stretching the quadriceps by gently pressing the foot toward the buttock often reproduces the pain in the patellar tendon.

is frequently present in Osgood-Schlatter disease. Occasionally this inflammatory process is so intense as to suggest an infection—a rare condition at this location in a child or adolescent.

Flexion may be limited in any of the conditions. Attempting to place the heel against the buttock (Fig. 9–26) reproduces the discomfort that characterizes the specific problem. Knee tightness should be viewed as distinct from quadriceps tightness. If flexion of the knee is limited (in the position illustrated), the athlete should be asked if the pain is in the knee or in the anterior aspect of the thigh (rectus femoris portion of the quadriceps). Quadriceps tightness is usually present with patellar tendinitis.

An increased Q angle (see part B) and high-riding patella (patella alta) may also predispose to patellofemoral dysfunction.[48] The latter is best defined as patellar tendon length greater than the length of the patella.

RADIOGRAPHIC EXAMINATION

None of these conditions is diagnosed by radiographic examination. Although patellofemoral malalignment, as seen in the patellar views, is reported by many authors as a consistent finding in patellofemoral dysfunction, our experience supports that of Hughston—that is, radiographic findings are of only confirmatory value.[27]

Fragmentation of the bony attachment of the tendon and bone formation within the patellar tendon are often seen in both patellar tendinitis and Osgood-Schlatter disease. Only in recalcitrant cases do such findings play a role in the management of these conditions.

OTHER DIAGNOSTIC TESTS

Radionuclide bone scans sometimes reveal increased uptake within the patellar subchondral bone, perhaps indicative of a specific type of patellofemoral dysfunction. Likewise, soft tissue abnormalities evident with computerized axial tomography or MRI might point one in the direction of surgical management in recalcitrant cases of patellar tendinitis. We have experienced difficulty correlating abnormalities seen on MRI with findings at the time of surgical exploration; thus MRI evidence of abnormality *alone* does not serve as an indication for surgical intervention.

Arthroscopy is of no value in patellar tendinitis or Osgood-Schlatter disease and of only limited value in patellofemoral dysfunction. With the latter condition, abnormalities of the articular surface of the patella do not correlate well with signs and symptoms.

INITIAL TREATMENT

Initial treatment of all these conditions is aimed at decreasing the symptoms in order that a rehabilitative program can be instituted. The first step is to temporarily discontinue the pain-producing activities. Often this does not mean discontinuing the sport, but rather discontinuing activities within the sport. (For example, the gymnast with patellofemoral dysfunction might have only to limit vaulting.)

If the problem has progressed to the point that walking and other activities of daily living are painful—often the case of the athlete who hopes the pain will disappear if ignored—then the use of a knee immobilizer may be necessary for a few days. It is important to remember that all these problems are associated with, if not caused by, inadequate quadriceps strength. Any decrease in activities further reduces muscular strength, strength that must ultimately be recovered before treatment is completed. It is rarely necessary to immobilize the knee for more than a few days in any of these problems.

Treatment with ice, anti-inflammatory medications, and quadriceps isometric exercises is started immediately and continued until symptoms have subsided.

REFERRAL

Referral is necessary only when symptoms persist despite adequate nonoperative treatment.

In patellofemoral dysfunction, arthroscopy may prove helpful in eliminating the presence of a pathological plica as the cause of the symptoms (see part I). Surgical procedures such as a lateral retinacular release may be helpful in patellofemoral dysfunction by redirecting the pull of the quadriceps mechanism. We have generally been unimpressed with the results of procedures aimed at altering the articular surface of the patella—patellar shaving, facetectomy, or abrasion arthroplasty.

Occasionally a resistant case of patellar tendinitis requires surgical exploration of the patellar tendon. This procedure has a high rate of success if it is possible to identify an unhealed, inflamed, intrasubstance tear of the tendon.

Much has recently been written regarding the role of foot pronation (flat feet) and patellofemoral dysfunction and patellar tendinitis. Our practice, regardless of how pathological the pronation appears, is first to utilize the rehabilitation program outlined in this section. If the program fails and if Low-Dye taping (see Fig. 12–4) alleviates the symptoms, we refer the patient so the condition can be evaluated for the use of orthoses.

DEFINITIVE TREATMENT

In most cases, relative rest, standard knee rehabilitation, correction of biomechanical problems such as hyperpronation, and very gradual resumption of activity are all that is required. In all cases the mainstay of treatment is restoration of normal quadriceps strength, endurance, and flexibility.[10, 51, 59]

Stretching should be undertaken as many times during the day as is realistically possible. The quadriceps should be stretched (see Fig. 9–14) to the point of discomfort, the stretch held for a minimum of 20 seconds, and the procedure repeated two or three times. At a minimum, stretching should be done upon awakening, before and after athletic activities, and at bedtime.

Isometric strengthening should also be done many times during the day. The muscle is contracted, the contraction is held for 6 to 8 seconds and relaxed for 2 seconds, and the procedure is repeated three or four times. The sequence should be repeated at least hourly throughout the day. The exercise is best accomplished while the patient sits with the knee fully extended (see Fig. 9–16A). The athlete should palpate the vastus medialis with the fingertips to ensure that the contraction is including the vastus medialis. It is not enough merely to tell the athlete to set or contract the quadriceps. The athlete must be shown how to do the exercise and be able to demonstrate a solid contraction before leaving the office.

Some individuals have a great deal of difficulty in producing a satisfactory quadriceps contraction. If painful, the exercise can be done either with the knee flexed in a comfortable position (see Fig. 9–16B) or with fingertip pressure on the lateral aspect of the patella. If these methods fail it may be necessary to stimulate the vastus medialis externally to familiarize the athlete with the sensation accompanying a contraction of this muscle. Most physical therapists have the appropriate equipment available.

Occasionally even zealous performance of the rehabilitative exercises fails to alleviate symptoms. Before we advise complete cessation of the symptom-producing activities or consideration of surgical intervention, it is our practice to prescribe the use of a portable EMS unit. A physical therapist can instruct the athlete in the proper use of the unit. We suggest that both electrodes be placed over the vastus medialis (see Fig. 9–17) and that the unit be used for up to 2 hours a day for a minimum of 1 month. The EMS units are usually available for lease periods of 1 month or more.

The use of knee "sleeves" is often helpful in managing both patellofemoral dysfunction and patellar tendinitis. The common denominator of these devices is their ability to hold the patella medially, usually by pressure from a laterally placed pad (see Fig. 9–19). There is a myriad of products, each differing slightly in design and all claiming equal efficacy. Our impression is that a simple sleeve—knitted or neoprene—with a lateral pad suffices in the vast majority of instances.

The sleeve is worn during all potentially pain-producing activities. It should not be worn during long periods of sitting or at night. Care must be taken that it not be fitted so tightly as to produce edema distally. We usually suggest that use of the sleeve be continued for at least a few weeks after return to the athletic activity and find that most athletes continue to wear it long after their symptoms have disappeared.

A variation of the patellar stabilizing sleeve is McConnell taping. With only a single strip of tape the patella is pulled medially, often resulting in an appreciable decrease in discomfort. If the pain relief is immediately obvious

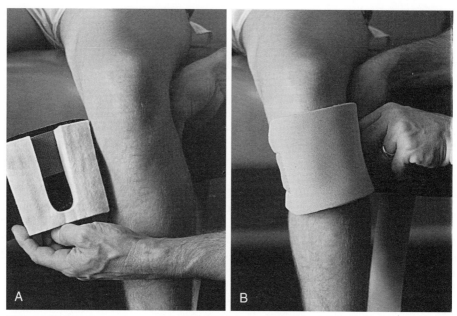

Figure 9–27. The Osgood-Schlatter pad protects the tibial tuberosity from direct pressure by redistributing the blow around the bony prominence.

the patients are taught to apply the tape themselves and to use the technique during activities that usually produce discomfort. Generally this technique cannot be used for long periods of time because of skin irritation from the tape. Most physical therapists are familiar with this taping method.

A slightly different appliance is used for Osgood-Schlatter disease. Much of the discomfort associated with Osgood-Schlatter disease is the result of direct pressure on the swollen and prominent tibial tuberosity (from kneeling or falling on the anterior aspect of the knee). An *Osgood-Schlatter pad* is a device that places a felt horseshoe around the prominence of the tibial tuberosity, thus protecting it from direct pressure (Fig. 9–27). These pads are easily fitted, comfortable, readily accepted by athletes, and very effective.

Athletic activities are gradually resumed. We use a program that progresses from rapid walking to jogging, sprinting, cutting, and finally jumping. Weight lifting (knee extensions) is resumed only if it can be done painlessly. In some cases of patellofemoral dysfunction the athlete may never be able to resume heavy weight lifting. Contrary to the belief of many coaches, most athletes can return successfully to nearly any sport without doing repetitive, heavily weighted, knee extensions. Rigorous cycling (if painless) is an excellent quadriceps-strengthening or maintenance exercise.

A dancer or cyclist with persistent symptoms despite adequate rehabilitation should be observed for improper technique (Fig. 9–28), and the bicycle should be checked for proper adjustment (see Fig. 3–2).

K. CHRONIC INSTABILITY

Instability is a symptom that can accompany a variety of knee complaints. It is frequently the chief, and perhaps only, complaint of an athlete with a knee

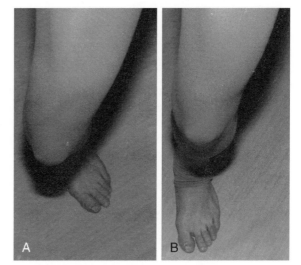

Figure 9–28. *A*, Forcing turnout is a common cause of knee pain in dancers. The ballet dancer with inadequate external rotation at the hips will try to achieve the desired turned-out placement of the feet by external rotation at the knee. Observe that as this dancer does a plié (i.e., knee bend), her knee moves medially to her foot (i.e., in front of the foot when viewed from the front). *B*, Proper technique places the feet beneath the knees. With less turnout, the knee remains directly above the foot as the dancer does a plié and the torque at the knee is less.

problem. Management requires determination of the type, and thus the cause, of the instability and then treatment of the underlying condition.

Most complaints of instability fall into one of three categories: (1) instability from (quadriceps) *muscle weakness*, (2) instability from *ligamentous laxity* with or without muscle weakness, and (3) instability from *impingement*. The first is usually due to quadriceps insufficiency; the second to laxity of the anterior cruciate ligament, and the last to a torn meniscus or loose body.

HISTORY

MECHANISM OF INJURY. Instability from weakness usually occurs with fatigue or during activities demanding high levels of quadriceps strength such as climbing or descending hills or stairs. These episodes often occur with straight-ahead activities. Ligamentous instability usually occurs during twisting, cutting, or landing maneuvers. Impingement instability can occur anytime, often the first moment weight is borne on the leg.

SYMPTOMS. Weakness instability is often described as the knee *giving way.* The knee may collapse into flexion, often causing a fall, or may abruptly snap into hyperextension. These episodes are rarely painful and seldom result in swelling or effusion.

Instability from ligamentous laxity is often described as the knee *going out.* The knee is described as shifting in position—a description usually emphasized by the athlete showing with the hands how the shift occurred. Careful questioning reveals that the knee shifted in position and then collapsed. After this shift in position, an effusion usually results. With subsequent recurrences, the episodes often occur more easily, become less painful, and are less likely to produce effusions.

Impingement instability is characterized by sudden, sharp pain followed by collapse. This may be described as a pinching or painful catching sensation. An effusion/hemarthrosis usually results after the initial episodes but is less likely with subsequent occurrences.

Examination and treatment follow the schemes presented with the underlying diagnoses.

L. POPLITEUS TENDINITIS

Popliteus tendinitis is an occasional cause of knee pain in runners and hikers. It seldom seems to afflict other athletes. Its clinical significance is twofold. It can be absolutely disabling, particularly to the serious distance runner, and it can be difficult to differentiate from other causes of posterolateral knee pain, such as lateral meniscus injury and biceps tendinitis.

ANATOMY

The popliteus is a small, flat muscle that underlies the gastrocnemius in the lower part of the popliteal fossa. Its tendon of origin arises from the lateral femoral condyle and passes between the lateral meniscus and the capsule of the knee joint. Its insertion is directly onto the proximal posterior aspect of the tibia.

Two functions of the popliteus have been demonstrated by electromyography:[3] (1) As an internal rotator of the tibia with respect to the femur or as an external rotator of the femur with respect to the fixed tibia, the popliteus unlocks the knee at the initiation of knee flexion. (2) As a dynamic stabilizer of the knee, it assists the quadriceps and the posterior cruciate ligament in preventing anterior displacement of the femur with respect to the tibia.

By its attachments to the lateral meniscus, the popliteus may also function to prevent impingement of the meniscus between the femur and tibia as the knee is flexed.

HISTORY

MECHANISMS OF INJURY. Popliteus tendinitis is characteristically associated with downhill running and backpacking. The pathomechanics are probably related to the previously noted function of the muscle in resisting anterior displacement of the femur on the tibia at foot strike.

In our experience, extreme fatigue of the quadriceps seems particularly predisposing to popliteus overuse. A distance runner, for example, is likely to describe the onset of symptoms on resuming training too abruptly after having completed a marathon or ultramarathon race. A triathlete is likely to have first noted symptoms during a run following an exhausting bicycle ride.

Excessive pronation of the foot also seems to predispose to the development of popliteal tendinitis.

SYMPTOMS. The hallmark symptom is *viselike, running-related posterolateral knee pain*.

Not uncommonly, the runner is able to run for a short distance without pain but has a rather abrupt onset of symptoms at a predictable distance into the run and is then forced to stop and walk. The abrupt onset of pain is sometimes quite graphically described as something tightening up in the knee.

PHYSICAL EXAMINATION

Point tenderness may be elicited over the popliteus tendon on either side of the lateral collateral ligament or over the muscle's insertion along the medial border of the tibia, just anterior to the medial head of the gastrocnemius. However, because of the proximity of other possibly injured structures, neither finding is very specific. A small effusion may be present, but this, of course, is also a nonspecific finding. We have found provocation of *pain with popliteus-specific muscle testing* to be the most reliable sign of popliteus tendinitis (Fig. 9–29). With the knee flexed to 90 degrees, the examiner fully internally rotates the leg. The athlete is then asked to resist the examiner's attempt to rotate the leg externally. If the tendon is inflamed, pain will be reproduced by this maneuver. Passive stretching of the popliteus by externally rotating the leg maximally may also reproduce the pain.

Popliteus muscle testing should not be confused with McMurray's test, which involves fully flexing the knee and attempting to elicit pain as the flexed and rotated knee is extended (see part B). Signs of lateral meniscus impingement are most likely to be found when the test is performed with the leg internally rotated. This is the position of least tension on the popliteus tendon.

Important normal findings are the absence of impingement pain, a negative McMurray's test, the absence of point tenderness over the biceps tendon or iliotibial band, and the absence of pain with resisted knee flexion or hip abduction.

RADIOGRAPHIC EXAMINATION

Radiographic study and other diagnostic tests are not required.

INITIAL TREATMENT

The initial treatment consists primarily of *relative rest*. Ice massage to the posterolateral aspect of the knee, and ice and electrogalvanic stimulation therapy may be useful adjuncts.

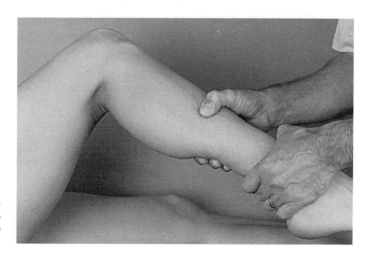

Figure 9–29. Popliteus muscle testing. The athlete is asked to resist the examiner's attempt to rotate the leg externally.

REFERRAL

Referral is not required.

DEFINITIVE TREATMENT

In most cases, relative rest, standard knee rehabilitation, correction of biomechanical problems such as hyperpronation, and very gradual resumption of running are all that is required. The serious runner will be able to maintain a high level of fitness for running by training on an exercycle or bicycle (see Chapter 3, part D).

As popliteus overuse seems to be almost always secondary to quadriceps overuse, rehabilitation comprises mostly quadriceps strength, endurance, and flexibility training. It seems logical also to carry out a popliteus-specific stretching and strengthening program using the techniques described earlier for popliteus testing. However, we have seldom found this to be necessary.

PREVENTION

Runners and backpackers should be cautioned about the risks of downhill running and hiking, especially when the quadriceps muscles are noticeably fatigued. Competitive runners should adequately rest after long races and only gradually resume hill running. Triathletes should include bike/run workouts in their training, with gradually increasing hill running if they plan to race hilly courses. As with all overuse syndromes, abrupt changes in training regimens should be avoided.

M. OSTEONECROSIS

Osteonecrosis is a condition found three times more commonly in women, usually beyond the age of 60 years.[15] It is included here because of the increased level of sports and fitness participation among older individuals as well as its frequent confusion with meniscal abnormality. Like osteochondrosis dissecans in the younger population, osteonecrosis involves an apparent loss of the blood supply to a section of the joint surface, usually the medial femoral condyle.

HISTORY

The onset is often spontaneous without an associated traumatic event. The pain is usually medial and present at both weight bearing and rest. It often awakens the patient at night. The pain is frequently associated with an effusion, usually described by the patient as a sense of "tightness" or "fullness." The pain may be sharp, resulting in giving-way episodes.

EXAMINATION

Often the only positive findings are the presence of a modest effusion, tenderness over the medial femoral condyle or joint line, and (secondary) quadriceps atrophy. The extremes of both flexion and extension are often limited.

RADIOGRAPHIC EXAMINATION

In the early stages, standard x-ray examinations are often normal. Later one might see a defect or flattening of the weight-bearing portion of the medial femoral condyle, often superimposed on some evidence of degenerative joint disease.

OTHER DIAGNOSTIC TESTS

Radioisotope bone scanning or MRI definitively documents the presence of the osteonecrotic lesion. MRI may also reveal the presence of a degenerative meniscus, a not uncommon incidental finding in this age group. If both meniscal abnormality and an osteonecrotic lesion are found, the osteonecrotic lesion *takes precedence* as the cause of the problem.

INITIAL TREATMENT

Pain-producing activities should be restricted, often necessitating the use of a cane. It this age group, crutches should be employed with caution. A quadriceps-strengthening program should be instituted.

REFERRAL

Once the diagnosis of osteonecrosis is made, the patient should be referred to an orthopedist.

DEFINITIVE TREATMENT

In some cases limitation of activities, with or without the use of a brace, results in healing of the lesion. This may require months or even years—a significant period of time for the older patient. Temporizing surgical procedures such as arthroscopic débridement are usually of little long-term help. More often than not these patients undergo replacement arthroplasty. As a general rule, lesions that involve over half the width of the femoral condyle are unlikely to heal.

N. DEGENERATIVE JOINT DISEASE (OSTEOARTHRITIS)

Degenerative joint disease is seen with increasing frequency among sports and fitness participants, not because the activities cause this particular problem but rather because older individuals are participating in these activities in increasing numbers. Whether post-traumatic (more common in men) or idiopathic (women), the salient clinical issues are the same: activity-related pain and swelling accompanied by (often substantial) radiographic changes in patients reluctant to give up those activities causing the symptoms.

HISTORY

The typical history is one of a gradual onset of activity-related pain. The symptoms often follow the introduction of a new activity such as fitness classes or increased participation in some ongoing activity such as golf after retirement. Although the problem may be bilateral, the initial symptoms are usually unilateral. The pain is often accompanied by swelling and limitation of motion, although both may have been gradually occurring previously without the patient's noticing. Difficulty with stairs and a positive "theater" symptom (the inability to sit comfortably for prolonged periods with the knees flexed) are frequent early complaints. Later, weakness, "instability," and "catching" are noted, and crepitation becomes more striking.

PHYSICAL EXAMINATION

The knee is usually swollen and exhibits some deformity, often in the form of enlargement (osteophytosis) of the joint margins, varus or valgus, and a loss of full extension. Less obvious but equally frequent is a loss of flexion. Virtually all exhibit quadriceps atrophy particularly of the vastus medialis. Medial or lateral ligamentous laxity accompany the joint space collapse responsible for the varus or valgus deformity. Joint line tenderness is common but probably emanates from the osteophytes rather than damaged menisci.

RADIOGRAPHIC EXAMINATION

All gradations of degenerative changes may be evident. It is important to obtain a semiflexed, weight-bearing anteroposterior view (Rosenberg's) to appreciate the degree of joint space collapse, which appears to correlate better with symptoms than the presence of even very large osteophytes.

It is important to remember that the patient, not the radiographs, is being treated. It is usually evident that the radiographic abnormalities have long preceded the symptoms and that sometimes truly dreadful radiographs are unaccompanied by complaints. Osteochondral loose bodies, often seen in the suprapatellar pouch or posterior aspect of the joint, are often unaccompanied by symptoms.

INITIAL TREATMENT

Avoidance of specific pain-producing activities—even to the extent of using a cane if mere walking is painful—cautious use of nonsteroidal anti-inflammatory drugs, and isometric quadriceps strengthening are the mainstays of nonoperative management of this problem. We frequently institute the use of an EMS unit on the initial visit with older patients. As with patellofemoral dysfunction, the electrodes are placed on the vastus medialis portion of the quadriceps muscle. The units can be employed for up to 2 hours per day.

REFERRAL

Orthopedic referral is indicated when the initial management regimen fails to result in significant improvement or in the presence of symptomatic loose bodies or true locking episodes.

DEFINITIVE TREATMENT

Definitive treatment is aimed at the symptoms, which initially are often the result of quadriceps weakness. Thus the regimen suggested for chronic anterior knee pain is followed. Additional means include the use of heel wedges to "unload" the more symptomatic or collapsed side of the joint. (With medial compartment collapse, a lateral wedge is employed and vice versa. Varus or valgus wedges are commercially available or can be fabricated from cork heel lifts.) Varus or valgus knee braces are now available. They, like heel wedges, result in a reduction of symptoms in nearly half the patients with unicompartmental disease.

Ultimately many of these patients will require knee replacement procedures. Even though substantially beneficial in 85% to 90% of patients older than 60 years, many of the athletically active put off such an operation for as long as possible, for it will spell the end of such activities as tennis and alpine skiing.

REFERENCES

1. Albright JP: Personal communication, 1986.
2. Arendt EA, Teitz CC: The lower extremities. *In* Teitz CC (ed): The Female Athlete. Rosemont, Ill, American Academy of Orthopaedic Surgeons, 1997, pp 45–61.
3. Basmajian JV, De Luca CJ: Muscles Alive, Their Functions Revealed by Electromyography, 5th ed. Baltimore, Williams & Wilkins, 1985.
4. Bechtel SL et al: Skier's knee: The "cruciate connection." Physician Sportsmed 12:51–54, Nov 1984.
5. Bronkhim B et al: The synovial shelf syndrome. Clin Orthop 142:135–138, 1979.
6. Buchbinder MR et al: Relationship of abnormal pronation to chondromalacia of the patella in distance runners. J Am Podiatr Assoc 69:159–162, 1979.
7. Casscells SW: Arthroscopy: Diagnostic and Surgical Practice. Philadelphia, Lea & Febiger, 1984.
8. Cross MJ, Powell JF: Long-term follow-up of posterior cruciate ligament rupture: A study of 116 cases. Am J Sports Med 12:292–297, 1984.
9. Daniel DM: Fate of the ACL-injured patient. A prospective outcome study. Am J Sports Med 22:632–644, 1994.
10. DeHaven KE: Chondromalacia patellae in athletes: Clinical presentation and conservative management. Am J Sports Med 7:5–11, 1979.

11. DeHaven KE: Diagnosis of acute knee injuries with hemarthrosis. Am J Sports Med 8:9–14, 1980.
12. DeHaven KE: Rationale for meniscus repair or excision. Clin Sports Med 4:267–273, 1985.
13. Derscheid GL, Garrick JG: Medial collateral ligament injuries in football: Nonoperative management of grade I and grade II sprains. Am J Sports Med 9:365–368, 1981.
14. Donaldson WF III et al: Comparison of acute anterior ligament examinations: Initial versus examination under anesthesia. Am J Sports Med 13:5–10, 1985.
15. Ecker LE et al: Spontaneous osteonecrosis of the knee. J Am Acad Orthop Surg 2:173–178, 1994.
16. Ellsasser JC et al: The non-operative treatment of collateral ligament injuries of the knee in professional football players. An analysis of 74 injuries treated surgically. J Bone Joint Surg Am 56:1185–1190, 1974.
17. Feagin JA Jr et al: The isolated tear of the anterior cruciate ligament. J Bone Joint Surg Am 54:1340–1341, 1972.
18. Fetto JF, Marshall JL: The natural history and diagnosis of anterior cruciate ligament deficiency. Clin Orthop 147:29–38, 1980.
19. Galway HR, MacIntosh DL: The lateral pivot shift. A symptom and sign of anterior cruciate ligament insufficiency. Clin Orthop 147:45–50, 1980.
20. Galway HR et al: Pivot shift: A clinical sign of symptomatic anterior cruciate ligament deficiency. J Bone Joint Surg Br 54:763–764, 1972.
21. Garrick JG: Knee problems in adolescents. Pediatr Rev 4:235–244, 1983.
22. Garrick JG: Characterization of the patient population in a sports medicine facility. Physician Sportsmed 13:73–90, Oct 1985.
23. Garrick JG, Requa RK: Medical care and injury surveillance in the high school setting. Physician Sportsmed 9:115–120, Feb 1981.
24. Giove TP et al: Nonoperative treatment of the torn anterior cruciate ligament. J Bone Joint Surg Am 65:184–192, 1983.
25. Grace TG et al: Isokinetic muscle imbalance and knee joint injuries: A prospective blind study. J Bone Joint Surg Am 66:734–740, 1984.
26. Hardaker WT et al: Diagnosis and treatment of the plica syndrome of the knee. J Bone Joint Surg Am 62:221–225, 1980.
27. Hughston JC et al: Patellar Subluxation and Dislocation. Philadelphia, WB Saunders, 1984.
28. Hume EL, McKeag DB: The complexities of diagnosing acute soft-tissue knee injuries. Emerg Med Rep 6:1–8, 1985.
29. Ireland J et al: Arthroscopy and arthrography of the knee. J Bone Joint Surg Br 62:3–6, 1980.
30. Jokl P et al: Nonoperative treatment of severe injuries to the medial and anterior cruciate ligaments of the knee. J Bone Joint Surg Am 66:741–744, 1984.
31. Katz JW, Fingeroth RJ: The diagnostic accuracy of ruptures of the anterior cruciate ligament comparing the Lachman test, the anterior drawer sign, and the pivot shift test in acute and chronic knee injuries. Am J Sports Med 14:88–91, 1986.
32. Kennedy JC, Hawkins RJ: "Breaststroker's knee." Physician Sportsmed 2:33–38, 1974.
33. Kennedy JC et al: The anatomy and function of the anterior cruciate ligament. As determined by clinical and morphological studies. J Bone Joint Surg Am 56:223–235, 1974.
34. Kennedy JC et al: Orthopedic manifestations of swimming. Am J Sports Med 6:309–322, 1978.
35. Keskinen K et al: Breaststroker swimmer's knee. Am J Sports Med 8:228–231, 1980.
36. Larson RL: Physical examination in the diagnosis of rotatory instability. Clin Orthop 172:38–44, 1983.
37. Losee RE et al: Anterior subluxation of the lateral tibial plateau. A diagnostic test and operative repair. J Bone Joint Surg Am 60:1015–1030, 1978.
38. Lysholm J et al: The effect of a patella brace on performance in a knee extension strength test in patients with patellar pain. Am J Sports Med 12:19–112, 1984.
39. McDaniel WJ Jr, Dameron TB Jr: Untreated ruptures of the anterior cruciate ligament. J Bone Joint Surg Am 62:696–705, 1980.
40. McDaniel WJ Jr, Dameron TB Jr: The untreated anterior cruciate ligament rupture. Clin Orthop 172:158–163, 1983.
41. Marshall JL, Warren RF: The all-American knee. Emerg Med Rep Aug:210–234, 1982.
42. Munzinger U et al: Internal derangement of the knee joint due to pathologic synovial folds: The mediopatellar plica syndrome. Clin Orthop 155:59–64, 1981.
43. Mysnyk MC et al: Prepatellar bursitis in wrestlers. Am J Sports Med 14:46–54, 1986.
44. Noyes FR et al: The symptomatic anterior cruciate-deficient knee. I: The long-term functional disability in athletically active individuals. J Bone Joint Surg Am 65:154–162, 1983.
45. Noyes FR et al: The symptomatic anterior cruciate-deficient knee. II: The results of rehabilitation, activity modification, and counseling on functional disability. J Bone Joint Surg Am 65:163–174, 1983.
46. Noyes FR et al: Advances in understanding of knee ligament injury, repair, and rehabilitation. Med Sci Sports Exerc 16:427–443, 1984.
47. O'Donoghue DH: Surgical treatment of fresh injuries to the major ligaments of the knee. J Bone Joint Surg Am 37:1–13, 1955.
48. Outerbridge RE: The etiology of chondromalacia patellae. J Bone Joint Surg Br 43:752–757, 1961.

49. Parolie JM, Bergfeld JA: Long-term results of nonoperative treatment of isolated posterior cruciate ligament injuries in the athlete. Am J Sports Med 14:35–38, 1986.
50. Patel D: Arthroscopy of the plical-synovial folds and their significance. Am J Sports Med 6:217–225, 1978.
51. Percy EC, Strother RT: Patellalgia. Physician Sportsmed 13:43–59, July 1985.
52. Renstrom P et al: Strain within the anterior cruciate ligament during hamstring and quadriceps activity. Am J Sports Med 14:83–86, 1986.
53. Rosenberg TD, Rasmussen GL: The function of the anterior cruciate ligament during anterior drawer and Lachman's testing: An in vivo analysis in normal knees. Am J Sports Med 12:318–322, 1984.
54. Rovere GD, Nichols AW: Frequency, associated factors, and treatment of breaststroker's knee in competitive swimmers. Am J Sports Med 13:99–104, 1985.
55. Rubin BD, Collins HR: Runner's knee. Physician Sportsmed 8:49–58, June 1980.
56. Saktu K et al: Posterior cruciate ligament injuries. Acta Orthop Scand 55:26–29, 1984.
57. Slocum DB, Larson RL: Rotatory instability of the knee. Its pathogenesis and a clinical test to demonstrate its presence. J Bone Joint Surg Am 50:211, 1978.
58. Slocum DB et al: Clinical test for anterolateral rotatory instability of the knee. Clin Orthop 118:63–69, 1976.
59. Steadman JR: Nonoperative measures for patellofemoral problems. Am J Sports Med 7:374–375, 1979.
60. Stiell IG et al: Derivation of a decision rule for the use of radiography in acute knee injuries. Ann Emerg Med 26:405–413, 1995.
61. Stoker DJ et al: Value of arthrography in the management of internal derangement of the knee. The first 1000 are the worst. Clin Radiol 32:557–566, 1981.
62. Stulberg SD et al: Breaststroker's knee: Pathology, etiology, and treatment. Am J Sports Med 8:164–171, 1980.
63. Torg J, Quedenfeld T: The shoe-surface interface and its relationship to football knee injuries. Am J Sports Med 2:261, 1974.
64. Torg JS et al: Clinical diagnosis of anterior cruciate ligament instability in the athlete. Am J Sports Med 4:84–93, 1976.
65. Walla DJ et al: Hamstring control and the unstable anterior cruciate ligament–deficient knee. Am J Sports Med 13:34–39, 1985.

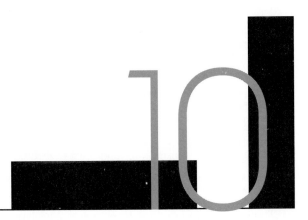

Leg Injuries

Of the anatomical regions involved with athletic injuries, the leg is the fourth most frequently involved.[10] Although injuries involving all the musculotendinous structures in the leg have been reported as occurring in athletes, the vast majority of the problems involve the calf musculature and Achilles tendon. Beyond the calf, only shin splints occur with enough frequency to merit detailed consideration.

Although two of the *acute* injuries considered here involve the same musculotendinous unit, they present an interesting contrast in severity and disability. A strain of the gastrocnemius is often accompanied by severe symptoms but should be of little ultimate medical consequence. Rupture of the Achilles tendon, on the other hand, may be a relatively painless injury but involves a minimum of 6 months of substantially curtailed athletic activities and an equally substantial commitment to an arduous rehabilitation program.

The *overuse* problems occurring in the leg are studies in frustration. With Achilles tendinitis the frustrations are associated with the frequently protracted course of the injury. With shin splints, our inability precisely to define both the cause and the pathophysiology of the condition results in frustration.

A.   GASTROCNEMIUS STRAIN (TENNIS LEG)

Tennis leg is a strain involving the musculotendinous junction of the medial head of the gastrocnemius and the Achilles tendon.[2, 30] It usually occurs in athletes older than 30 years and, in our experience, seems to occur more frequently in women. Although the vast majority of these injuries are associated with tennis, we have encountered the problem in a variety of activities, including hiking, basketball, and various forms of dance. If unrecognized or inappropriately managed, it can result in months of significant disability.

Interesting is the fact that this injury never involves the lateral head of the gastrocnemius or the soleus. The latter should come as no surprise as the soleus crosses only a single joint, thus rendering it relatively immune to strains. We are unaware of any similarly clear-cut explanation of the protection enjoyed by the lateral head of the gastrocnemius.

For many years this condition was erroneously diagnosed as a rupture of the plantaris (muscle/tendon). Despite surgical evidence to the contrary,[2] this "diagnosis" continues to be found in discussions of leg injuries in athletes, particularly tennis players.

HISTORY

MECHANISM OF INJURY. The injury is usually the result of a vigorous propulsive movement (i.e., plantar flexion of the ankle), as with a jump or sudden start. Like strains elsewhere in the body, the injury is often associated with fatigue, such as occurs with playing an extra hour of tennis or playing more consecutive days than usual. Occasionally the injury follows a bout of Achilles tendinitis or an ankle injury or sprain that has resulted in relative weakness with secondary tightness of the calf. Occasionally the injury occurs in two parts: a minor strain that is ignored, followed minutes later by complete rupture of the musculotendinous unit.

SYMPTOMS. The athlete feels or hears a *pop* in the medial upper aspect of the calf. Often, as with a ruptured Achilles tendon, the patient thinks he or she has been struck in the calf by a tennis ball or partner's racquet. The first response is invariably to look over the shoulder to find the source of the blow.

The injury is instantly *painful. Spasm* of the calf musculature occurs rapidly, plantarflexing the foot and leaving the athlete with the prospect of attempting to walk notwithstanding an inability to bring the heel to the ground or bear weight on the toes.

Swelling and ecchymosis, frequently not apparent the first few hours after the injury, are often significant enough at 24 to 48 hours to prompt the patient to seek medical care. Because of the effect of gravity, the ecchymosis may "surface" distally about the ankle or even the foot.

PHYSICAL EXAMINATION

The single most important diagnostic feature is exquisite *point tenderness* toward the medial side of the junction of the middle and proximal thirds of the calf (Fig. 10–1). *Swelling and ecchymosis* are usually present distal to the site of injury and may involve the ankle and even the foot.

Motion is limited, and the foot is held in plantar flexion. Although often uncomfortable, the athlete is forced to walk on the toes. If the athlete's knee is held fully extended, both passive dorsiflexion of the ankle and active plantar flexion against resistance will produce pain at the site of injury.

Occasionally it is possible to palpate a defect in the muscle at the site of the tear, but usually the defect fills rapidly with blood, obscuring this sign.

RADIOGRAPHIC EXAMINATION

Radiographic study is not required.

OTHER DIAGNOSTIC TESTS

It is not necessary to perform other diagnostic tests.

INITIAL TREATMENT

If the athlete is seen within a few hours of the injury, the ankle should be gently and gradually brought into a neutral (i.e., right angle to the leg) position and maintained there with a padded *posterior plaster splint*. This maneuver not only prevents contraction of the remaining intact portion of the gastrocnemius but also tightens the enveloping fascia, thus discouraging continued bleeding.

Swelling is also discouraged by the elastic wrap used to hold the splint in place. If the ankle cannot be moved from its plantarflexed position, one

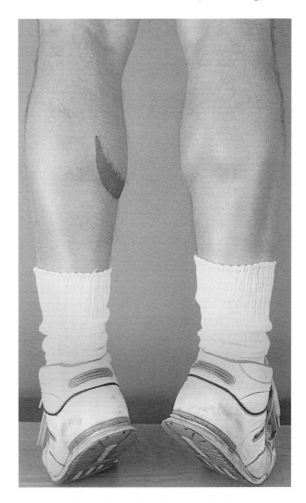

Figure 10–1. Location of maximal pain and tenderness in tennis leg.

must be content with repeated icing and the application of focal compression over the site of injury.

Efforts to regain ankle motion (mainly dorsiflexion) *must* be started at 24 hours after injury. Although gentle active and passive stretching of the calf are important, motion seems to be most quickly gained by forcing the athlete to walk, even though this is uncomfortable. Even more uncomfortable is climbing stairs, but it too helps appreciably in regaining motion. We tell patients that forced walking will be unpleasant, but in a day or two motion will be comfortable enough to allow a heel-to-toe gait.

Unfortunately the injury is usually first seen days or weeks after its occurrence, and the patient presents with an ankle that is rigidly held in plantar flexion by spasm of the calf musculature and a leg/foot that is chronically swollen. A *compression wrap* should be applied from toes to knee.

In these "neglected" cases non–weight-bearing crutch walking should be used for the first few days after the initial visit until the patient is capable of ambulating with a more-or-less painless heel-to-toe gait. In either case, oral administration of anti-inflammatory medications should be started immediately.

REFERRAL

Referral is not required.

DEFINITIVE TREATMENT

The goals of treatment are recovery of normal strength and flexibility of the calf musculature; they should be pursued aggressively. A series of three to five daily physical therapy sessions appreciably enhances the early return of motion. These sessions should include use of high-intensity galvanic stimulation, ice, and active and passive stretching of the gastrocnemius muscle. Crutches, non–weight bearing, and compression for the first 24 hours should be sufficient to quell bleeding. After that, aggressive, usually uncomfortable, active and passive gastrocnemius stretching should be employed multiple times during waking hours. The ankle should be immobilized at night with a right angle posterior splint. This regimen coupled with forced walking with a heel-to-toe gait usually results in a striking diminution of symptoms within 48 to 72 hours. Failure to stretch the Achilles mechanism early in the course of this injury prolongs the recovery time by weeks or months.

A ¾- or 1-in. heel lift can be used to enhance weight-bearing ambulation, which can be started as soon as it is tolerated. The patient is encouraged to walk with the toes pointed straight ahead rather than using the externally rotated gait favored by those with this injury. With short steps and a slow gait, ambulation is usually possible within a few days of the injury.

Calf strengthening is begun by using the resistance provided by a Theraband for three sets of 10 slow repetitions, at least three times daily, both with the knee fully extended and with it partially flexed. Single-leg toe raises are started as soon as tolerated. The toe raises are started with the knee flexed 15 to 20 degrees; with time, the knee is gradually fully straightened.

The athlete is taught to do contract-relax stretching either by sitting with the legs extended to the front, using a towel as a stirrup (Fig. 10–2), or by

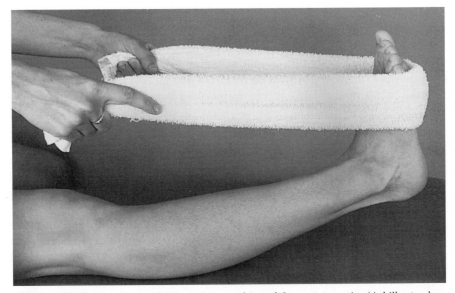

Figure 10–2. Use of a towel for passive stretching of the gastrocnemius/Achilles tendon.

standing (in a shoe with a raised heel) with the knee extended and alternately attempting to rise onto the toes, holding this position for 15 to 20 seconds, and then letting the heel drop and leaning forward as with a normal gastrocnemius stretch (Fig. 10–3).

Twenty minutes of icing following the exercise periods is often helpful in controlling swelling and discomfort. A compression wrap should be employed throughout the course of active treatment.

When comfortable, the athlete should begin rapid walking and progress through a walk-to-run program (see Chapter 2, part A).

When strength and flexibility appear almost normal, a series of isokinetic workout sessions may hasten the return to athletic activities. These are done to exhaustion at speeds of 180, 240, and 300 degrees per second and repeated at least twice during the exercise session. Because of the profound fatigue that follows such workouts, postexercise stretching should be thorough and the athlete cautioned to avoid vigorous exercises or activities for at least 12 hours.

Recurrences are nearly always the result of incomplete rehabilitation, usually inadequate restrengthening. Simple tests to assess strength include balancing on the toes of the involved side for at least as long as is possible on the uninvolved side, or being able to hop on the toes of the involved side for at least 10 to 20 repetitions without allowing the heel to come in contact with the floor.

In the past this injury has been managed by casting or prolonged periods of rest and non–weight bearing. We believe that this leads to needlessly long periods of disability. Nonetheless, if such an initial treatment regimen is chosen, the previously described rehabilitation program can be employed after removal of the cast.

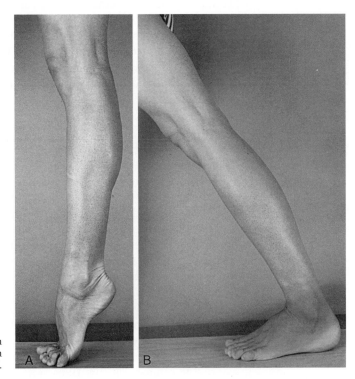

Figure 10–3. *A,* Toe raise with knee fully extended. *B,* Calf stretch (gastrocnemius) with knee extended.

B. ACHILLES TENDON STRAIN (RUPTURE)

In spite of the fact that this injury involves one of the largest tendons in the body and usually occurs in an abrupt, dramatic fashion, Achilles tendon rupture is frequently misdiagnosed. Thus the first item of medical importance is establishing the diagnosis.

The second aspect of medical importance is the controversy surrounding treatment of this injury. Although we recommend that all patients with a ruptured Achilles tendon be referred to an orthopedic surgeon, it nonetheless seems appropriate to discuss briefly the management of this injury.

HISTORY

MECHANISM OF INJURY. The usual mechanism of injury is a *push-off with the forefoot* (forceful plantar flexion of the ankle from a fully dorsiflexed position) *while extending the knee.* Basketball, racquetball, softball, and tennis are the sports most often associated with the injury, although it can be seen in any propulsive athletic activity. The injury may also occur as a result of *unexpected or forced dorsiflexion of the plantarflexed ankle.*

The injury often occurs at a time of relative fatigue, that is, late in a game or match or after a few days of unaccustomed, increased activity.

Achilles tendon ruptures usually occur in athletes older than 30 years, with the incidence appearing to peak in the 40s. The injury is less common in women.

SYMPTOMS. The most striking symptom is the *sensation of being struck* in the region of the tendon. This is usually accompanied by an audible pop or snap. Although sometimes painful, the discomfort is usually overshadowed by the sensation of something letting loose. The patients often think they have sprained an ankle and note dysfunction only to the extent that the ankle does not feel right. The more observant athlete notes an inability to rise onto the toes of the involved side.

PHYSICAL EXAMINATION

The most important finding on examination is a *lack of reflex plantar flexion when the calf is sharply squeezed—a positive Thompson test* (Fig. 10–4).[38]

There is also substantial *loss of strength in plantar flexion,* resulting in an inability to rise onto the toes, and often even to balance, on the affected leg. The athlete can usually demonstrate a modicum of active plantar flexion by using the accessory plantar flexors—the peroneal, posterior tibial, and toe flexor muscles—but lacks the strength to stand on the toes.

Careful palpation usually reveals a gap or *loss of continuity* in the tendon. Bleeding and swelling may be substantial and, in 24 to 48 hours, obscure this sign. Tenderness and pain with motion are variably present and not indicative of the severity of the injury.

Gait is *antalgic and apropulsive.* Typically, the athlete walks with the foot and leg externally rotated, as this does not require push-off with the calf muscles.

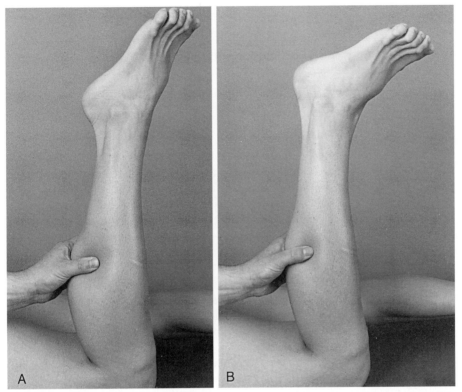

Figure 10–4. Thompson's test for Achilles tendon integrity.[38] The calf is sharply squeezed. *A,* An intact tendon allows plantar flexion of the ankle. *B,* A lack of plantar flexion indicates disruption of the Achilles tendon.

RADIOGRAPHIC EXAMINATION

Radiographic study is not indicated.

OTHER DIAGNOSTIC TESTS

Although other diagnostic tests are not required, magnetic resonance imaging (MRI) may be useful to demonstrate the extent and exact location of disruption of the tendon. Sonography may also be useful in assessing the extent and location of the tear. Unfortunately, even though far less expensive than MRI, sonography is often not readily available in the United States.

INITIAL TREATMENT

The leg, from knee to toes, should be placed in a *compression wrap*. The ankle should be in a position of gravity-assisted plantar flexion, as occurs when the athlete sits on an examining table with the legs hanging over the side. A *posterior plaster splint* applied over the compression dressing helps maintain the plantarflexed position and the approximation of the torn tendon ends.

REFERRAL

Patients with any evidence suggesting rupture of the Achilles tendon should be referred to an orthopedic surgeon.

DEFINITIVE TREATMENT

The decision concerning treatment should be left to the treating orthopedist. Regardless of whether operative or nonoperative management is used, the patient will probably be immobilized in a cast or removable cast-brace for 2 to 3 months, followed by another 2 to 3 months of active rehabilitation. Innovations for immobilization include the use of prefabricated braces that allow plantar flexion but block various degrees of dorsiflexion, usually 20 degrees for the first 4 weeks. Running and jumping activities are usually prohibited for at least 9 months from the time of injury.

The literature is replete with reports "comparing" the results of surgical and nonsurgical management of Achilles tendon ruptures.[8, 13, 15, 18–21] In our estimation, however, there is only one study that compared the results in two essentially randomized groups of patients in which neither physician nor patient controlled the method of treatment.[34] In this particular study it was concluded that the treatment of choice should be nonsurgical. Obviously the results of this investigation have been viewed as less than compelling by a significant number of orthopedic surgeons. At the present time we estimate that the majority of patients younger than 40 years with Achilles tendon rupture are treated with surgical repair. Likewise, there appears to be an even greater leaning toward surgical intervention in the athletic individual regardless of age.

The proponents of surgical repair cite two major issues: (1) that direct reapproximation of the torn tendon fibers is necessary to preserve the normal length/tension relationship of the musculotendinous unit and thereby allow reattainment of normal strength and (2) that rerupture occurs less frequently in those injuries that have been surgically repaired.

Those espousing the cause for nonsurgical management cite the (sometimes appalling) occurrence of surgical complications, such as infections and skin necrosis, and appreciably lower medical costs of nonsurgical management. They further point out that if rehabilitation is approached with the same zeal regardless of whether the patient has undergone a surgical procedure, there is no reason that strength and muscle function should differ.[21, 23, 24, 34]

Our personal preference is for the nonoperative management of many of these injuries. We believe that the sophistication with which rehabilitation is approached is a much more important determinant of success than is the initial surgical or nonsurgical management.

C. ACUTE COMPARTMENT SYNDROMES

A compartment syndrome is a condition in which the tissues within an osteofascial compartment are compromised by increased pressure within that compartment. Of the four osteofascial compartments in the leg (anterior, lateral or peroneal, and superficial and deep posterior), the anterior is by far the most commonly involved.

Acute compartment syndromes are uncommon but do occur in sports. Anyone involved in the primary care of athletes should be aware of this diagnosis. A high index of suspicion and timely intervention may prevent permanent nerve and muscle injury.

Chronic or exertional compartment syndromes are relatively more common but do not require as urgent intervention. These syndromes are discussed along with other causes of chronic leg pain in part E.

HISTORY

MECHANISM OF INJURY. Virtually any macrotrauma or microtrauma, including fractures, tendon ruptures, muscle strains, contusions, and "acute" overuse, that is associated with *bleeding or edema formation within an unyielding osteofascial compartment* can produce a compartment syndrome.[1, 7, 16, 22] Especially in acute injury, a tightly applied *circumferential cast or bandage* may also produce a compartment syndrome.

SYMPTOMS. The hallmark symptom is severe *pain*, disproportionate to the apparent severity of injury. *Paresthesias* may also be noted.

PHYSICAL EXAMINATION

Swelling and *tenderness* over the compartment are early signs. Pain is also typically exacerbated by *specific compartmental muscle testing*, e.g., resisted dorsiflexion of the ankle with anterior compartment syndrome. *Paresis, pallor, and pulselessness* are late and ominous signs.

DIAGNOSTIC TESTS

The clinical diagnosis of acute compartment syndrome should be confirmed by direct measurement of intracompartmental pressure (see part E for further discussion).[31, 32]

INITIAL TREATMENT

Initial treatment consists mainly of *rest and the application of ice*. The athlete should not be allowed to bear weight on the involved leg. Compression is contraindicated; any constricting clothing, bandages, casts, and the like should be removed or split. In the severe case in which the intracompartmental pressure exceeds the intra-arterial pressure, elevation is also probably contraindicated. Continual careful monitoring is essential.

REFERRAL

If the clinical diagnosis of acute compartment syndrome cannot be ruled out by direct measurement of intracompartmental pressure, if intracompartmental pressure exceeds 30 mm Hg, or if there are any signs or symptoms of neurovascular impairment, referral to an orthopedic surgeon on an emergent basis is indicated.[37]

DEFINITIVE TREATMENT

Mild cases may be treated expectantly. If symptoms, signs, and intracompartmental pressures improve with rest and icing, definitive treatment may not be required. More severe cases, in which intracompartmental pressure exceeds 30 mm Hg and which are associated with neurovascular impairment, require urgent decompression, i.e., *fasciotomy*. Multiple compartment syndrome may be treated by proximal fibulectomy, but in our experience, it has not been necessary to do so.

D. ACHILLES TENDINITIS

Inflammation of the Achilles tendon may be among the most common forms of tendinitis in athletes. Like many overuse injuries, it is often initially ignored. Once established, it can result in long periods of disability and even predispose to later rupture.

The problem associated with treating this condition is twofold: (1) The injury is often seen only when it has become chronic and (2) adequate rehabilitation is a time-consuming and frustrating process—difficult to supervise in the driven, high-intensity athlete in whom the injury seems so prevalent.

The pathoanatomy of this condition includes examples of chronically inflamed partial rupture, stenosis of the surrounding soft tissues, and calcification within the tendon. These conditions are usually associated with chronicity and ignored or expediently treated symptoms. Whether the tendon or surrounding soft tissues are involved matters only when surgical management is being considered.

HISTORY

MECHANISM OF INJURY. This condition is usually the result of too much of an unaccustomed activity such as hill running, changing of heel height on the running shoe, or repetitive jumping. Occasionally the condition can be the result of direct trauma such as pressure from the top of the heel counter of a shoe, a poorly fitting skating boot, or improperly tied ribbons on a ballet pointe shoe.

The injury may be associated with a high-arched foot, a flat or pronated foot, or a "tight" Achilles tendon. Although pathomechanics of the foot or leg often seem to play some role in the creation of this problem, it is difficult to imagine how abnormal mechanics can be solely responsible for a condition occurring in a 40-year-old athlete who had run comfortably for the 20 years preceding the injury.

Careful and precise history taking almost always reveals an activity change preceding the onset of the condition.[5]

SYMPTOMS. Pain and stiffness are the usual initial complaints. These symptoms are first noted a few hours or the next day after bouts of athletic activity. Initially, stretching loosens the tendon, allowing the athlete to continue comfortable participation. Later, symptoms occur during the activity and ultimately go on to precede it. Occasionally, especially when the condition has had a particularly rapid onset, the athlete notices the presence of crepitation, often of the squeaking or snowball type.

Athletes often report they are more comfortable in shoes with higher heels and that they are unable to walk barefoot, especially on soft ground or sand.

PHYSICAL EXAMINATION

Palpation or squeezing the tendon produces *tenderness*. Because *swelling* is often minimal, its presence should be sought by comparing ipsilateral and contralateral sides with the patient lying prone (Fig. 10–5).

Passively dorsiflexing the ankle with the knee extended often produces pain in the inflamed tendon. Likewise, resisted plantar flexion of the ankle often results in pain.

Palpable and visible masses within the tendon, representing swollen, poorly healed partial ruptures, can occasionally be observed. A diffusely, grossly enlarged, dense, tender tendon usually indicates the presence of peritendinous fibrosis and scarring.

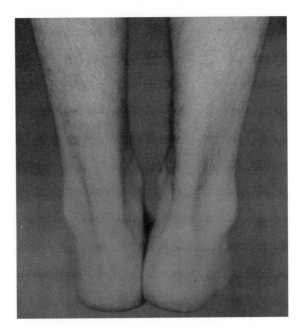

Figure 10–5. Swelling associated with Achilles tendinitis (left leg).

RADIOGRAPHIC EXAMINATION

Radiographic study is not routinely necessary. In chronic cases a lateral view of the leg (tibia/fibula) may reveal the presence of calcification or ossification within the tendon.

OTHER DIAGNOSTIC TESTS

In the presence of recalcitrant tendinitis and ossification/calcification within the tendon, a radionuclide bone scan reveals whether the process is still active. A "hot" scan is an indication for continued rest and avoidance of surgical intervention.

MRI, and to a lesser degree sonography, is becoming increasingly popular as a means of studying Achilles tendon abnormality. Visualization of partial ruptures might prompt earlier referrals or at least an increased modicum of caution concerning the return to athletic endeavors. On the other hand, studies demonstrating a "normal" tendon encased in a thickened, fibrotic paratenon might allay some anxiety concerning the likelihood of future rupture. As a general rule we believe such tests should be ordered *after* the referral and not serve as the cause for it.

INITIAL TREATMENT

The *avoidance of pain-producing activities* is the most important phase of initial management. This may involve anything from complete cessation of weight bearing and the use of crutches to mere avoidance of running. Regardless, athletes must understand that if they cannot become pain free they will not get well. The use of a ½-in. heel lift, nonsteroidal anti-inflammatory drugs, and repeated applications of ice may help alleviate symptoms. Sleeping in a right-angle, "Achilles" ankle brace usually alleviates the early morning stiffness and pain so often present.

If the condition has occurred relatively suddenly and the examiner is confident that a (partial or complete) rupture is not present, a burst of oral corticosteroids may abruptly alleviate the symptoms (see Chapter 5, part F).

As is true for any tendon subject to great tensile loads, local corticosteroid injection into or about the Achilles tendon may well predispose to rupture and is probably contraindicated.[17, 36]

Referral to a physical therapist is often appropriate during the initial management. High-intensity galvanic stimulation, ultrasonography, cryotherapy, and even transverse friction massage often aid in lessening the symptoms.

REFERRAL

Failure to alleviate the initial symptoms or an unsuccessful comprehensive rehabilitative program is indication for referral. An orthopedic surgeon should be consulted if symptoms continue and there is chronic nodular or diffuse enlargement of the tendon. In the absence of these anatomical changes, an evaluation for a trial of orthotics may be appropriate.

DEFINITIVE TREATMENT

Chapter 3 covers the management of overuse injuries involving musculotendinous units. Because of the potentially enhanced likelihood of rupture and the severity of this complication, it is particularly important to alleviate the symptoms first. Occasionally in the case of long-standing problems, immobilization in a cast may be necessary. This option should, however, be reserved as a last resort, because reversing the muscle weakness and atrophy that follow immobilization substantially increases the time required for rehabilitation.

Stretching exercises should be performed repeatedly throughout the day and should always both precede and follow strengthening exercises. Stretching should be done in each of the two positions necessary to affect both the soleus and the gastrocnemius (Fig. 10–6; see also Fig. 10–3B). It is important that the patients demonstrate how they are doing the stretching exercises, as small variations in technique, such as externally rotating the foot, may render them worthless.

Likewise, strengthening exercises should be done in both the extended- and flexed-knee positions. When weakness is profound, Theraband or surgical tubing can be used to provide the resistance. (The elastic material should be wrapped once around the forefoot to decrease the likelihood of its slipping off during the exercise. Furthermore, the patient should not face the foot

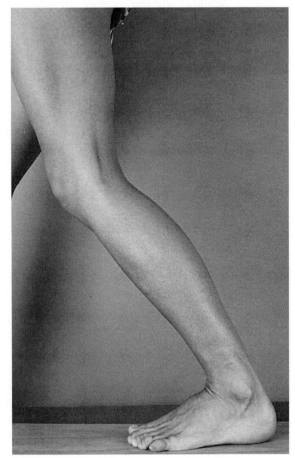

Figure 10–6. Soleus is stretched with the knee partially flexed.

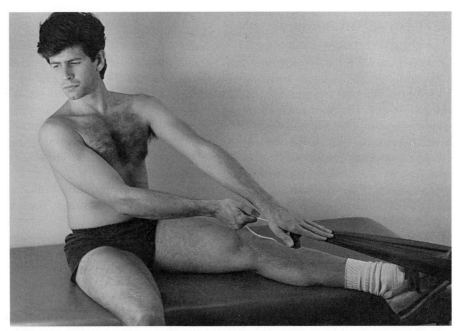

Figure 10–7. Theraband exercises should always be done with the face turned away from the elastic material to avoid injury should the material break or slip off the foot.

while doing the exercise, thus lessening the likelihood of injury should the elastic material slip [Fig. 10–7].) Strengthening exercises should employ only the painless range of motion, which early in the course of rehabilitation may involve only a 10-degree arc.

We have found it most effective, and least likely to cause exacerbation of symptoms, to do 10 repetitions of each (i.e., gastrocnemius and soleus) exercise many times during the day. If the athlete attempts to do all the strengthening exercises at one time, fatigue lessens their effectiveness, and recurrence of symptoms is much more likely the following day.

Toe raises are begun as soon as they can be comfortably tolerated. The exercises are initiated with the majority of weight on the uninjured side, with more weight gradually being shifted to the injured extremity. Ultimately these exercises should be done on a block or slant board (Fig. 10–8), using a full range of dorsiflexion and plantar flexion, but some weeks may be required before this can be accomplished comfortably. Toe raises should also be undertaken in two positions—knee straight and slightly flexed.

Isokinetic exercises should be instituted just before the beginning of unsupported weight-bearing ambulation. These exercises should never be done at speeds less than 90 to 120 degrees per second. Because the exercises are done to the point of exhaustion, the patient should thoroughly stretch after the workout and should be warned of the subsequent fatigue and enhanced chance of re-injury associated with too vigorous activity immediately after the exercise session.

Unsupported ambulation is begun with short steps and with the involved foot pointed forward—not externally rotated as most patients are prone to do. The stride length is increased consistent with comfort. Running should not be attempted until the patient is able to (1) balance at least 20 seconds on the toe of the involved side, (2) hop painlessly 10 times on the involved side without allowing the heel to touch the floor, and (3) walk 20 minutes briskly

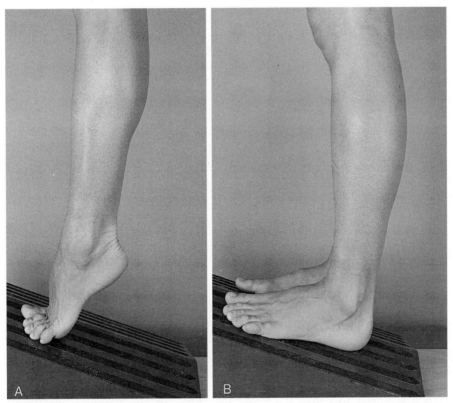

Figure 10–8. Use of the slant board for calf strengthening and stretching. *A,* Toe raise on the slant board. *B,* Calf stretch on the slant board.

with a normal stride and no limp. A ½-in. heel lift can be used as ambulation is initiated, and then gradually smaller lifts can be used as full activity is regained.

The patient with recalcitrant tendinitis might be a candidate for evaluation for the possible use of orthotics. Unfortunately, many of these patients have a rigid, high-arched (cavus) foot that may defy effective correction with orthotic appliances. Likewise, the athlete with true chronic, unassailable tendinitis may be a candidate for surgical intervention. Incising constricting paratendinous tissues or excising focal areas of chronic inflammation that have resulted from limited, unhealed ruptures is often successful.

Calcaneal apophysitis (Sever's disease) might properly be viewed as a variant of Achilles tendinitis seen in the skeletally immature. In our experience its onset is often associated with rapid growth spurts; thus prophylactic calf stretching in the growing child may help to prevent this problem. Additionally, the use of a ¼-in. heel lift in flat-heeled soccer-style tennis or basketball shoes relieves tension on the Achilles tendon. Otherwise Achilles tendinitis is managed as in the adult.

E. CHRONIC ANTERIOR LEG PAIN (SHIN SPLINTS)

Athletes, coaches, trainers, and physicians have for years used the term *shin splints* in referring to virtually any case of pain between the knee and the ankle not involving the calf/Achilles tendon. As a diagnosis, shin splints is a wastebasket term, but at least the wastebasket is becoming smaller. The differential diagnosis includes stress fractures, chronic (exertional) compartment syndromes, periostitis, tibialis posterior syndrome, and other specific entities that can be accurately diagnosed.[4, 6, 9, 11, 14, 25, 26, 28, 33, 35] Nonetheless, there remain athletes with chronic leg pain for whom no specific diagnosis seems to apply.

The conditions considered in this section are all overuse injuries, primarily associated with running or jumping activities. Although the majority of these conditions are generally benign, there is one particular stress fracture that should be viewed with some degree of alarm: Transverse stress fracture of the anterior cortex of the midshaft of the tibia not only is especially slow to heal but also has a high likelihood of overtly fracturing and displacing.

HISTORY

MECHANISM OF INJURY. Virtually all these conditions are the result of unaccustomed activity or overuse. For the runner, increases in mileage, alterations in terrain, and a change of shoes are the most common causes. Specific tasks within an activity are often associated with these problems. Among these causes are vaulting in gymnastics, grands jetés (large jumps) in ballet, and wind sprints in football.

As is true with nearly all overuse injuries, the better the athlete, the less change required to cause the problem. Thus, for the national-level figure skater, a mere additional 10 minutes a day of practicing a new jump can result in a stress fracture of the fibula.

Biomechanical abnormalities, such as hyperpronation of the foot, are often noted but have not been shown to have predictive importance. Thus, for example, in treating a runner with tibialis posterior syndrome and excessive foot pronation, we might prescribe orthoses, but we certainly would not suggest that all runners with pronation should have orthoses to prevent this condition.

SYMPTOMS. The primary symptom for all these conditions is *pain*. Initially present after the activity, the painful period gradually intrudes into the workout, ultimately preceding, and precluding, the activity. In many cases, at the time the athlete presents for treatment, symptoms are present during the activities of daily living.

The location of the pain is important (Fig. 10–9). Pain in the distal lateral aspect of the leg often indicates a fibular stress fracture. Pain in the entire anterior lateral area of the leg may indicate the presence of a chronic compartment syndrome. Pain over the anterior surface of the tibia in the midleg indicates a tibial stress fracture, and medial pain in the distal third of the leg can indicate either tibialis posterior syndrome or a tibial stress fracture.

The timing of the occurrence of the pain is particularly important. Pain that is present early in the workout but disappears with continued activity only to return after the workout is completed suggests tibialis posterior syndrome. Pain that always occurs at the same time or mileage during the workout suggests a chronic compartment syndrome.

Localized *swelling* may accompany stress fractures. Diffuse swelling, often described as a tense sensation, in the anterolateral aspect of the leg suggests a compartment syndrome, as does the presence of small, well-localized areas

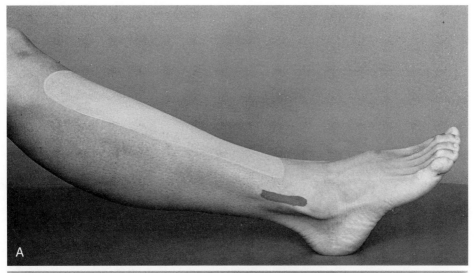

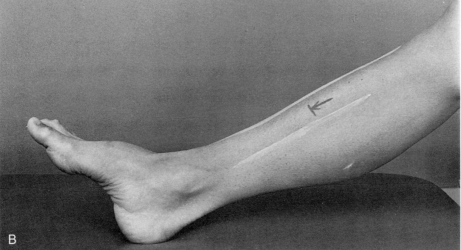

Figure 10–9. Characteristic areas of pain/tenderness with various conditions. *A,* Distal lateral aspect of leg—fibular stress fracture (dark); and anterolateral area of leg—anterior compartment syndrome (light). *B,* Distal medial third of the leg—tibialis posterior syndrome or tibial stress fracture (light); and midtibia—transverse stress fracture (arrow).

of soft tissue swelling—fascial hernias. Paresthesia or hypesthesia is occasionally described by patients with chronic compartment syndromes.

PHYSICAL EXAMINATION

The major effort in the examination is directed toward precisely locating the areas of maximal *tenderness*, which are generally present in the same location as the pain described in the history. Tenderness over either the tibia or the fibula, localized to an area less than 1½ in. in diameter, is very suggestive of a stress fracture. Diffuse tenderness along either the medial or the lateral border of the tibia means little. Tenderness along the distal third of the medial border of the tibia suggests tibialis posterior syndrome.

Muscle testing is helpful in some conditions (Fig. 10–10). Pain with resisted dorsiflexion may be noted with chronic anterior compartment syn-

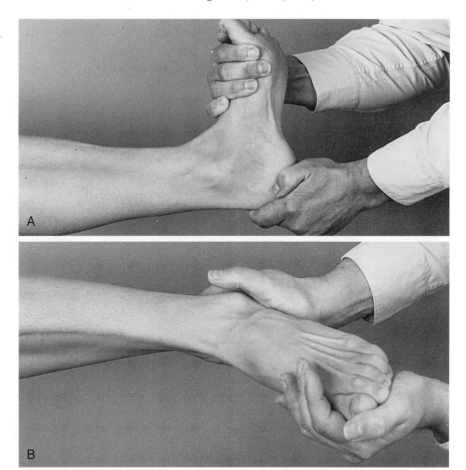

Figure 10–10. Muscle testing. *A,* In chronic anterior compartment syndrome, resisted dorsi-flexion is often painful. *B,* In tibialis posterior syndrome, resisted inversion and plantar flexion is often painful.

drome. Pain with resisted plantar flexion and inversion suggests tibialis posterior syndrome.

Careful palpation of the anterior compartment may reveal increased tightness, sometimes accompanied by tenderness. Fascial hernias are identified as small, focal prominences in the muscle, usually in the lower half of the leg and most often in the anterior compartment. The hernias are noted only after exercise, as a result of muscle swelling. When the athlete is rested they appear as small indentations or defects in the fascia and are best palpated by covering that portion of the leg with mineral oil or K-Y jelly.

Tight Achilles tendons, the presence of a high-arched (cavus) foot, or significant pronation may all be associated with these conditions.

RADIOGRAPHIC EXAMINATION

Anteroposterior and lateral radiographs of the leg often reveal stress fractures that have been symptomatic for more than 3 to 4 weeks. The presence of these areas of focal periosteal thickening is sometimes seen only with oblique radiographs (see Chapter 3, part C). An actual fracture line is rarely seen except in transverse fractures of the anterior midshaft of the tibia (Fig. 10–11).

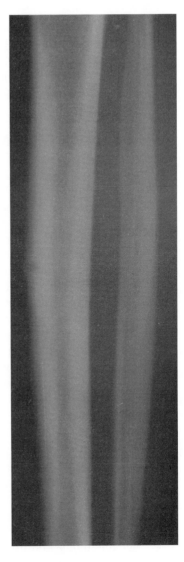

Figure 10–11. Lateral radiograph demonstrating a transverse stress fracture of the anterior aspect of the midtibia, the dreaded black line.

OTHER DIAGNOSTIC TESTS

Confirmation of the clinical diagnosis is often necessary to convince athletes and others of the need to curtail pain-producing activities. *Radionuclide bone scanning* provides the most accurate, though not infallible, means of proving the presence of stress fractures.[12, 27, 29] We routinely order the test early, even before obtaining standard radiographs (see Chapter 3, part C).

A triple-phase bone scan can be used to differentiate periostitis from stress fracture.[27] Periostitis appears as linear, vertically oriented increased uptake seen only on the delayed images, whereas stress fractures are evidenced by intense, round or fusiform "hot spots" and may be seen on the flow, blood pool, and delayed images.

Measurements of *pre-exercise and postexercise intracompartmental pressures* can be used to confirm the diagnosis of chronic compartment syndromes. The necessary equipment is currently available in kit form, and measurement of anterior compartment pressures is technically rather straightforward. Proper catheter placement, instrument calibration, and so on are confirmed by appropriate pressure changes with specific compartmental muscle testing. Treadmill running or isokinetic workouts may be used to reproduce the athlete's symptoms. A positive compartment test requires provocation of symptoms and correlation of symptoms with prolonged elevation of intracompartmental pressure after the provocative exercise.[33]

INITIAL TREATMENT

With any of these conditions the most important aspect of treatment is *discontinuation of the pain-producing activity* or activities. If the condition has progressed to the point that mere walking is painful, then non–weight-bearing crutch ambulation is indicated. On the other hand, with a condition that was diagnosed early, only a specific activity, such as vaulting in gymnastics, may have to be discontinued.

With any of the inflammatory conditions, such as periostitis and tibialis posterior syndrome, initial treatment may also include the use of modalities such as icing, ultrasonography, and high-intensity galvanic stimulation, as well as nonsteroidal anti-inflammatory medication.

Recent reports suggest that the use of an extended, air-filled ankle splint (Aircast) results in a shortened healing time for stress fractures of the tibia and fibula. Those wearing the brace were able to return to pain-free athletic activities some weeks earlier than those not using the brace.

REFERRAL

Athletes with a transverse stress fracture of the anterior cortex of the tibia who are unwilling or unable to undergo a long period of attenuated, pain-free activity should be referred to an orthopedic surgeon. Percutaneous drilling of the fracture line appears to hasten healing of what may be viewed as nonunion of a stress fracture. Some authors have advocated prophylactic intramedullary rodding of the tibia for this condition. We believe this to be overzealous in most instances.

Athletes with positive exercise compartment tests should be referred for consideration of fasciotomy. Those in whom compartment syndrome is suspected, but not confirmed, should be referred for evaluation and treatment of the condition. We suggest that particularly those with suspected multiple or deep posterior compartment syndromes be referred to an experienced examiner for testing.

Patients with recalcitrant nonspecific symptoms, periostitis, tibialis posterior syndrome, and so on may be referred to a podiatrist for further evaluation of gait and the need for orthoses.[39]

DEFINITIVE TREATMENT

Stress fractures are managed as discussed previously and in Chapter 3, part C.

Chronic compartment syndromes may be treated operatively or nonoperatively, by fasciotomy or by simply avoiding pain-producing levels of activity. The prospect of possibly having to modify an activity on a permanent basis often makes the option of operative treatment more attractive to the athlete.

Treatment of tibialis posterior syndrome should include specific stretching and strengthening exercises (see Chapter 11, part A).

Management of any of these conditions, including nonspecific chronic leg pain, may include any or all of the following:

STRETCHING AND STRENGTHENING EXERCISES. Calf stretching and strengthening are employed before and after each period of athletic activity, as well as on awakening and just before retiring at night. Both the gastrocnemius and soleus must be used in these exercises; thus, both stretching and strengthening must be undertaken with the knee fully extended as well as flexed 20 degrees or more. If the condition is bilateral, stretching combined with toe raises is best undertaken using a slant board (see Fig. 10–8). The strengthening exercises are performed to the point of fatigue and followed—immediately—by at least three repetitions of 20-second stretches in each of the two positions (see Figs. 10–3*B* and 10–6).

A dorsiflexion-strengthening board can be made by nailing surgical tubing, a Theraband, or a piece of inner tube to a section of plywood. The foot is then placed beneath the elastic material, and three sets of 10 slow repetitions are done at least three times daily. Placing the foot on the board in increasing degrees of plantar flexion increases both the difficulty and the range of motion necessary to accomplish the exercise.

The intrinsic muscles of the foot can be strengthened by towel pulling with the curled toes or by picking up marbles with the toes. Either of these exercises should be carried to the point of exhaustion (or cramping) two to three times daily.

ARCH SUPPORTS. Commercially available arch supports such as those made by Spenco or Dr. Scholl's often provide relief for patients with shin splints. Unfortunately the use of foot appliances is nearly impossible in some sports such as gymnastics and ballet. In these circumstances we suggest that the appliance be worn during all nonathletic daily activities.

BAND OR COUNTERFORCE BRACING. As with tennis elbow, the use of a taut, circumferential band often lessens the symptoms associated with shin

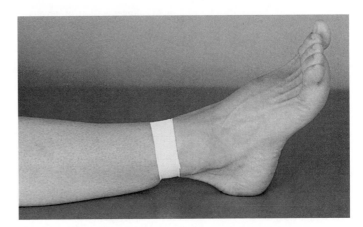

Figure 10–12. Circumferential adhesive tape band sometimes used to alleviate pain associated with shin splints.

splints.[3] A tennis elbow band or ring of tautly applied adhesive tape should be placed 2 to 4 in. proximal to the malleoli (Fig. 10–12).

REFERENCES

1. Arciero RA et al: Acute anterolateral compartment syndrome secondary to rupture of the peroneus longus muscle. Am J Sports Med 12:366–367, 1984.
2. Arner O, Lindholm A: What is tennis leg? Acta Chir Scand 116:73–77, 1958.
3. Beekman S: Shinsplints taping. Physician Sportsmed 10:209–211, Oct 1982.
4. Boyd AM et al: Intermittent claudication, a clinical study. J Bone Joint Surg Br 31:325–355, 1949.
5. Clement DB et al: Achilles tendinitis and peritendinitis: Etiology and treatment. Am J Sports Med 12:179–184, 1984.
6. Davey JR et al: The tibialis posterior muscle compartment. An unrecognized cause of exertional compartment syndrome. Am J Sports Med 12:391–397, 1984.
7. Davies JAK: Peroneal compartment syndrome secondary to rupture of peroneus longus: Case report. J Bone Joint Surg Am 61:783–784, 1979.
8. Denstad TF, Roaas A: Surgical treatment of partial Achilles tendon rupture. Am J Sports Med 7:15–17, 1979.
9. Detmer DE et al: Chronic compartment syndrome: Diagnosis, management, and outcomes. Am J Sports Med 13:162–170, 1985.
10. Garrick J, Requa R: Injuries in high school sports. Pediatrics 61:465, 1978.
11. Gironi G et al: Muscle compartment syndrome of the leg. Ital J Sports Traumatol 1:227, 1979.
12. Holder LE, Michael RH: The specific scintigraphic pattern of "shin splints in the lower leg": Concise communication. J Nucl Med 25:865–869, 1984.
13. Inglis AE et al: Ruptures of the tendo Achillis. An objective assessment of surgical and nonsurgical treatment. J Bone Joint Surg Am 58:990–993, 1976.
14. Jackson DW: Shin splints: Update. Physician Sportsmed 6:51–62, Oct 1978.
15. Jacobs D et al: Comparison of conservative and operative treatment of Achilles tendon rupture. Am J Sports Med 6:107–111, 1978.
16. Kennedy JD, Roth JH: Major tibial compartment syndromes following minor athletic trauma: Two case reports. Am J Sports Med 7:201–203, 1979.
17. Kleinman M, Gross AE: Achilles tendon rupture following steroid injection: Report of three cases. J Bone Joint Surg Am 65:1345–1346, 1983.
18. Kouvalchouk JF, Monteau M: Bilan du traitement chirurgical des ruptures du tendon d'Achille. Rev Chir Orthop 62:253–266, 1976.
19. Kouvalchouk JF et al: Rupture of the tendo Achillis: A comparison of operative and nonoperative treatment. Rev Chir Orthop 70:473–478, 1984.
20. Kristensen JK, Andersen PT: Rupture of the Achilles tendon: A series and review of literature. J Trauma 12:794–798, 1972.
21. Lea RB, Smith L: Rupture of the Achilles tendon: Nonsurgical treatment. Clin Orthop 60:115–118, 1968.
22. Leach RE, Corbett M: Anterior tibial compartment syndrome in soccer players. Am J Sports Med 7:258–259, 1979.
23. Lipscomb PR, Wakim KG: Regeneration of severed tendons: An experimental study. Proc Staff Meet Mayo Clin 36:271–276, 1961.
24. Lipscomb PR, Wakim KG: Further observations in the healing of severed tendons: An experimental study. Proc Staff Meet Mayo Clin 36:277–282, 1961.
25. Lysens RJ et al: Intermittent claudication in young athletes: Popliteal artery entrapment syndrome. Am J Sports Med 11:177–179, 1983.
26. Martens MC et al: Chronic leg pain in athletes due to a recurrent compartment syndrome. Am J Sports Med 12:148–151, 1984.
27. Martire JR: The role of nuclear medicine bone scans in evaluating pain in athletic injuries. Clin Sports Med 6:713–737, 1987.
28. Michael RH, Holder LE: The soleus syndrome. A cause of medial tibial stress (shin splints). Am J Sports Med 13:87–94, 1985.
29. Milgrom C et al: Negative bone scans in impending tibial stress fractures: Report of three cases. Am J Sports Med 12:488–491, 1984.
30. Millar AP: Strains of posterior calf musculature (tennis leg). Am J Sports Med 7:172–174, 1979.
31. Mubarak SJ et al: The wick catheter technique for measurement of intramuscular pressure. A new research and clinical tool. J Bone Joint Surg Am 58:1016–1020, 1976.
32. Mubarak SJ et al: Acute compartment syndromes: Diagnosis and treatment with the aid of a wick catheter. J Bone Joint Surg Am 60:1091–1095, 1978.
33. Mubarak SJ et al: The medial tibial stress syndrome: A cause of shinsplints. Am J Sports Med 10:201–205, 1982.

34. Nistor L: Surgical and non-surgical treatment of Achilles tendon rupture. J Bone Joint Surg Am 63:394–399, 1981.
35. Orava S, Puranen J: Athletes' leg pains. Br J Sports Med 13:92–97, 1979.
36. Smart GW et al: Achilles tendon disorders in runners—A review. Med Sci Sports Exerc 12:231–243, 1980.
37. Subcommittee on Advanced Trauma Life Support (ATLS) of the American College of Surgeons (ACS) Committee on Trauma: Advanced Trauma Life Support Course. Instructor Manual. Chicago, American College of Surgeons, 1984.
38. Thompson TC, Doherty JH: Spontaneous rupture of tendon of Achilles: A new diagnostic clinical test. J Trauma 2:126–129, 1962.
39. Viitasalo JT, Kvist M: Some biomechanical aspects of foot and ankle in athletes with and without shin splints. Am J Sports Med 11:125–130, 1983.

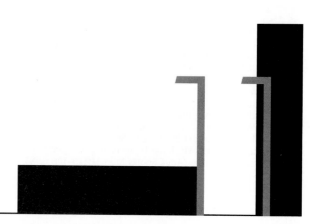

Ankle Injuries

T r i a g e

Indications for Referral

◆ **Acute**

History

Obvious deformity

Immediate onset of numbness or hypesthesia

Crepitation with attempted motion

Eversion mechanism of injury

Examination

Obvious deformity

Neurological deficit

Tender, swollen, or displaced peroneal tendons, or all of these

Achilles tendon defect or positive Thompson's test, or both

X-ray films

Malleolar fractures (experienced practitioners can care for nondisplaced fractures)

Proximal fibular fracture

Diastasis

Talar dome fracture

◆ **Gradual onset**

History

Unpredictable, sharp lancinating pain with or without momentary locking

Abrupt flattening of arch (unilateral pronation)

Examination

Asymmetrical significant pronation and loss of tibialis posterior tendon function

X-ray films

Talar dome defect (osteochondritis dissecans)

Indications for X-ray (Always Anteroposterior, Lateral, and Mortise Views)

◆ **Acute**

History

Inability or unwillingness to bear weight and walk three steps

Examination

Bony tenderness (over malleoli or proximal fibula)

◆ **Gradual onset**

History

Recurrent locking or sudden lancinating pain ("something getting caught"), or both

Reproducible pain with extremes of plantar flexion or dorsiflexion

Examination

Posterior pain with extreme of plantar flexion

Anterior pain with extreme of dorsiflexion

Ankle injuries are probably the most ubiquitous of sports injuries. Among sports requiring ballistic movements such as football, basketball, and gymnastics, acute injuries—mostly sprains—are common[16] and can usually be managed in a relatively straightforward manner. Overuse injuries, more common in endurance activities such as running, often present greater diagnostic and treatment challenges.

In this chapter we discuss our approach to the athlete who presents with acute injury, chronic instability, and chronic pain. We also separately discuss lateral ligament sprains, peroneal tendon strains, peroneal tendon dislocations, tibialis posterior tendinitis, anterior impingement syndrome, and posterior impingement syndrome.

A. ACUTE INJURY

Approximately 85% of acute ankle injuries are sprains,[16] and approximately 85% of these involve the lateral ligaments only.[7] Uncomplicated lateral ligament sprains can be expected to respond well to the type of treatment and rehabilitation program presented later.[8, 13] This holds true as well for acute strains of the peroneal tendons and avulsion fractures of the base of the fifth metatarsal.[25]

Although the vast majority of acute ankle injuries can thus be managed nonoperatively, certain acute injuries and structurally significant fractures may very well require operative treatment for best results.[10, 12, 24, 30] A logical approach to acute ankle injury in the athlete must therefore differentiate those injuries that generally merit orthopedic evaluation and treatment from those that do not.

HISTORY AND PHYSICAL EXAMINATION

Athletes are asked about prior injury to the ankle, the mechanism of injury, their perception of the severity of injury, the extent of the disability, and the postinjury course. Initial physical examination consists of systematic inspection and palpation of possibly injured structures, i.e., the medial malleolus, deltoid ligament, base of the fifth metatarsal, lateral malleolus, calcaneofibular ligament, anterior talofibular ligament, posterior tibial tendon, tibiofibular ligaments, peroneal tendons, and superior peroneal retinaculum (Fig. 11–1).

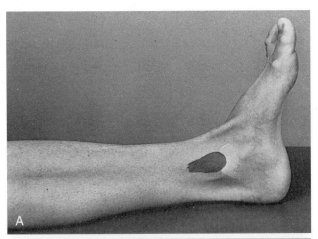

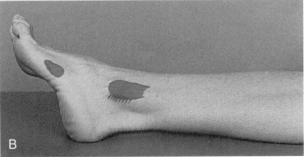

Figure 11–1. Surface anatomy of ankle indicating specific sites at which point tenderness is sought: *A,* medial aspect—medial malleolus (dark) and deltoid ligament (light). *B,* Lateral aspect—base of the fifth metatarsal (dark), lateral malleolus (dark), anterior talofibular and calcaneofibular ligaments (light), and superior peroneal retinaculum (hatched).

Assessment of the skin and the neurovascular status of the foot is particularly important if severe swelling or deformity is present. Any manipulation of the injured ankle is usually deferred until indicated radiographic examination has been carried out.

Some caution is advised in making inferences from the clinical findings alone. Both inversion and eversion mechanisms can result in injury to both medial and lateral structures. Perceived severe injury, immediate and severe pain, rapid and diffuse swelling, and significant disability (i.e., the inability or unwillingness to bear weight) obviously increase the index of suspicion for severe injury but are not necessarily diagnostic. A mild to moderate sprain treated initially with hot soaks can appear identical to a structurally significant fracture. Conversely, the ability to bear weight does not always rule out the possibility of fracture. The most discriminating finding, point tenderness over the injured structure, may be obscured by time and inappropriate initial treatment. However, the finding of both an ability to bear weight and localization of tenderness anteroinferior to the lateral malleolus does adequately discriminate lateral ligament sprains from fractures.[28] Also, a history of a dorsiflexion mechanism of injury is very specific for peroneal tendon dislocation.[12, 22, 25] Localization of tenderness posterosuperior to the lateral malleolus is also highly specific for this diagnosis, and the finding of palpably dislocated tendons is pathognomonic. But by 2 hours after injury, neither finding is likely to be present.[12]

RADIOGRAPHIC EXAMINATION

Radiographic examination is indicated not as a matter of routine, but rather for specific indications.[6, 18, 28] Anteroposterior, lateral, and mortise (an anteroposterior view taken with the leg in 20 degrees of internal rotation) views of the ankle are indicated if the clinical findings do not permit differentiation of lateral ligament sprain from ankle fracture (Fig. 11–2). If there is obvious injury to the medial aspect of the ankle and no apparent injury to the lateral aspect, then tibia/fibula films are also indicated to rule out fibular fracture proximal to the ankle (Fig. 11–3). If tenderness over the fifth metatarsal is present, foot films are indicated to rule out a true Jones fracture (Fig. 11–4).

Appropriate radiographic examination obviously confirms or does not confirm the diagnosis of ankle fracture. If the previously described indications are used for radiographic examination, the only fractures likely to be missed are those that may be appropriately managed as sprains.[6, 28, 29] With fractures the extent of injury can usually be inferred from the clinical and radiographic findings, although the radiographic examination taken by itself can underestimate the extent of injury (see Fig. 11–3).

A possible exception to the "fracture rules" (described earlier) may exist in the skeletally immature child. Nondisplaced fractures of the physis ("epiphyseal fractures") of the Salter I, II, V, and VI types are often not apparent on x-ray films. Our practice is to treat ankle injuries accompanied by bony tenderness overlying the physeal line as epiphyseal fractures and immobilize them for 3 to 4 weeks.

With peroneal tendon dislocation, a characteristic avulsion fracture of the lateral malleolar cortex is found in about 13% of cases and can be considered pathognomonic (Fig. 11–5).[12] This finding should not be confused with avulsion flakes off the tip of the lateral malleolus or talus, which signify nothing more than lateral ligament injury.

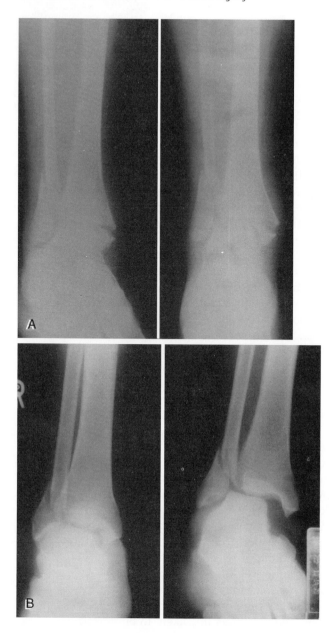

Figure 11–2. *A,* Anteroposterior (AP) and mortise radiographs of the ankle showing a bimalleolar fracture. *B,* AP and mortise radiographs of the ankle showing a typical fracture of the lateral malleolus. Injury to the deltoid ligament can be inferred from the widening of the ankle mortise.

OTHER DIAGNOSTIC TESTS

Stress testing can ideally differentiate severe (third-degree) sprains from mild and moderate (first- and second-degree) sprains. However, as all lateral ligament sprains can be treated the same,[8, 13, 18] stress testing these ligaments in acute cases is not required. Gentle stress testing may be useful in confirming the diagnosis of peroneus brevis strain, in which case passive inversion and resisted eversion produce pain localized to the lateral aspect of the foot. With acute peroneal tendon dislocation, any attempt at manipulation may be poorly tolerated by the patient. However, intense retromalleolar pain on resisted eversion and dorsiflexion is quite specific for the diagnosis.[1, 21] If radiographic examination reveals a fracture, stress testing is generally not indicated. Stabil-

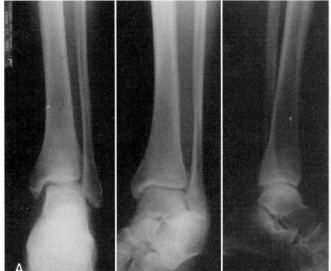

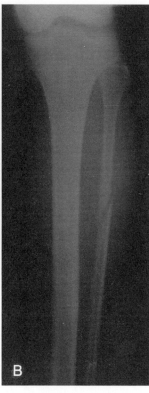

Figure 11–3. *A,* AP, mortise, and lateral views of the ankle. Clinically there was obvious injury to the medial aspect of the ankle, but no fracture is revealed radiographically. *B,* AP view of the leg of the same patient revealing a Maisonneuve fracture. The mechanism of injury was eversion with external rotation. The involved structures, in the order in which they were injured, are the deltoid ligament, the interosseous ligaments, the interosseous membrane, and the fibular shaft.

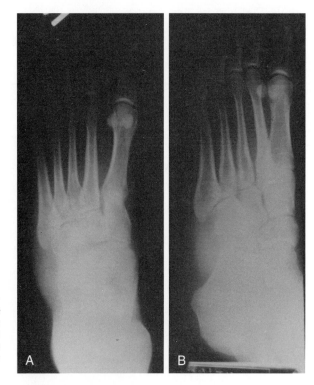

Figure 11–4. *A,* Radiograph demonstrating a typical avulsion fracture of the base of the fifth metatarsal. This injury can be satisfactorily treated as a sprain, whereas a true Jones fracture[20] *(B),* a fracture of the proximal shaft of the fifth metatarsal, may require operative treatment.

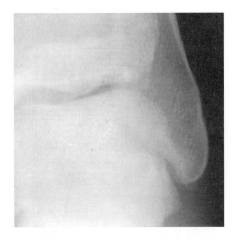

Figure 11–5. Radiograph of the ankle showing an avulsion fracture of the lateral malleolar cortex characteristic of peroneal tendon dislocation.

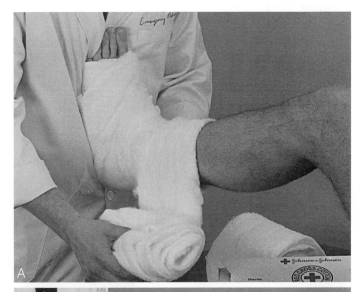

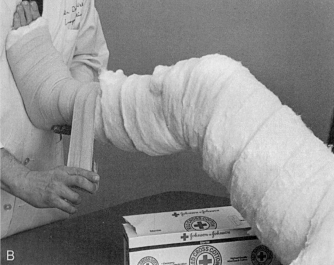

Figure 11–6. *A* and *B,* Application of Jones compression dressing: 2 in. of cotton batting is wrapped firmly with elasticized plaster, as shown. Alternatively, the cotton batting may be first wrapped with a roll of gauze (Kerlix or Kling), then a posterior plaster splint applied and held in place with a snug elastic wrap.

ity of ankle fractures can usually be inferred from the other clinical and radiographic findings.

Recurrent acute injuries, often consisting of painful, momentary "locking" episodes, should give rise to suspicions of talar dome fractures. Often not seen in the standard x-ray views described previously, they can usually be illustrated on radioisotope bone scans.

INITIAL TREATMENT

Urgent treatment is required if there is any neurovascular or cutaneous impairment. This may entail correction of gross malalignment, which can usually be accomplished by gentle manipulation with gentle in-line traction on the ankle. It may be necessary to attempt this if orthopedic consultation is not readily available. It is important to assess and record the neurovascular status after any such attempt.

Splint immobilization is indicated for ankle fractures and peroneal tendon dislocation. It is rarely indicated for other ankle injuries, if the athlete can be relied on not to abuse the injury. Immobilization and compression can be readily achieved with a Jones compression splint (Fig. 11–6) or a three-quarter round posterior splint.

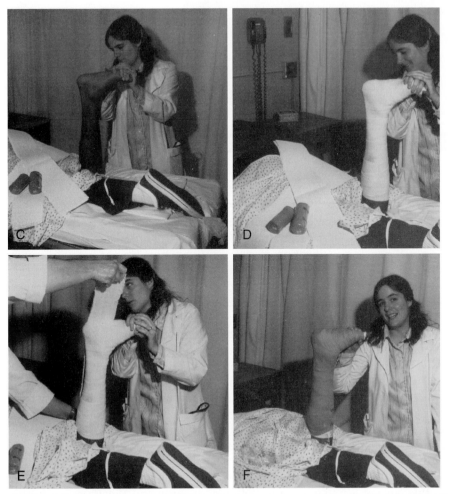

Figure 11–6 *Continued. C–F,* Application of a three-quarter round plaster splint. Each "slab" is 12 layers in thickness. Having the athlete lie prone facilitates holding the ankle in a neutral position.

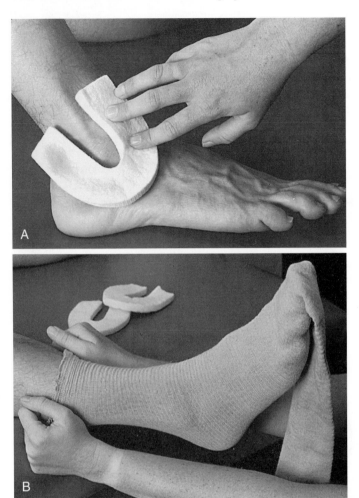

Figure 11–7. Application of elasticized stockinette over felt horseshoe padding ½ in. thick.

The *RICE* mnemonic, indicating rest, ice, compression, and elevation, applies in all cases. In the case of ankle injury, *rest* initially implies no weight bearing. When immobilization is not required, non–weight-bearing crutch ambulation is advanced to partial–weight-bearing ambulation with heel-to-toe gait as tolerated. *Ice* implies the application of crushed ice for 20 minutes at least once every 4 waking hours. It can and should be employed over any splints applied. Ice treatment is continued until the swelling stabilizes. When immobilization is not required, *compression* is achieved with an elasticized stockinette (Tubi-Grip) over felt horseshoe padding around the malleoli (Fig. 11–7). (The simple application of an elastic wrap *will not suffice*. Compression must be focused on the depressions adjacent to the malleoli—areas overlying the capsule and ligaments where swelling will result in a loss of motion and function. The horseshoes "fill in the depressions.") As dependent accumulation of extravasated blood is prevented, a pattern of ecchymosis may appear proximal to the malleoli. This finding is not a cause for concern but rather is an indication that the compression dressing has been properly applied. *Elevation* implies keeping the injured ankle at or above waist level at all times when the athlete is not actively using it. Both compression and elevation are continued until all swelling is resolved. At first, elevation may be intuitive, as the

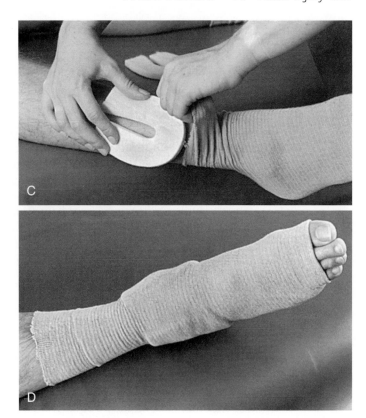

Figure 11–7 *Continued*

athlete soon realizes the ankle hurts more when it is dependent. Later, however, the athlete may have to be reminded to keep it elevated.

REFERRAL

Orthopedic referral is generally indicated for the definitive treatment of ankle fractures and medial ligament sprains, true Jones fractures, ruptures of the posterior tibial tendon, and peroneal tendon dislocations. Positive radiographs, medial greater than lateral localization of ecchymosis, swelling, tenderness, the abrupt emergence of significant pronation (flattening of the arch), or any of the specific findings for peroneal tendon dislocation may reasonably be considered indications for referral.

Some primary care physicians may choose to manage some ankle fractures themselves. Fractures that are minimally displaced and stable, as defined by Yablon,[29] can be satisfactorily treated by cast immobilization alone. Minimal displacement implies less than 1 mm displacement of the fracture fragments and less than 1 mm widening of the ankle mortise. Stable fractures include fractures of the lateral malleolus without evidence of medial injury, isolated fractures of the medial malleolus, isolated sprains of the deltoid ligament, and marginal fractures of the tibia involving less than 25% of the articular surface. Unstable fractures include fractures of the lateral malleolus with lateral displacement of the talus, bimalleolar fractures, fractures of the fibular shaft with evidence of medial injury, and marginal fractures of the tibia involving more than 25% of the articular surface. Fractures not meeting these criteria of displacement and instability should be referred for orthopedic evaluation and treatment.

REHABILITATION

Rehabilitation begins with the initial treatment of the acute injury and continues until the athlete is fully recovered.[17] Specific measures are used to achieve the following specific objectives: the prevention of swelling, the reduction of swelling, the restoration of motion, the maintenance and restoration of strength, the restoration of proprioception, and the maintenance of fitness. Concomitantly there is progression of functional use of the ankle, during which time it must be appropriately protected from further injury. Decisions relating to the initiation and discontinuation of specific measures and to the progression of functional use of the ankle are rather straightforward. They are further discussed later.

PREVENTION OF SWELLING. Measures to prevent swelling are discussed earlier under Initial Treatment.

REDUCTION OF SWELLING. Measures to reduce swelling include relative rest, elevation, compression, electrogalvanic stimulation, and contrast baths with active range-of-motion exercises. Unless immobilization precludes their use, those measures not already begun can be started as soon as the swelling has stabilized—usually 24 hours after the injury. Otherwise they can be started as soon as immobilization is discontinued. It is important to emphasize to the patient that range-of-motion exercises be done during the warm phase of the contrast baths. These measures are continued until the swelling has resolved.

RESTORATION OF MOTION. Measures to restore motion are begun as soon as the swelling has stabilized or immobilization is discontinued. All these measures are active range-of-motion exercises, which for the most part implies alphabet writing. In this exercise, the patient traces the capital letters of the alphabet with the large toe, using motions as large as possible. We have found patient understanding of and compliance with alphabet writing to be better than with the standard inversion, eversion, plantar flexion, and dorsiflexion exercises.

Motion exercises are continued until a full range of motion has been achieved. If a full range of motion, particularly in dorsiflexion, has not been restored with alphabet writing alone, then other specific stretching exercises are used (see Figs. 10–2, 10–3*B*, and 10–8).

MAINTENANCE AND RESTORATION OF STRENGTH. Measures to maintain and restore strength are also begun as soon as swelling has stabilized or as soon as immobilization is discontinued. Initially, manual resistance isometric exercises are used. Subsequently, Theraband exercises are started and advanced as tolerated. Ankle Theraband exercises are shown in Figure 11–8. When the athlete is easily able to handle three sets of 20 repetitions of the strongest Theraband, isokinetic exercises can be started. Proprioceptive training (see later) consisting of balancing on the toes of the injured extremity can be used if isokinetic equipment is not readily available. Specific strengthening exercises are continued until full strength has been restored.

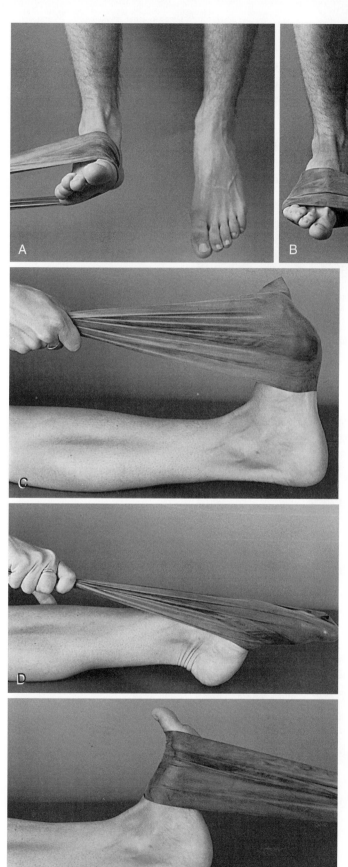

Figure 11–8. Theraband exercises for inversion *(A)*, eversion *(B)*, plantar flexion (*C* and *D*), and dorsiflexion *(E)*.

AMBULATION. Partial–weight-bearing (crutch) ambulation is permitted as soon as a normal heel-to-toe gait is possible. The crutches may be discarded as soon as painless weight bearing is possible. However, the ankle must then be protected as ambulation progresses. We use taping or the Malleoloc, Aircast, or other commercially available ankle brace for this purpose (Fig. 11–9). Ambulation progresses sequentially as indicated in Figure 11–10, with the criterion for advancement being the absence of pain and swelling with the attempted activity. A reasonable predictor of the ability to start running

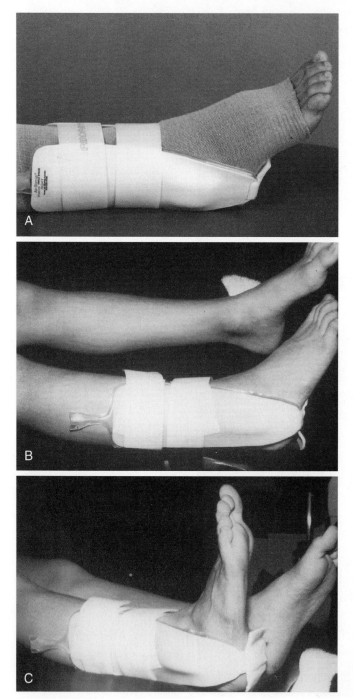

Figure 11–9. *A,* Aircast brace applied over a compression dressing. *B* and *C,* Plantar flexion and dorsiflexion of the ankle are permitted.

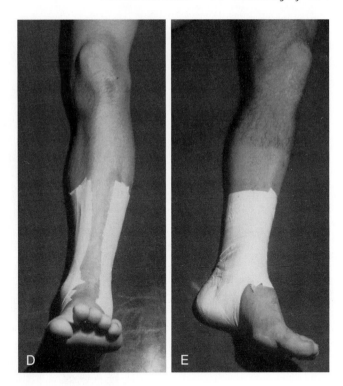

Figure 11–9 *Continued. D* and *E,* Ankle supported by adhesive taping—open to accommodate swelling *(D)* and closed after swelling has stabilized *(E).*

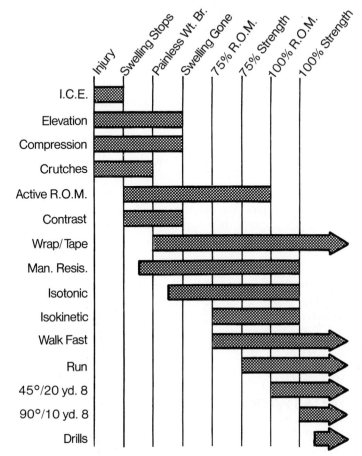

Figure 11–10. Ankle rehabilitation. I.C.E., ice, compression, elevation; R.O.M., range of motion; Man. Resis., manual resistance; Wt. Br., weight bearing. (Adapted from Garrick JG: A practical approach to rehabilitation of the ankle. Am J Sports Med 9:67–68, 1981.)

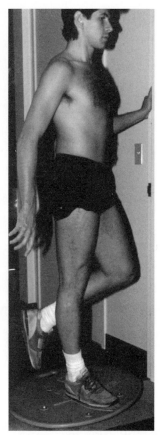

Figure 11–11. Athlete using BAPS board.

is the ability to stand on the toes and to hop up and down on the side that has been injured. It is usually apparent to athletes that if they are unable to do this they are not yet ready to run.

RESTORATION OF PROPRIOCEPTION. The importance of restoring proprioception has been emphasized in the literature.[15, 27] We begin tilt-board (biomedical ankle platform system [BAPS]) (Fig. 11–11) or toe-balancing exercises as soon as 75% motion and strength have been achieved and advance these exercises (greater tilt) as tolerated. We let the athlete start running 20-yd figure of eights and make 45-degree cuts when full motion has been achieved and advance to 10-yd figure of eights and 90-degree cuts as full strength is achieved.

MAINTENANCE OF FITNESS. Measures to maintain fitness while the athlete's injury precludes the usual training regimen are begun as soon as tolerated. Strength of the uninvolved limbs can be maintained with appropriate weight training. Endurance fitness can be maintained or even improved with swimming or stationary bicycling, which, as a rule, can be started well before the athlete is able to run.

RETURN TO SPORTS PARTICIPATION

Ideally, return to sports participation is simply the final step in the sequence of rehabilitation. For the athlete whose sport makes lesser demands on the ankle, return to the sport occurs before completion of the full rehabilitation program just discussed. However, for the athlete whose sport places great demands on the ankle, e.g., football, basketball, or tennis, completion of all steps of the rehabilitation program is recommended.

This recommendation notwithstanding, the physician is often asked to consider letting the athlete return to a sport before full rehabilitation has been achieved. The physician must then weigh the risks of re-injury and the consequences of re-injury against the athlete's desire to return to play.

In the case of ankle sprains, whatever the risk of re-injury, the consequences are not much more than having to start all over with a fresh injury.[8] Athletes are not at increased risk for incurring other acute injury because they are playing with a taped ankle.[19] Accordingly, if the athletes, and their parents, as the case may be, are accepting of some increased risk of re-injury, and if they are functionally able to play, then they should probably be allowed to do so.

Rehabilitation efforts should not abruptly cease with the return to athletic activities. The previously injured ankle will continue to be "favored," often resulting in a gradual loss of strength and a return of symptoms or even an increased likelihood of a recurrence of the sprain. Strengthening exercises should be continued for at least 4 to 6 weeks after the resumption of sports activities.

B. LATERAL LIGAMENT SPRAINS

The two inversion injuries, sprains of the lateral ligaments and strains of the peroneal tendons, account for more than 85% of all acute ankle injuries and are entirely amenable to treatment by rehabilitation alone. They are discussed separately.

HISTORY

MECHANISM OF INJURY. The mechanism of injury in isolated lateral ligament injuries is *inversion*. This may occur in running, especially on uneven surfaces; cutting; or landing from a fall or jump. Because up to 25% of ankle sprains are recurrences of previous injuries, an important historical fact may be the presence of a similar previous (but perhaps incompletely rehabilitated) injury.

SYMPTOMS. Athletes may report a cracking or popping sensation at the time of injury. They may be unable to continue the activity. but usually are able to ambulate, with or without limping. Early, there may be discrete goose-egg swelling laterally. Subsequently the pain and swelling may become more diffuse, particularly if the ankle is kept dependent or if heat is applied.

PHYSICAL EXAMINATION

Early on, *swelling and tenderness* are usually well localized over the anterior talofibular ligament and sometimes also over the calcaneofibular ligament. Palpation reveals *no bony tenderness* other than at the attachments of these ligaments. Subsequently, however, there is likely to be more diffuse swelling and tenderness with dependent ecchymosis.

Well-localized, exquisite tenderness over the anterior inferior tibiofibular ligament, the hallmark of the "high ankle sprain," should alert the examiner to the possibility of diastasis (spreading apart of the tibia and fibula) of the ankle mortise. Without radiographic abnormalities these injuries can be treated like any other lateral sprain, but the athlete should be warned that the likelihood of a very slow recovery is appreciable.

RADIOGRAPHIC EXAMINATION

Radiographic study is not indicated if the clinical findings are specific for isolated lateral ligament injury.[6, 18, 28] With the combined findings of an ability to bear weight and point tenderness anteroinferior to the lateral malleolus, there is a 97% probability of soft tissue injury only.[28] Furthermore, those fractures that are likely to be missed clinically are small avulsion fractures or nondisplaced hairline fractures of the lateral malleolus.[6] As such fractures may be satisfactorily managed as sprains,[6] the cost of misdiagnosing them as sprains is nil.

OTHER DIAGNOSTIC TESTS

Stress testing of the ligaments can ideally differentiate severe (third-degree) sprains of the anterior talofibular and calcaneofibular ligaments from mild and moderate (first- and second-degree) sprains. Stress testing has been emphasized by those orthopedists who advocate primary repair of acute third-degree sprains.[4, 5] As our practice has been to treat all lateral ligament sprains the same, we do not attach great importance to stress testing these ligaments in the acute setting. Although stress testing may be fairly well tolerated in the very acute setting, e.g., on the sidelines immediately after injury, it is usually not well tolerated after significant swelling has occurred. We certainly do not advocate anesthesia for stress testing of these ligaments. Nor do we believe that radiographic documentation of the stress-testing procedure provides any additional useful information. The technique of stress testing the lateral ligaments is discussed in the sections on chronic conditions of the ankle.

INITIAL TREATMENT

Initial treatment consists of *rest, ice, compression, and elevation*, as discussed earlier.

REFERRAL

Referral is not required.

DEFINITIVE TREATMENT

Definitive treatment as such is not required. Initial treatment is followed immediately by mobilization and rehabilitation, as discussed previously.

The treatment of severe sprains by early mobilization and rehabilitation is not without some controversy. It has been correctly pointed out that the achievement of mechanical stability is more likely with surgery than with other methods of treatment.[4, 5, 8, 13] In our opinion, however, the functional outcome, rather than the talar tilt test or the anterior drawer test, represents the appropriate "bottom line." Mechanical stability or a lack thereof has not been found to correlate closely with the functional outcome.[8, 14] Moreover, none of the advocates of surgical treatment have been able to show a priori which patients are at risk for functionally significant mechanical instability and would therefore presumably benefit from primary repair. It has been shown, however, that delayed repair or simple reconstruction of the anterior talofibular ligament is as simple and effective as primary repair in achieving mechanical stability.[9] Even if the cost and logistics were of no consideration, the data would not be sufficiently compelling for us to commit all our patients with acute third-degree lateral ligament sprains to operative treatment. (The decision of whether to repair these ligaments primarily is formally analyzed in Chapter 13.)

Not much controversy remains regarding immobilization as a treatment option for moderate and severe sprains, there being little to recommend it. The achievement of mechanical stability is no better than with early mobilization, and the duration of disability after injury is as prolonged as with surgical treatment.[8, 13]

C. PERONEUS BREVIS STRAIN/AVULSION FRACTURE OF BASE OF FIFTH METATARSAL

HISTORY

MECHANISM OF INJURY. The mechanism of injury is *inversion*.

SYMPTOMS. Athletes may report a cracking or popping sensation at the time of injury. They may be unable to continue the activity but usually are able to ambulate, with or without limping. Pain and swelling tend to be mild to moderate and localized to the lateral aspect of the foot.

PHYSICAL EXAMINATION

Swelling and tenderness are usually well localized over the peroneus brevis tendon just proximal to its insertion or over the base of the fifth metatarsal. Dependent ecchymosis and crepitation may also be noted.

RADIOGRAPHIC EXAMINATION

If bony tenderness is present, foot films are indicated to rule out the possibility of a true Jones fracture, a fracture of the proximal diaphysis of the fifth metatarsal. Whereas an avulsion fracture of the base of the fifth metatarsal is appropriately treated the same as a strain, a Jones fracture should be referred for orthopedic evaluation and treatment, as open reduction and internal fixation are sometimes required.[20]

OTHER DIAGNOSTIC TESTS

If radiographic examination is not indicated or is negative, the diagnosis of tendon injury may be confirmed with gentle muscle testing. Passive inversion and resisted eversion produce pain localized to the lateral aspect of the foot.

INITIAL TREATMENT

Rest, ice, compression, and elevation constitute the initial treatment, as discussed previously.

REFERRAL

Referral is not required.

DEFINITIVE TREATMENT

Definitive treatment as such is not required. Initial treatment is followed immediately by mobilization and rehabilitation, as discussed earlier, with emphasis on restrengthening the ankle evertors.

D. ACUTE PERONEAL TENDON DISLOCATION

Peroneal tendon dislocations probably account for no more than 2% of all acute ankle injuries. These dislocations are not amenable to treatment by rehabilitation alone and may be difficult to differentiate from lateral ligament sprains.

HISTORY

MECHANISM OF INJURY. By far the most common mechanism is *forceful passive dorsiflexion*, as may occur when a skier catches a tip and falls forward over the ski.[12, 22, 25]

SYMPTOMS. Patients may report a cracking sensation, accompanied by an intense flash of pain.[12] They are usually unable to continue the activity and often unable to ambulate.[1, 12]

PHYSICAL EXAMINATION

Immediately after injury, *swelling and tenderness* may be well localized *postero-superior to the lateral malleolus*. However, after 2 hours or more, pain, swelling, ecchymosis, and tenderness become more diffuse.

Palpation may reveal *frankly dislocated tendons*, reducible by plantar flexion of the ankle.[22] By the time the ankle is examined, however, the dislocated tendons are usually obscured by swelling[1, 12] or, more likely, have spontaneously reduced.

Examination of the contralateral ankle may reveal *congenital dislocation of tendons*[22] or *shallow support.*[12]

RADIOGRAPHIC EXAMINATION

Ankle films are indicated if the clinical findings are suggestive of the diagnosis. A characteristic avulsion fracture of the lateral malleolar cortex is found in about 13% of cases and can be considered pathognomonic (see Fig. 11–5).[12] This finding should not be confused with avulsion flakes off the tip of the lateral malleolus or talus, which signify nothing more than lateral ligament injury.

OTHER DIAGNOSTIC TESTS

Any attempt at manipulation may be poorly tolerated by the patient. However, *intense retromalleolar pain on resisted eversion and dorsiflexion* is quite specific for the diagnosis.[1, 21] There should be no instability or (before the onset of diffuse swelling and tenderness) pain on varus stress.[22] Postinjury ecchymosis, appearing 24 to 48 hours later, often extends 3 to 4 in. proximally along the posterior border of the fibula—much higher than seen with lateral ankle sprains.

INITIAL TREATMENT

The initial treatment consists of *rest, ice, compression* (a Jones compression splint is appropriate), *and elevation.*

REFERRAL

Referral to an orthopedic surgeon is indicated.

DEFINITIVE TREATMENT

The definitive treatment of choice is primary surgical repair, which is followed by rehabilitation, as discussed earlier.

Definitive treatment is not without some controversy. All authors agree that treatment as for a sprain results in chronic or recurrent instability. Some have advocated treatment by immobilization initially with subsequent surgical reconstruction for failures of closed treatment.[21, 25] Others have advocated immediate operative treatment,[1, 12] and we concur. The primary repair is technically much easier than the reconstructive procedures, and the results are superior.

E. CHRONIC INSTABILITY

Chronic functional instability of the ankle, whatever its cause, presents in a characteristic way. There is complaint of a weak ankle, an unstable ankle, giving way, a chronic sprain, frequent sprains, and so on and a past history of a prior severe sprain, often not properly treated or rehabilitated. Limited dorsiflexion,[2] peroneal weakness,[3, 26] loss of proprioception,[14, 15] mechanical instability,[4, 26] and recurrent peroneal tendon dislocation[1, 22] have been implicated as etiological factors. Of these, the first three are amenable to treatment by rehabilitation alone, whereas the latter two may require surgical treatment.

In our experience, functional instability is most often the result of incomplete rehabilitation of a prior ankle injury. Mechanical instability may or may not correlate with functional instability. Chronic instability requires specific treatment only if the ankle remains functionally unstable despite adequate rehabilitation. Chronic peroneal tendon dislocation is unlikely to respond well to rehabilitation alone;[1, 22] however, there is little to lose and much possibly to be gained by attempting rehabilitation before considering reconstructive sur-

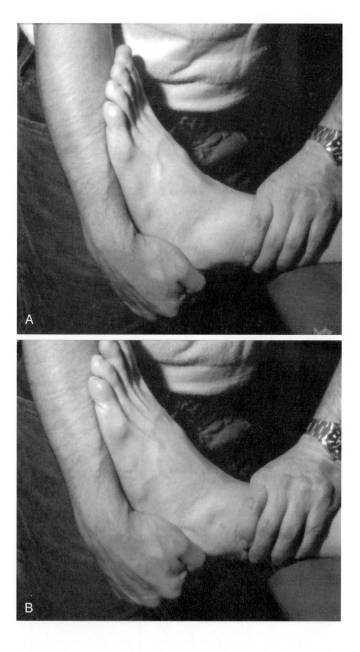

Figure 11–12. *A* and *B,* Demonstration of a positive anterior drawer test.

gery. Our recommended approach to chronic functional instability in the athlete involves assessment of the possible etiological factor, a trial of rehabilitation as indicated, and subsequent referral if indicated.

The athlete is first asked about prior injury to the ankle, any previous treatment and its results, the circumstances that reproduce the symptoms, and any associated symptoms. A snapping sensation associated with the instability episodes is characteristic but not diagnostic of peroneal tendon dislocation.[1] Sharp, lancinating pain just preceding the instability episode might suggest momentary, mechanical impingement from an ununited talar dome fracture.

Next, ankle motion, strength, proprioception, and mechanical stability are systematically assessed. Strength is initially assessed by manual resistance. Proprioception and strength can be assessed both by having the patient balance or hop on the affected foot and by observing the athlete on a tilt board. Mechanical stability can be adequately assessed by the anterior drawer test[9] and by varus and valgus stressing of the ankle (Fig. 11–12).

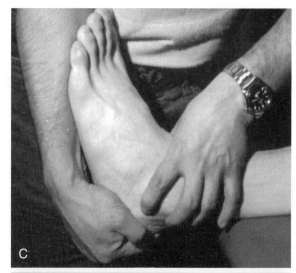

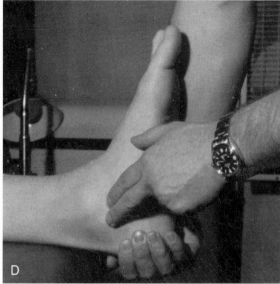

Figure 11–12 *Continued.* Varus *(C)* and valgus *(D)* testing of the ankle.

Finally, the specific physical findings of peroneal tendon dislocation are sought. In the absence of acute recurrence of injury, the tendons may be anteriorly dislocatable with either gentle pressure[22] or active dorsiflexion and eversion and reducible with plantar flexion. When pain and swelling preclude adequate examination of the symptomatic ankle, examination of the contralateral ankle may show congenital dislocation of the tendons.[22] After an acute recurrence, localization of pain, swelling, and tenderness posterosuperior to the lateral malleolus would be a specific, but not often present, finding.[1, 12, 22]

Ankle rehabilitation, as discussed in part A, is then begun. It is continued until motion, strength, and proprioception have been fully restored.

As a matter of practicality, functionally significant mechanical instability is most often treated with external support during athletic activity.[19, 27] If the ankle remains functionally unstable after full rehabilitation and the athlete desires definitive treatment for it, the athlete should be referred for further evaluation. When the mechanical instability is due to prior sprains of the lateral ligaments, delayed repair can be easily carried out.[9]

When the functional instability is due to recurrent peroneal tendon dislocation, this condition has not responded satisfactorily to rehabilitation, and the athlete desires definitive treatment, the athlete should be referred for orthopedic evaluation.

F. CHRONIC PAIN

Chronic, activity-related ankle pain is the bane of many athletes who run or jump. It is the usual presenting symptom of tendinitis, ankle impingement syndrome, degenerative joint disease, osteochondral fracture, and osteochondrosis dissecans. It may be a prominent feature of those conditions discussed previously that characteristically present as functional instability. Differentiation among the various conditions that can cause chronic ankle pain provides the basis for subsequent treatment and referral.

HISTORY

The athlete is asked about prior injury to the ankle, any previous treatment and its results, the character and localization of the pain, the circumstances that produce the pain, and any associated symptoms. A history of a bad sprain preceding the onset of the chronic pain is characteristic of osteochondral fracture and peroneal tendon dislocation. Pain in the front of the ankle with extreme dorsiflexion is characteristic of anterior talotibial impingement. Pain in the back of the ankle with extreme plantar flexion is characteristic of posterior talotibial impingement. Episodes of lateral ankle pain associated with a snapping sensation are characteristic of recurrent peroneal tendon dislocation.[1, 22] Pain, swelling, and instability, not necessarily related to activity and not well localized, often characterize osteochondrosis dissecans as does recurrent, sharp, unpredictable, lancinating, momentary pain within the ankle.

PHYSICAL EXAMINATION

Physical examination includes inspection and palpation, as discussed in part A, and assessment of stability, as discussed in part E. In addition, the anterior and posterior joint lines are palpated with the ankle in positions of plantar flexion, neutral, and dorsiflexion. Joint line tenderness is characteristic of talotibial impingement, osteochondral fracture, osteochondrosis dissecans, and advanced degenerative joint disease. With anterior and posterior impingement, pain is reproduced by forced passive dorsiflexion and plantar flexion, respectively.

RADIOGRAPHIC EXAMINATION

If the ankle pain can be attributed just to tendinitis, then radiographic examination is not required. In all other cases, at least anteroposterior, mortise, and lateral views of the ankle are indicated. If either osteochondral fracture or osteochondrosis dissecans is suspected, then additional mortise views with the ankle fully dorsiflexed and fully plantarflexed are indicated to permit more complete visualization of the dome of the talus.

With degenerative joint disease there are characteristic radiographic changes if the condition is moderately advanced. This also holds true for the talotibial impingement syndromes, which may be considered special cases of degenerative joint disease. If the lateral radiograph reveals some degenerative changes, then additional lateral views in dorsiflexion (for anterior impingement) and plantar flexion (for posterior impingement) may help determine the extent of bony impingement.

OTHER DIAGNOSTIC TESTS

Tomography, computed tomography (CT), or magnetic resonance imaging (MRI) of the talus can reveal osteochondral fractures and osteochondrosis dissecans not seen on plain radiographs (Fig. 11–13). They may also be useful in determining the extent of these lesions. Radionuclide bone scanning will reveal whether an osteochondral fragment may be amenable to closed treatment (hot spot) or whether it is not (cold spot). We have not found other tests to be particularly useful in the work-up of chronic ankle pain. Whether the primary care physician orders any of these special tests or defers their ordering to a consultant depends on individual circumstances.

INITIAL TREATMENT

The initial treatment for tendinitis, impingement syndrome, or symptomatic degenerative joint disease may include relative rest, nonsteroidal anti-inflammatory medication, ice massage, contrast baths, and ice and electrogalvanic stimulation treatments. Of these measures, relative rest is the most important.

Relative rest implies only avoidance of those activities that produce pain and swelling. The specific activities to be avoided depend on the specific problem and the individual athlete.

REHABILITATION

Any motion, strength, or proprioceptive deficits are rehabilitated as discussed previously. With anterior impingement, strengthening the ankle plantar flex-

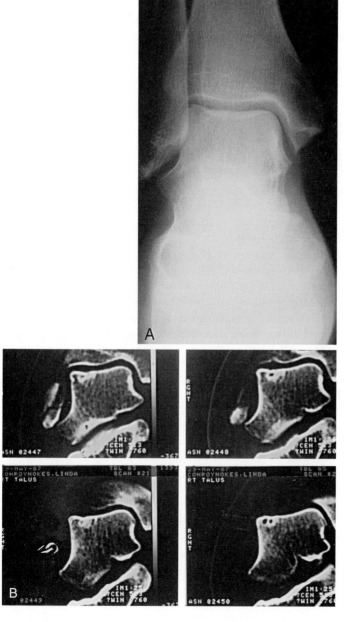

Figure 11–13. AP radiograph (A) and computed axial tomograms (B) of the right ankle of a dancer, both demonstrating an osteochondral fracture of the lateral corner of the dome of the talus.

ors is particularly important; similarly, with posterior impingement, strengthening the ankle dorsiflexors is particularly important.

REFERRAL

Orthopedic referral is indicated for the management of osteochondral fractures and osteochondrosis dissecans. Referral may be considered for advanced degenerative joint disease that has not responded satisfactorily to symptomatic measures, activity modification, and rehabilitation. This also holds true for impingement syndromes with evidence of bony impingement.

RETURN TO SPORTS PARTICIPATION

Ideally there is a gradually progressive return to full activity as symptoms permit. The absence of pain and swelling with an attempted level of activity is the criterion for advancement to that level of activity.

Sometimes, however, the athlete is unable to resume a desired level of activity without a recurrence of symptoms. In this case, the athlete should be counseled regarding the risks of continuing the activity, e.g., acceleration of degenerative joint disease and development of secondary overuse syndromes. The recreational or fitness athlete should be advised of alternative activities, such as swimming and bicycling, which do not place as much stress on the ankle as do weight-bearing activities.

G. ANTERIOR (TALOTIBIAL) IMPINGEMENT SYNDROME

Of the various conditions that account for chronic ankle pain in athletes, the two talotibial impingement syndromes are unique to both athletics and the ankle. They are discussed separately.

HISTORY

MECHANISM OF INJURY. The mechanism of injury is *repetitive, forced dorsiflexion*, such as may occur when gymnasts land short on dismounts or when dancers land jumps in grands pliés. The syndrome has also been reported in baseball, basketball, and tennis players.[23]

SYMPTOMS. The athlete complains of *pain in the front of the ankle*. Initially the pain may be present only during athletic activity in which the ankle is forcibly dorsiflexed. Subsequently there may be pain with activities of daily living in which the ankle is dorsiflexed, as in walking uphill. Eventually there may be constant pain.

PHYSICAL EXAMINATION

Physical examination reveals tenderness over the anterior joint line of the ankle. Dorsiflexion may be limited, and forced passive dorsiflexion reproduces the impingement pain. A small effusion may be palpable. Osteophytes may be palpable on the anterior margin of the tibia and the corresponding part of the talus.

RADIOGRAPHIC EXAMINATION

Radiographic examination is indicated to determine the extent of bony impingement. Talar osteophytes may be present but may be too far anterior to contribute to impingement. In addition to standard ankle views, a lateral view with the ankle in full dorsiflexion helps determine the extent of bony impingement.

OTHER DIAGNOSTIC TESTS

If the clinical and radiographic findings are inconclusive, a *radionuclide bone scan* may be indicated to rule out navicular stress fracture. This is especially the case if the anterior ankle pain is not just dorsiflexion-related, or if there is point tenderness over the tarsal navicular.

INITIAL TREATMENT

Relative rest and other measures to reduce pain, swelling, and inflammation make up the initial treatment. *Nonsteroidal anti-inflammatory drugs, ice massage, and contrast baths* are routinely used. Relative rest may imply simply avoidance of forced dorsiflexion. For example, the gymnast refrains from practicing dismounts and the dancer refrains from jetés and grands pliés. Alternatively, taping the ankle to limit dorsiflexion may permit continuation of training without pain.

REHABILITATION

Any motion, strength, or proprioceptive deficits are rehabilitated, as discussed previously. With anterior impingement, strengthening the ankle plantar flexors is particularly important, as this may help limit the hyperdorsiflexion.

REFERRAL

Referral is not required unless there is evidence of *bony impingement* and the problem does not respond satisfactorily to symptomatic treatment. In that case, surgical débridement (osteophytectomy) may be necessary.

H.   POSTERIOR (TALOTIBIAL) IMPINGEMENT SYNDROME

HISTORY

MECHANISM OF INJURY. The mechanism of injury is *repetitive, forced plantar flexion*, such as may occur with practicing karate kicks or dancing en pointe. The initial symptomatic episode may be preceded by a lateral ankle sprain.

SYMPTOMS. The athlete complains of *pain in the back of the ankle*. Initially the pain may be present only during the athletic activity in which the ankle is forcibly plantarflexed. Subsequently there may be constant pain.

PHYSICAL EXAMINATION

Tenderness anterior to the Achilles tendon, which itself is nontender, is revealed by the physical examination. Resisted plantar flexion is not painful, but the range of plantar flexion may be limited, and *forced passive plantar flexion reproduces the impingement pain*. A small joint effusion may be palpable.

RADIOGRAPHIC EXAMINATION

Radiographic study is indicated to determine the extent of bony impingement. In addition to the standard ankle views, a lateral view with the ankle in full plantar flexion may help with this determination. A normal os trigonum should not be mistaken for posterior impingement that has progressed to the point of stress fracture (Fig. 11–14), although a "normal os trigonum" may be the cause of the symptoms in an activity such as ballet that requires *hypernormal* plantar flexion.

Occasionally posterior impingement occurs in the *absence* of either a posterior process of the talus or an os trigonum. We have encountered a fibrocartilaginous, labrum-like structure posterior to the articular margin of the talus that appeared to block plantar flexion in a ballet dancer.

OTHER DIAGNOSTIC TESTS

Other diagnostic tests are not required.

INITIAL TREATMENT

Relative rest and other measures to reduce pain, swelling, and inflammation make up the initial treatment. *Nonsteroidal anti-inflammatory drugs, ice massage,*

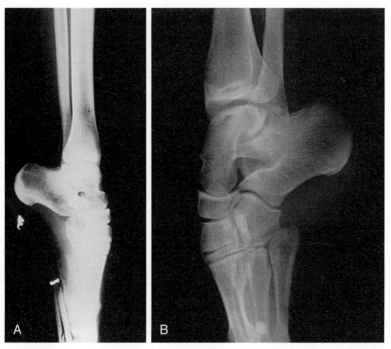

Figure 11–14. Lateral radiographs of the ankle in full plantar flexion showing a normal ankle *(A)* and an os trigonum *(B)*.

and contrast baths are routinely used. Relative rest may imply simply avoidance of forced plantar flexion. For example, the dancer refrains from dancing en pointe or demi-pointe, or the ankle is taped to limit plantar flexion.

REHABILITATION

Any motion, strength, or proprioceptive deficits are rehabilitated, as discussed previously. With posterior impingement, strengthening the ankle dorsiflexors is particularly important, as this may help to limit the hyperplantar flexion.

REFERRAL

Referral is required if there is evidence of bony impingement and the problem does not respond satisfactorily to symptomatic treatment. In that case, surgical débridement (osteophytectomy) may be necessary.

I. TALAR OSTEOCHONDROSIS

Osteochondrosis dissecans of the talus is a condition in which a small area of the weight-bearing portion of the talus loses its blood supply. Usually located on either the posteromedial or anterolateral aspect (corner) of the talus, this condition can heal spontaneously, remain dormant—and thus asymptomatic—for long periods, or result in chronic ankle problems usually associated with failure of the avascular fragment to heal or unite with the underlying bone. The problem may in some instances represent nonunion of a talar dome fracture resulting from an ankle "sprain." In other cases the lack of a preceding episode of trauma suggests that the condition may arise a priori.

The condition is considered here in some detail because the symptoms are often vague, intermittent, and unaccompanied by the signs usually associated with chronic ankle injuries. The indistinct history and examination often lead to the erroneous conclusion that the athlete is a complainer or malingerer. We have encountered a number of patients with this condition who have been sent to pain clinics, one of whom was undergoing psychotherapy.

HISTORY

MECHANISM OF INJURY. The condition may arise from either a medial or lateral ankle sprain, presumably the result of the edge of the tilted talus coming in contact with the lateral or medial malleolus, respectively. More often the onset of the symptoms is unassociated with any specific incident of trauma.

SYMPTOMS. Pain is the primary complaint. It may be sudden and lancinating, accompanied by *locking*, which may be only momentary or may require manipulation for relief. (The sudden onset of pain and locking usually indicates that the avascular fragment has broken free, creating a loose body within the joint.) More often the pain is vague, diffuse, and aching, unassociated with activity. An effusion is often present but is not diagnostic.

PHYSICAL EXAMINATION

Physical examination usually reveals little more than the presence of an effusion or synovitis of the ankle joint. Occasionally a loose body is palpable in the anterior aspect of the ankle. There may or may not be weakness of the muscles crossing the ankle, depending on the duration and severity of the symptoms.

RADIOGRAPHIC EXAMINATION

In all instances of unexplained, recurrent ankle pain, radiographic study should be carried out. If the three standard ankle views fail to reveal any abnormality, we order the mortise view taken in maximal plantar flexion, neutral, and maximal dorsiflexion. This permits viewing the "profile" of the posterior, middle, and anterior surfaces of the dome of the talus, respectively.

OTHER DIAGNOSTIC TESTS

In the event of negative radiographs, tests such as CT or MRI often reveal the presence of the lesion as well as its exact size and location (see Fig. 11–13). Radionuclide bone scanning, if "hot," suggests the potential of healing.

INITIAL TREATMENT

A program aimed at re-establishing normal strength of the muscles crossing the ankle, especially the peroneals and tibialis anterior and posterior, should be included in the initial treatment. Although restrengthening muscles obviously has no influence on an osteochondritic lesion, the symptoms may be associated with an unrehabilitated ankle sprain, with the osteochondrosis dissecans representing a "chance" finding. Nonsteroidal anti-inflammatory drugs may be helpful in controlling any associated synovitis.

REHABILITATION

Rehabilitation is undertaken to rule out the possibility that the signs and symptoms arise from a cause unrelated to the osteochondrosis dissecans lesion. Both range-of-motion and strengthening exercises should be carried out only if painless.

REFERRAL

Referral to an orthopedic surgeon is indicated with documentation of an osteochondrosis dissecans lesion.

DEFINITIVE TREATMENT

Immobilization is considered by some to enhance the likelihood of healing but in our experience has been less than rewarding. Avoidance of the activities that produce either pain or effusion is, in our estimation, an equally successful and more palatable alternative.

Surgical management includes efforts directed toward aiding the lesion to reunite with the underlying fragment (internal fixation of the fragment) or removal of the osteochondritic fragment with curettage of the base of the defect to promote filling of the defect. The latter procedure can often be carried out arthroscopically.

J. POSTERIOR TIBIAL TENDON DYSFUNCTION

Posterior tibial tendon dysfunction is generally considered to be an affliction seen in women older than 50 years and is rarely described in the sports medicine literature. With the desire for enhanced fitness in the older population we are seeing this condition with increased frequency, usually associated with hiking or walking activities.

We include this problem not because of its frequency but because of its potential for producing severe disability and the difficulty of management.[11]

HISTORY

The history is usually benign, rarely preceded by a traumatic episode, and more often associated with deformation of the foot or difficulty walking rather than pain. Indeed, the first indication of trouble may be the appearance of a collapsed arch.

PHYSICAL EXAMINATION

Unilateral collapse of the arch is often the most striking finding. Swelling and tenderness posterior and inferior to the medial malleolus are often present. As the patient attempts to arise on the toes, the hindfoot fails to invert as it should normally. Resisted eversion may be painful and nearly always reveals weakness of the posterior tibial muscle.

OTHER DIAGNOSTIC TESTS

Although MRI studies are reported as best being able to characterize the status of tendons, we have had difficulty correlating those findings with the clinical picture and, more importantly, have not found MRI helpful in making decisions about treatment.

INITIAL TREATMENT

The initial management consists of discontinuing all pain-producing activities (including weight bearing if necessary), the use of an arch support or orthosis, and a 2- to 3-week course of nonsteroidal anti-inflammatory medications. If this regimen fails, then a short leg cast should be applied and worn for a minimum of 3 weeks.

REHABILITATION

Rehabilitation ultimately involves regaining the strength and flexibility of the posterior tibial muscle tendon unit. Stretching and strengthening programs should not be instituted until they can be accomplished in an absolutely painless manner.

REFERRAL

This condition should be referred to an orthopedic surgeon after diagnosis or, at the outside, after failure to resolve after 3 weeks of anti-inflammatory medication and activity attenuation.

REFERENCES

1. Arrowsmith SR, Fleming LL, Allman FL: Traumatic dislocations of the peroneal tendons. Am J Sports Med 11:142–146, 1983.
2. Balduini FC, Tetzlaff J: Historical perspectives on injuries of the ligaments of the ankle. Clin Sports Med 1:3–12, 1982.
3. Bosien WR, Staples OS, Russell SW: Residual disability following acute ankle sprains. J Bone Joint Surg Am 37:1237–1243, 1955.
4. Brand RL, Black HM, Cox JS: The natural history of inadequately treated ankle sprain. Am J Sports Med 6:248–249, 1977.
5. Brand RL, Collins MDF: Operative management of ligamentous injuries to the ankle. Clin Sports Med 1:117–130, 1982.
6. Brooks SC, Potter BT, Rainey JB: Inversion injuries of the ankle: Clinical assessment and radiographic review. Br Med J 282:607–608, 1981.
7. Brostrom L: Sprained ankles. I: Anatomic lesions in recent sprains. Acta Chir Scand 128:483–495, 1964.
8. Brostrom L: Sprained ankles. V: Treatment and prognosis in recent ligament ruptures. Acta Chir Scand 132:537–550, 1966.
9. Brostrom L: Sprained ankles. VI: Surgical treatment of chronic ligament ruptures. Acta Chir Scand 132:551–565, 1966.
10. Burwell NH, Charnley AD: The treatment of displaced fractures at the ankle by rigid internal fixation and early joint movement. J Bone Joint Surg Br 47:634–660, 1965.
11. Cracchiolo A: Posterior tibial tendon dysfunction. Contemp Orthopaed 28:4; 368–371, 1994.
12. Eckert WD, Davis EA Jr: Acute rupture of the peroneal retinaculum. J Bone Joint Surg Am 58:670–673, 1976.
13. Freeman MAR: Treatment of ruptures of the lateral ligament of the ankle. J Bone Joint Surg Br 47:661–668, 1965.
14. Freeman MAR: Instability of the foot after injuries to the lateral ligament of the ankle. J Bone Joint Surg Br 47:669–677, 1965.
15. Freeman MAR: The etiology and prevention of functional instability of the foot. J Bone Joint Surg Br 47:678–685, 1965.
16. Garrick JG: The frequency of injury, mechanism of injury, and epidemiology of ankle sprains. Am J Sports Med 5:241–242, 1977.
17. Garrick JG: A practical approach to rehabilitation of the ankle. Am J Sports Med 9:67–68, 1981.
18. Garrick JG: The athlete's ankle and other injuries. Emerg Med Aug 15, pp 178–209, 1982.

19. Garrick JG, Requa RK: Role of external support in the prevention of ankle sprains. Med Sci Sports 5:200–203, 1973.
20. Kavanaugh JH, Brower TD, Mann RV: The Jones' fracture revisited. J Bone Joint Surg Am 60:776–782, 1978.
21. McLennan JG: Treatment of acute and chronic luxations of the peroneal tendons. Am J Sports Med 8:432–436, 1980.
22. Marti R: Dislocation of the peroneal tendons. Am J Sports Med 5:19–22, 1977.
23. Parkes JC II et al: The anterior impingement syndrome of the ankle. J Trauma 20:895, 1980.
24. Ramsey PL, Hamilton W: Changes in tibiotalar area of contact caused by lateral talar shift. J Bone Joint Surg Am 58:356–357, 1976.
25. Scheller AD, Kasser JR, Quigley TB: Tendon injuries about the ankle. Orthop Clin North Am 11:801–811, 1980.
26. Staples OS: Ruptures of the fibular collateral ligaments of the ankle. J Bone Joint Surg Am 57:101–107, 1975.
27. Tropp H: Prevention of ankle sprains. Am J Sports Med 13:259–262, 1985.
28. Vargish T, Clarke WR: The ankle injury—Indications for the selective use of x-rays. Injury 14:507–512, 1983.
29. Yablon IG: Which ankle fractures can be managed conservatively? J Musculoskel Med 1(13):19–26, Dec 1984.
30. Yablon IG, Heller FG, Shouse, L: The key role of the lateral malleolus in displaced fractures of the ankle. J Bone Joint Surg Am 59:169–173, 1977.

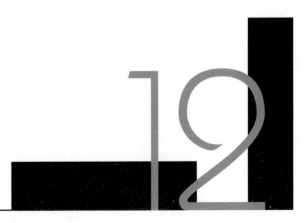

Foot Injuries

Conditions to Be Referred

- **Jones fracture**
- **Displaced metatarsal fractures**
- **Lisfranc's fracture/dislocation**

Triage

Indications for Referral	Indications for X-ray

Indications for Referral

- **Acute**
  History
  Examination
    Plantar ecchymosis of midfoot
    (Lisfranc's injury)
  X-ray films
    Transverse fracture of base of
    fifth metatarsal
- **Gradual onset**
  History
  Examination
  X-ray films

Indications for X-ray

- **Acute**
  History
    Pain at base of fifth metatarsal
    Hyperplantar flexion injury
  Examination
    Tenderness at base of fifth
    metatarsal
    Tenderness/swelling midfoot
    Ecchymosis of plantar aspect of
    midfoot
- **Gradual onset**
  History
    Localized metatarsal shaft pain
    Pain at base of fifth metatarsal
  Examination
    Focal tenderness of metatarsal
    shaft
    Focal tenderness at base of fifth
    metatarsal

The stable base of support provided by the foot is essential to the vast majority of sports and recreational activities. Although the foot functions differently in running and in aerobic dance, it is nonetheless the final interface between the athlete and the playing surface. Perhaps the most compelling evidence supporting the variety of ways the foot functions is the availability of the differing shoe designs for various of sports.

As is true with other anatomical areas, acute injuries involving the foot are usually diagnostically straightforward. Although their consequences may be devastating in an athletic sense—a fractured talus, for example—there are few unique "sports medicine" considerations necessary for their management.

Overuse injuries of the foot present greater diagnostic and therapeutic challenges. Thorough familiarity with the demands (on the foot) of various activities is often necessary to allow resolution of the problem.

Although any foot problems/injuries can be associated with athletic activities, we have limited this discussion to those that occur most commonly in our practice. We have, in addition, included a section dealing with foot problems unique to certain endeavors such as ballet.

A. METATARSOPHALANGEAL JOINT INJURIES (TURF TOE)

Turf toe is a sprain of the plantar aspect of the capsule of the metatarsophalangeal joint of the great toe. It is typically the result of forced hyperextension (dorsiflexion) of the joint, as might occur in a football pile-up. It may also be the result of repeated maneuvers requiring push-off from the dorsiflexed great toe. It is seen more often on synthetic playing surfaces.

The metatarsophalangeal joint is painful, swollen, and tender. Active or passive dorsiflexion is especially painful and causes the athlete to use a flatfooted (apropulsive) gait in an attempt to avoid push-off.

The injury is treated like any other sprain with the initial use of ice, compression, elevation, and relative rest. Contrast baths are helpful in reducing the swelling. Limitation of dorsiflexion can be achieved by the use of a stiff-soled shoe or by placing a semirigid plate in the shoe (Fig. 12–1).

Turf and shoe manufacturers and athletes themselves must share the blame for the occurrence of this problem. The unyielding characteristics of synthetic turf would be less devastating if the soles of the shoes were less flexible.[1] However, the pliability of the shoes is a result of the demands placed on the manufacturers by athletes. A lightweight, flexible shoe simply offers less protection to the great toe.

B. PLANTAR FASCIITIS

The plantar fascia is a dense, fibrous sheet extending from the anterior border of the os calcis forward into the flexor apparatus of the toes (Fig. 12–2). Simplistically, and functionally, it might be viewed as the bowstring that helps maintain the "bow" or longitudinal arch of the foot. It functions passively in

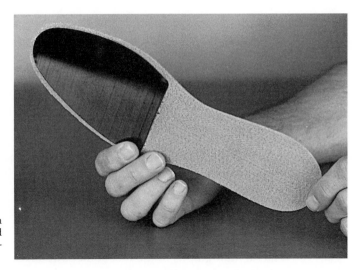

Figure 12–1. Protection from turf toe is afforded by a semirigid insole that restricts metatarsophalangeal joint excursion.

concert with the muscles of both inversion and eversion (of the ankle) that actively support or enhance the arch.

HISTORY

MECHANISM OF INJURY. The majority of injuries are of the overuse variety, associated with training errors such as an abrupt increase in hill running or sprinting, either of which emphasizes push-off or toe running. The injury may also be associated with incomplete rehabilitation (strengthening) following a previous ankle injury, usually a sprain. Weak peroneal muscles may inadequately support the arch, thus placing additional stress on the plantar fascia. Plantar fasciitis has been associated with abnormal pronation, as well as with the relative rigidity of the high-arched, cavus foot.

Both partial and complete ruptures of the plantar fascia have been reported. These acute injuries are often associated with pre-existing plantar fasciitis, often previously treated with corticosteroid injections.

SYMPTOMS. Pain, the most prevalent symptom, is usually of gradual onset. It may occur along the entire medial border of the fascia or can be well localized to the origin of the fascia on the anteromedial aspect of the os calcis (see Fig. 12–2). In the latter location it is often mistaken for a stone bruise.

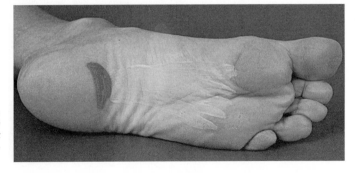

Figure 12–2. The plantar fascia. The darkened area represents the origin on the os calcis, the most frequent site of pain and tenderness.

Initially the pain is usually sport related, but later it may be present with all ambulatory endeavors. Rising onto the toes often increases the pain.

PHYSICAL EXAMINATION

Tenderness is usually present along the medial border or origin of the fascia (see Fig. 12–2). Occasionally a small defect in the medial border of the fascia is palpable. Swelling, if present, is usually localized to the area just anterior to the os calcis. Pain is often prompted by dorsiflexing the great toe.

RADIOGRAPHIC EXAMINATION

Lateral radiographs of the foot sometimes reveal spur formation at the antero-inferior border of the os calcis, seemingly the result of new-bone formation at the site of repeated, minor avulsion of the origin of the fascia (Fig. 12–3). Abnormal radiographs are not necessary for establishment of the diagnosis, and in our experience, the size or presence of the anterior calcaneal spur has little prognostic value.

OTHER DIAGNOSTIC TESTS

Low-Dye taping may serve as a diagnostic test, as it may result in striking, abrupt reduction of the pain present with ambulation (Fig. 12–4).

INITIAL TREATMENT

Initial management should include local application of ice, administration of nonsteroidal anti-inflammatory drugs, and cessation of pain-producing activities, including non–weight bearing with crutches if mere walking is painful.

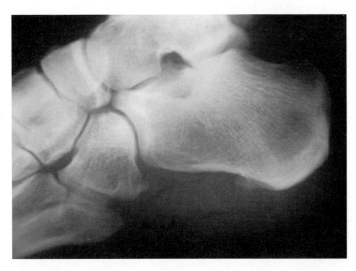

Figure 12–3. Lateral radiograph of the foot, showing a calcaneal spur often associated with plantar fasciitis.

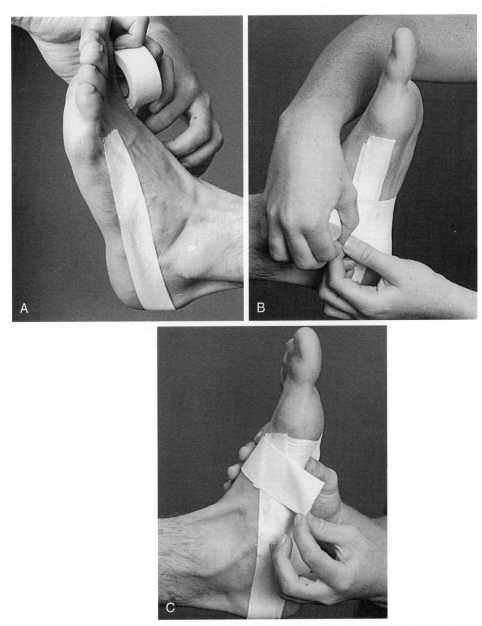

Figure 12–4. Low-Dye taping technique: The foot and ankle are held in inversion to accentuate the longitudinal arch. *A,* Three horseshoe strips of 1-in. tape are placed from the fifth metatarsal head around the heel to the first metatarsal head while the metatarsal head is depressed. *B,* Three strips of 1-in. tape are placed from lateral to medial to form a sling beneath the arch. *C,* The taping is finished with an anchor strip of 1-in. tape.

REFERRAL

Failure to resolve the condition within a reasonable period of conservative management should prompt referral for evaluation regarding the use of an orthotic appliance.[9] Podiatrists specializing in athletic injuries are often able to fabricate a device that relieves the symptoms and allows continued athletic participation.

Surgical intervention can include excision of the bursa often overlying the calcaneal spur or release of the plantar fascia from its origin, or both. We believe that surgical options should be considered only if orthoses fail to resolve the problem.

DEFINITIVE TREATMENT

Physical therapy modalities such as ultrasonography or high-intensity galvanic stimulation should be tried in recalcitrant cases. An adequate trial should include treatments two or three times weekly for at least 2 weeks.

Low-Dye taping often provides pain relief for the activities of daily living. The athlete must be cautioned that even though taping may allow comfortable walking, athletic activities should not be attempted. Protracted running or jumping while the foot is Low-Dye taped often results in blistering beneath the tape, thus further prolonging disability.

Exercise programs aimed at strengthening the peroneal, anterior tibial, and posterior tibial muscles should be instituted as soon as they can be performed comfortably (see Chapter 11, part A).

The use of a night splint is often helpful particularly in alleviating the pain encountered when first getting up in the morning. Such splints are commercially available or can be fashioned with posterior plaster or fiberglass splints holding the ankle at 90 degrees.

C. PLANTAR (MORTON'S) NEUROMA

Morton's neuroma is a focal enlargement of a plantar digital nerve usually located between the third and fourth metatarsals. Its importance lies in the fact that the accompanying pain can result in significant disability, and if the condition is allowed to become chronic, surgical intervention is often necessary. Although the problem is most commonly associated with wearing high-heeled shoes that are too narrow across the forefoot, it is not an uncommon problem among athletes and dancers.

HISTORY

MECHANISM OF INJURY. Although this particular nerve may be vulnerable to injury because of anatomical idiosyncrasies, the onset of symptoms is usually associated with footwear that is too narrow and tight across the forefoot. Activities that are often associated with this condition include those in which the body is propelled forward off the dorsiflexed toes, such as sprinting and running uphill. The dorsiflexion probably stretches the nerve, resulting in inflammation and swelling. Once swollen, its increased prominence renders it more likely to become repeatedly entrapped between the metatarsal heads, thus traumatizing it further. Finally the nerve becomes scarred and permanently enlarged.

SYMPTOMS. Sharp and sometimes severe *pain* with weight bearing while wearing footwear is the most common complaint. The pain is often described as an electrical shock extending into the fourth and third toes. Patients learn quickly that the pain can usually be alleviated by removing the shoe. The initial episode is often associated with wearing new shoes and with toe-running types of activity.

PHYSICAL EXAMINATION

The characteristic *pain* is usually elicited by gently compressing the forefoot from side to side while squeezing the tissue between the metatarsal heads with the fingertips (Fig. 12–5). Occasionally *hypesthesia* is present in the web space and the opposing sides of the adjacent toes. In a thin foot a *mass* may be palpable from the plantar aspect.

RADIOGRAPHIC EXAMINATION

Radiographs may be of value in differentiating this condition from degenerative joint disease involving the metatarsophalangeal joints or from a stress fracture of a metatarsal bone.

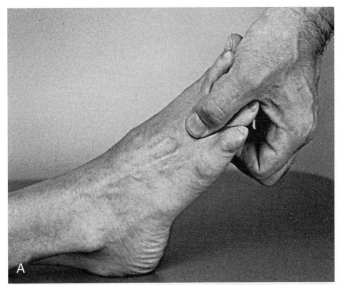

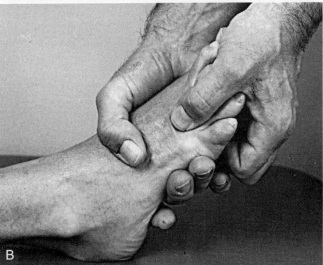

Figure 12–5. Provocative tests for Morton's neuroma: *A,* Thumb and forefinger compress the space between the third and fourth metatarsal heads. *B,* Metatarsal heads are compressed together transversely while the neuroma is entrapped.

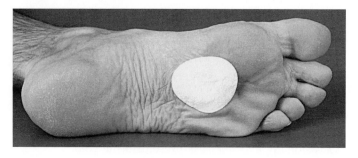

Figure 12–6. Metatarsal pad for Morton's neuroma. The dome of the pad is placed between the third and fourth metatarsals, just posterior to the metatarsal heads.

OTHER DIAGNOSTIC TESTS

Other diagnostic tests are not required.

INITIAL TREATMENT

Avoidance of the offending shoes, the application of ice after activity, and the use of contrast baths should be instituted immediately. Theoretically, if the problem can be dealt with while the nerve is merely edematous, the condition can be "cured."

REFERRAL

An increase in symptoms in spite of appropriate nonoperative management is an indication for referral. Surgical management involves excision of the neuroma and results in numbness of the web space and opposing surfaces of the involved toes. The surgical procedures are successful in approximately 85% of the cases.

DEFINITIVE TREATMENT

Relative rest (avoidance of pain-producing activities), avoidance of constrictive footwear, and utilization of local methods to control and alleviate inflammation and swelling should be tried. A small metatarsal pad or "cookie" should be placed in the shoe just proximal to the metatarsal heads. By enhancing the transverse arch, such a pad in effect narrows the foot, thus allowing more space in the shoe. Additionally, pressure is taken off the metatarsal heads by such a pad (Fig. 12–6).

If conservative management fails, a single local injection of a corticosteroid preparation may give relief. After such an injection the athlete should be warned not to abuse the foot for a week or 10 days, as some time will be required for the swelling to disappear.

D. STRESS FRACTURES

Stress fractures of the foot merit special consideration, not because they differ appreciably from those found elsewhere in the body, but rather because they can occur in so many varied locations, many of which defy easy radiographic documentation and thus may go undiagnosed, be inappropriately treated, and result in significant disability.[2–8, 10, 11] The clinical picture and management are described in the section dealing with stress fractures (see Chapter 3, part C).

The shafts of the second through the fifth metatarsals are the most common sites of injury. These injuries are perhaps most commonly seen in athletes involved in endurance running activities. Fractures of the base of the *second metatarsal* are seen in ballet dancers. Stress fractures of the proximal third of the *fifth metatarsal* seem to appear more commonly in sports that combine running with a rapid direction change, such as basketball. Jumping activities are frequently associated with stress fractures of the *tarsal navicular*. These injuries too seem more common in basketball players.

Like stress fractures elsewhere, these injuries are heralded by activity-related pain. Palpation, relatively easy to accomplish on the dorsum of the foot because of the lack of overlying soft tissues, usually reveals tenderness over the site of the injury. Occasionally, periosteal and soft tissue swelling can be palpated as well, especially if the injury involves the metatarsal shafts.

Radiographs, if abnormal, are most helpful in establishing a definitive diagnosis (Fig. 12–7). Two circumstances, however, deter the standard radiograph from being the diagnostic gold standard: (1) if the patient presents very early after the onset of symptoms before radiographic changes are present and (2) if fracture lines lie outside the plane usually traversed by the beam of radiographs.[4, 8] Our usual practice is immediately to order radionuclide bone scans rather than radiographs in multiple planes in an attempt to reveal a fracture site. Some specific examples in which the bone scan is particularly helpful include stress fractures of the tarsal navicular and base of the second metatarsal (Fig. 12–8), as well as any activity-related foot pain that eludes diagnosis.

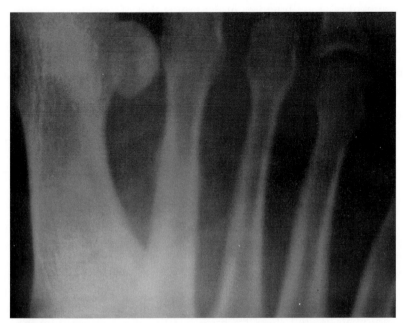

Figure 12–7. Anteroposterior (AP) radiograph of the foot demonstrating a classic stress (march) fracture of the shaft of the second metatarsal. Note the cortical thickening and the indistinct cortical surface.

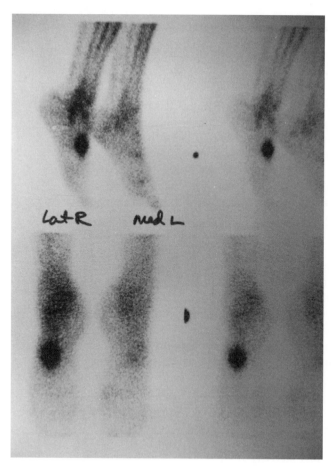

Figure 12–8. Radionuclide bone scan demonstrating stress fractures of the base of the second metatarsal.

Treatment of stress fractures of the foot is that of any stress fracture (see Chapter 3, part C), including reduction of activity until the athlete is pain free, followed by gradual resumption of activity but avoidance of *any* symptoms. In the cases of fractures of the navicular and proximal portion of the fifth metatarsal, this usually includes immobilization and non–weight bearing and, in some instances, might even involve surgical intervention.

E. SESAMOIDITIS

The sesamoid bones of the great toe are located within the tendons of the flexor hallucis brevis on the plantar aspect of the foot. During the propulsive or toe-off portion of gait, these bones help redistribute and attenuate force over the first metatarsal head.

Injuries to the sesamoids are important because they produce both diagnostic and therapeutic challenges. Diagnosis is complicated by the fact that these small bones can be the site of degenerative joint disease, osteochondrosis, chondromalacia, and stress fractures. Treatment is hampered by the difficulty of protecting the sesamoids from the forces of mere walking, to say nothing of sprinting or dancing.

HISTORY

MECHANISM OF INJURY. The sesamoids can be fractured as the result of landing a jump on the forefoot or of weight bearing on the hyperdorsiflexed great toe. Running and jumping can result in overuse injuries such as stress fractures and degenerative joint disease. The activities associated with either acute or overuse injuries are usually those emphasizing push-off from the forefoot such as sprinting, driving out of the stance of a football lineman, or doing a relevé in ballet. There is some suggestion that the highly arched (cavus), rigid foot is more commonly associated with sesamoid problems.

SYMPTOMS. *Pain and swelling* in the ball of the foot are characteristic of sesamoiditis. Rolling through the foot to stand on the toes is painful, as are running and, finally, walking. The athlete with chronic problems often has pain on the lateral aspect of the foot from ambulating in inversion in an attempt to protect the painful first metatarsophalangeal joint.

PHYSICAL EXAMINATION

Well-localized tenderness is usually present directly over the sesamoid on the plantar aspect of the foot. With dorsiflexion of the great toe, the sesamoids move distally, as does the area of maximal tenderness. Swelling may be present but is often difficult to appreciate because of the presence of the subcutaneous fat.

RADIOGRAPHIC EXAMINATION

Lateral and "sesamoid" projections should be obtained (Fig. 12–9). Evaluation of the radiographs is complicated by the fact that the sesamoids are often bipartite. This condition is usually bilateral and most often involves the tibial (medial) sesamoid, but nonetheless it is often mistaken for a fracture. Irregularity of the plantar surface or cyst formation is indicative of chondromalacia and degenerative joint disease.

OTHER DIAGNOSTIC TESTS

Radionuclide bone scanning is helpful in strengthening the diagnoses of both stress fractures and degenerative joint disease.[11]

INITIAL TREATMENT

The first order is to avoid the pain-producing activity and reduce the swelling and inflammation. Often a crescent-shaped ¼-in. felt pad can be fashioned to reduce pressure over the sesamoid (Fig. 12–10). If this is ineffective, then painful weight bearing must be avoided. Occasionally a stiff-soled shoe alleviates the pain with weight bearing. Nonsteroidal anti-inflammatory drugs, contrast baths, and physical therapy may be helpful in decreasing symptoms.

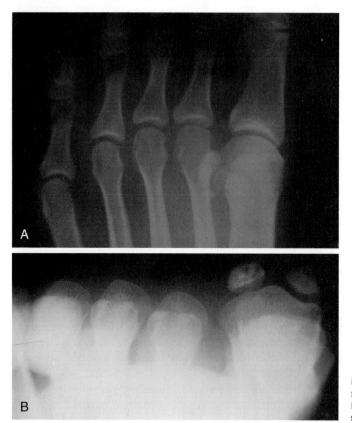

Figure 12–9. *A,* AP and *B,* "sesamoid-view" radiographs demonstrating cystic changes in lateral (fibular) sesamoid.

REFERRAL

Podiatric referral for evaluation and fabrication of orthoses is indicated if a short course of conservative management fails. Not only do orthoses often alleviate the symptoms, but they may also alter the biomechanics of the foot and reduce the likelihood of further recurrences.

Significant degenerative changes and resistance to conservative management are sometimes indications for excision of the sesamoid. This procedure should not be considered lightly, as it can result in biomechanical alterations that are as problematic as the original problem. In addition, with degenerative joint disease of the sesamoid, the opposing articular surface of the metatarsal head may also be involved, and this may result in continued symptoms.

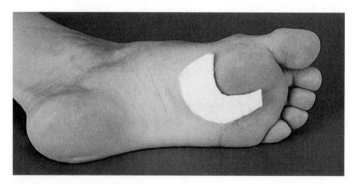

Figure 12–10. Felt pad used to alleviate pressure on the lateral sesamoid.

DEFINITIVE TREATMENT

If the problem is of short duration, the initial treatment may suffice. In the case of stress fractures, guarded weight bearing for weeks or months and even cast immobilization may be necessary.

F. BLISTERS

Blisters in athletes merit mention because they are preventable and because they often occur at particularly inopportune times, thus requiring "heroic" treatment. Blisters, like calluses, are the result of friction, except that with blisters the friction occurs *within* the skin. For this to occur the surface of the skin must (momentarily) stick to the material applied to it—the shoe, or even adhesive tape. Socks are worn to provide a bearing-like interface between the shoe and the foot, allowing the friction to occur between the sock and the shoe. The sock thus becomes an extension of the skin.

If identified early, the preblister stage consists of a "hot spot" of localized redness and tenderness. Treatment at this time should be aimed at reducing the pressure/friction over the traumatized area. This can be accomplished by surrounding the area with a doughnut pad or by covering the area with a material that will bear the brunt of the friction. We use Second Skin or Adhesive Knit material.

Once the blister forms, it exposes tender, intraepidermal tissue to pressure and friction and becomes painful. Small (<1-cm diameter) blisters can usually be treated as preblister problems. Larger blisters should be drained in a sterile fashion and covered by Second Skin, Adhesive Knit, or even adhesive tape if nothing else is available. If adhesive tape is used, its outer surface should be covered with petroleum jelly or silicone spray to enhance its capability to act as a bearing.

REFERENCES

1. Coker TP et al: Traumatic lesions of the metatarsophalangeal joint of the great toe in athletes. Am J Sports Med 6:326–334, 1978.
2. Delee JC et al: Stress fracture of fifth metatarsal. Am J Sports Med 11:349–353, 1983.
3. Drez D Jr et al: Metatarsal stress fractures. Am J Sports Med 8:123–125, 1980.
4. Grahame R et al: Use of scintigraphy in the diagnosis and management of traumatic foot lesions in ballet dancers. Rheumatol Rehabil 18:235–238, 1979.
5. Marymont JH Jr et al: Fracture of the lateral cuneiform bone in the absence of severe direct trauma: Diagnosis by radionuclide bone scan. Am J Sports Med 8:135–136, 1980.
6. Meurman KOA: Stress lesions of the talus. Fortschr Geb Roentgenstr Nuklearmed 132:469–471, 1980.
7. Pavlov H et al: Tarsal navicular stress fractures: Radiographic evaluation. Radiology 148:641–645, 1983.
8. Saunders AJS et al: Stress lesions of the lower leg and foot. Clin Radiol 30:649–651, 1979.
9. Taunton JE et al: Plantar fasciitis in runners. Can J Appl Sports Sci 7:41–44, 1982.
10. Torg JS et al: Stress fractures of the tarsal navicular: Retrospective review of 21 cases. J Bone Joint Surg Am 64:700–712, 1982.
11. Van Hal ME et al: Stress fractures of the great toe sesamoids. Am J Sports Med 10:122–128, 1982.

13

Decision Analysis

As clinicians, we must continually make decisions. Do we order a certain test? Do we treat now or wait for the test results? What treatment do we choose? Decision making is inevitable, and this is just as true in sports medicine as in other areas of clinical practice.

Sometimes the decision making is straightforward. Given certain key findings, the diagnosis is clear; given the diagnosis, there is a preferred treatment. Much of the time, however, decisions must be made despite uncertainties. Clinical findings are equivocal. A diagnostic test has false-positive and false-negative results. Even given an accurate diagnosis, authorities disagree how a given patient ought to be treated.

Decision analysis is a systematic approach to decision making under conditions of uncertainty.[15, 17, 22] It has been widely used in such diverse fields as business,* public policy, and, more recently, clinical medicine,[19, 22, 23] and we have found it to be a useful tool in our practice of sports medicine.

We hasten to point out, however, that decision analysis is intended only to enhance, not to substitute for, clinical judgment. It cannot predict an outcome for an individual patient, but it may suggest an optimal approach to a given clinical problem that, if consistently applied to a population of patients, will generally provide the best results (S. Crane, personal communication).

The method is based on mathematical logic and probability and, as illustrated later, comprises four basic steps.[22] The first step is to identify and to bound the decision problem. Bounding is a mathematical term meaning, for practical purposes, that there are definite beginning and end points and not an indefinite string of "what if's." The second step is to structure the problem as a temporal and logical sequence of decisions and outcomes, often represented schematically as a decision tree. The third step is to assign values to the possible outcomes. The fourth is to determine an optimal strategy, i.e., to decide which decision or decisions will maximize the probability of obtaining a desired outcome.

---

*A computer spreadsheet program, for example, is a common business application.

In this chapter we discuss two specific applications of decision analysis in sports medicine. We first consider a typical choice-of-treatment decision problem and show how the problem can be clarified using the method previously described. We next consider how the values assigned to possible outcomes affect the utility of a clinical decision.

A. ANALYSIS OF A SIMPLE OPERATE/DO NOT OPERATE DECISION PROBLEM[21]

A common and often controversial decision in sports medicine is whether primary operative treatment should be carried out for a given condition. This is a consideration not only for the surgeon who will do the operation, but also for the primary care physician who must decide how to evaluate the patient and whether the patient should be referred.

In this section we consider, as an example, the decision of whether to do primary repair of complete tears of the lateral ligaments of the ankle. The results of treating acute injury by primary repair, cast immobilization, and rehabilitation are available from the literature,[6, 9, 11, 13, 16] as are the results of treating chronic injury by delayed repair.[8] Intuitively, it might seem that if the results of primary repair were superior to both the results of nonoperative treatment and the results of delayed repair, then for optimal results one ought to carry out primary repair. Analysis of the decision reveals that this is not necessarily so.

A universal concern in the treatment of acute ankle injuries is the prevention of chronic functional instability.[1-3, 6, 8, 9, 11-14, 16, 20] Functional instability is characterized by *complaints* of a weak ankle, an unstable ankle, an untrustworthy ankle, giving way, difficulty in running on uneven surfaces, difficulty in cutting and jumping in athletic activities, a chronic sprain, frequent sprains, and the like and by a past history of prior severe sprain, often not properly treated or rehabilitated.

Arguments for primary operative treatment are largely based on the premise that complete ligamentous disruption leads to mechanical joint instability, which in turn leads to functional instability (which in turn may lead to accelerated degenerative joint disease). To prevent this undesirable chain of events, it seems important both to make the diagnosis of complete ligamentous disruption and to try to achieve mechanical joint stability.

A counterargument is that the benefit of achieving mechanical stability might not outweigh the cost of surgical treatment. Although it is generally agreed that mechanical stability of the ankle can best be achieved surgically, opinion is divided as to the correlation between mechanical and functional stability.[2, 3, 6, 11, 12, 14] It seems that certainly within a population of patients and probably for many individuals, the cause of functional instability is multifactorial. Indeed, limited dorsiflexion,[1] peroneal weakness,[2, 20] loss of proprioception,[11, 12] and internal derangement, as well as mechanical instability,[3, 6, 11, 20] have all been implicated.

Moreover, even the surgically aggressive acknowledge a "downside" to operative treatment. Although the financial cost might be no object to an injured superstar, the cost (to someone) and the logistics of operating on every athlete with a severe ankle sprain would be staggering. Athletes of all ages and abilities want to return to their sports as quickly as possible. However, with surgical treatment, as opposed to early mobilization, both the time away from the sport and the time away from the athlete's occupation are substantially prolonged.[6, 11] There is a small but finite risk of operative/ anesthetic complications, some of which would be considerably worse than functional instability. The possibility also exists that the athlete could undergo surgical treatment and, even barring complications, might still not achieve the desired outcome.[6, 11]

Whatever one might surmise on the basis of intuition or deductive reasoning, it seems important, if possible, to subject those conclusions to experimentation and inductive reasoning. In the case of ankle sprains, randomized, prospective studies comparing the results of surgery, immobilization, and rehabilitation have in fact been reported.[6, 9, 11, 13] At least within studies the results seem to have been consistently evaluated, and in one study[6] the sample size was very large indeed. Even so, except to discount immobilization, there was no consensus among the authors as to the "optimal" treatment.

Thus, as is often the case, whatever position one might choose to take, a rationale can be found for it in the literature. In such situations, rather than be dogmatic, we might do better first to "agree to disagree" and then to try to analyze how and why we disagree.

Before proceeding with formal analysis of the treatment of ankle sprains, let us briefly consider a hypothetical injury for which the reasonable treatment options are primary repair, rehabilitation, or delayed repair, and for which the results of the different treatment alternatives are available from the literature—85% excellent results with primary repair, 60% with rehabilitation, and 70% with delayed repair. Suppose that we all agree what constitutes an excellent result and that we all accept the reported results as accurate and applicable.

Let us then pose the following question: If obtaining an excellent result were the *only* concern, should we do primary repair? To the extent that we might answer the question differently, since we have already agreed about what data to accept and how to evaluate the possible outcomes, it seems that we must view the logic of the problem differently.

The logical structure of a decision problem may be represented schematically by a decision tree. By convention, the tree branches from left to right as a temporal sequence of events. Branch points representing decisions are designated by small squares. Branch points representing chance events, such as the consequences of those decisions, are designated by small circles. A simplified decision tree for the decision whether to operate for an acute injury is shown in Figure 13–1.

In the example we are considering, operating means doing primary repair, which has a spectrum of possible outcomes. Not operating means first rehabilitation, which also has a spectrum of possible outcomes (Fig. 13–2). Of these, some will be indications for delayed repair, which in turn has a spectrum of possible outcomes (Fig. 13–3). The complete logical structure of the decision problem of whether to do primary repair is thus represented by the decision tree shown in Figure 13–4. For purposes of analysis we may choose to dichotomize all the possible outcomes as either excellent or anything less, i.e., nonexcellent, in which case the logic structure of the decision problem would be as shown in Figure 13–5.

Were we then to consider only the probability of obtaining an excellent

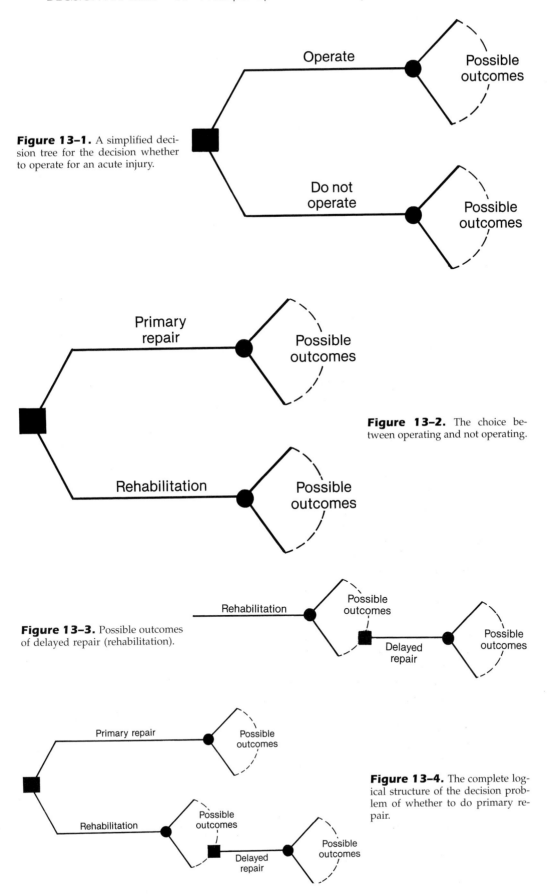

Figure 13–1. A simplified decision tree for the decision whether to operate for an acute injury.

Figure 13–2. The choice between operating and not operating.

Figure 13–3. Possible outcomes of delayed repair (rehabilitation).

Figure 13–4. The complete logical structure of the decision problem of whether to do primary repair.

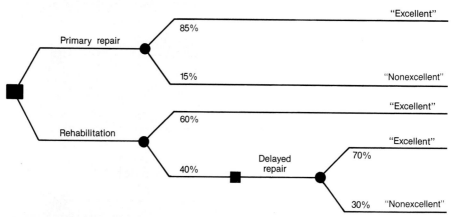

Figure 13–5. Dichotomization of all posible outcomes as either excellent or nonexcellent.

result depending on the initial decision made, we would see that there is not much difference between the two alternatives. The probability of obtaining an excellent result with primary repair is 85%. As can be inferred from Figure 13–5, the probability of obtaining an excellent result with rehabilitation and delayed repair if necessary is 88% (60% plus 70% of 40%).

As also can be inferred from Figure 13–5, the critical difference between the two competing strategies seems to be downtime. Not doing primary repair would result in the shortest downtime in the event that rehabilitation alone were successful, but in the longest downtime in the event that rehabilitation were unsuccessful and delayed repair were required.

Thus in the example given, possible indications for primary repair might be an unwillingness to wait and see what the results of initial rehabilitation would be or an ability to predict a priori who would not do well with rehabilitation alone. All things considered, however, we could probably all agree that primary repair would not be our usual treatment of choice.

Let us now proceed with our analysis of the decision whether to operate on lateral ankle sprains. Precisely identifying the problem is possible, largely because of the work of Broström.[4, 5, 7] In his series of hundreds of patients with sprained ankles, he found that about three fourths had arthrographically confirmed disruption of the joint capsule or ligaments, or both. Of these, approximately 85% were found at operation to have complete disruption of one or more of the lateral ligaments, and of these, all had complete disruption of the anterior talofibular ligament and about one third also had complete disruption of the calcaneofibular ligament.

Bounding the problem within the context of sports medicine would also seem to be straightforward. We might reasonably choose as a starting point the decision of how to treat an athlete who has just sustained a complete disruption (acute grade III sprain) of the anterior talofibular or calcaneofibular ligament, or both, and as an end point the ability or inability of the athlete to return safely and effectively to the chosen sport.

As a first approach the logical structure of the initial decision could be represented schematically as shown in Figure 13–6. The possible options would include primary repair, cast immobilization, rehabilitation, and nontreatment.

However, because we have agreed to bound the problem within the context of sports medicine, we can probably prune the decision tree. There is not much to be said for immobilization as a treatment option. The achieve-

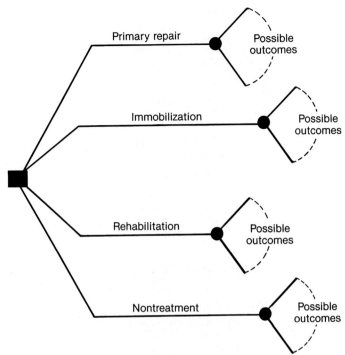

Figure 13–6. The logical structure of the initial decision.

ment of mechanical stability is no better than with early mobilization, and the
duration of disability after injury is as prolonged as with surgical treatment.[6, 9,
11, 13, 16] Since the whole point of decision analysis is to determine an optimal
strategy, it seems reasonable to exclude both immobilization and nontreatment
from further consideration. The logical structure of the decision problem
would then be the same as that shown in Figure 13–4.

Next we have to consider the question of the priority of the possible
outcomes. An ideal outcome might comprise all of the following: a return to
the sport, no functional impairment, no complications of treatment, a minimal
risk of re-injury, no long-term sequelae, no mechanical instability, a minimal
downtime, and a minimal cost. Obviously, such an outcome would be impossible to achieve. Choosing an optimal strategy, therefore, necessarily involves
some trade-offs and depends on how we value the *possible* outcomes.

To facilitate analysis, we might initially dichotomize the possible outcomes as either desired or anything less, equally valuing all undesired outcomes. The logical structure of the decision problem would then be the same
as that shown in Figure 13–7.

In the present context at least, it would seem appropriate to consider a
return to the sport *without functional impairment* as the desired outcome.[1] After
all, the usually given justification for surgery is, "In any other case, I would
treat conservatively, but because he (she) is a professional (elite, talented,
promising, or young) *athlete* (dancer), I would operate to give him (her) the
best possible chance of obtaining a good result."

We could then pose the following critical question: If achieving functional
stability of the ankle were the *only* concern, should we do primary repair? As
in the hypothetical previous example, given the results of primary repair,
rehabilitation, and delayed repair, we should be able to calculate the probabilities of obtaining the desired outcome for each of the competing strategies.

Again it seems appropriate to consider the work of Broström.[6, 8] Both

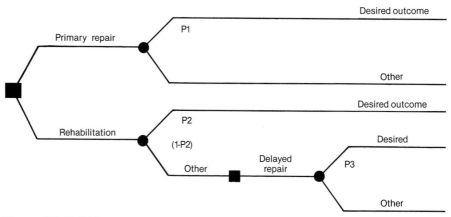

Figure 13–7. Dichotomization of all possible outcomes as either desired or anything less.

proponents and opponents of primary repair cite his studies. His is certainly the largest series of patients and the only series in which the same investigator evaluated the results of treating both acute and chronic injuries.

He reported the following: In 83 of 86 patients with acute injury treated by primary repair and in 67 of 85 patients with acute injury treated by strapping alone, there was no functional instability.[6] In 85 of 86 patients treated by primary repair and in 80 of 85 patients treated by strapping alone, there was no severe functional instability.[6] There was no functional instability in 43 of 60 patients with chronic injury treated by delayed repair and no severe or moderate functional instability in 57 of 60 of those patients.[8]

If one uses these data, the probability of having no functional instability would be 97% with primary repair, 79% with strapping alone, and 72% with delayed repair. With strapping and delayed repair if necessary, the probability of having no functional instability would be 94% (79% plus 72% of 21%).

Similarly, the probability of having no severe functional instability would be 99% with primary repair. It would also be 99% with strapping and delayed repair if necessary.

Thus even if achieving functional stability were the only concern, there would seem to be no compelling reason for primary repair. As discussed previously, a possible indication might be an unwillingness to wait to see.

We may not wish to accept this as the final analysis, however. Although no one seems to question the validity of Broström's data, it seems possible to question its applicability in the context of sports medicine. As discussed later, there are two biases of the study that seem to favor nonoperative treatment and one that seems to favor operative treatment.

Not all of Broström's patients were athletes. He admitted that "the prognosis was less good in young patients than in older patients in this series, presumably because the strains put on the foot were greater in the young patients who, moreover, tended to be more demanding as regards satisfactory function." However, he did not comment on whether this was a statistically significant finding, nor did he present the data to determine this.

Less severe injuries (single ligament, primary sprain) were lumped with more severe ones (double ligament, recurrent sprain). Broström did report that in his nonoperatively treated patients "the frequency of symptoms . . . seemed to be greater when both ligaments had been torn than when only the anterior talofibular ligament had been torn," but noted that "the difference is not statistically significant." He also stated that "the poorest results were observed in cases with concomitant rupture of the calcaneofibular ligament and the anterior talofibular ligament and a history of previous sprains," but again noted that "the higher frequency of symptoms is not statistically verified."

However, we believe that these considerations are more than offset by the fact that what Broström described as *strapping* was actually more akin to nontreatment than to rehabilitation. His strapping involved only an elastic wrap until the swelling subsided and elevation if there was severe swelling and ecchymosis. Patients were allowed to walk on the injured foot immediately. They were encouraged to do exercises such as toe rising and toe jumping, but "the help of a physiotherapist was seldom necessary."

The importance of complete rehabilitation in preventing chronic functional instability is probably best demonstrated by the work of Freeman.[11-13] His patients were for the most part athletically active, fit, young adult, male soldiers. In his initial study, at 1-year follow-up he found no functional instability in 10 of 16 patients (62%) treated by primary repair or in 7 of 12 patients (58%) treated by early mobilization.[11] In a subsequent study, he again found no functional instability in 8 of 16 patients (50%) treated by early mobilization or in 14 of 16 patients (88%) treated by complete rehabilitation including proprioceptive training.[13] As he observed, "Coordination exercises thus led to a significant ($p = 0.0088$) reduction in the incidence of functional instability." Were they to take Freeman's work to heart, the surgically inclined might actually argue, "Because he (she) is *not* a professional athlete (dancer) and may not have the time, motivation, or skills to complete a proper rehabilitation program, I would operate to give him (her) the best possible chance of obtaining a good result."

In any case, we believe that it is wrong, even though it is often done, to cite Broström's work as justification for primary repair in athletes. On the basis of the foregoing analysis, we conclude that even if the functional stability of the ankle were deemed to be the single most important outcome consideration, if Broström's data were accepted as true and applicable, then primary repair should not be considered as the usual treatment of choice for grade III lateral ankle sprains. Certainly, Freeman's data also support this conclusion.

A further implication of this analysis for the primary care physician is that the work-up of acute ankle injury need not discriminate between complete and incomplete sprains of the lateral ligaments. Treatment will be the same in either case, and neither the athlete nor the physician needs an anterior drawer test, talar tilt test, arthrography, or magnetic resonance imaging to know that it will take longer to recover from a more severe injury than from a less severe injury.

Other choice-of-treatment problems in sports medicine can be similarly analyzed. Although the literature often does not provide as good data as for lateral ankle sprains, we believe that consideration of the logical structure of the decision problem permits some generalizations (Fig. 13–8). In logical terms, that the results of primary operative treatment will be better than the results of nonoperative treatment *and* better than the results of delayed operative treatment is not a *sufficient*, but rather a *necessary*, condition for primary operative treatment even to be considered. The greater the chance of successful outcome with nonoperative treatment, the more the benefits/risks of primary operation must exceed those of delayed operation for primary operative treatment to be considered the treatment of choice.

When controversy remains, decision analysis may at least help clarify the issues. Is it just that we do not agree about what data to accept? If so, perhaps

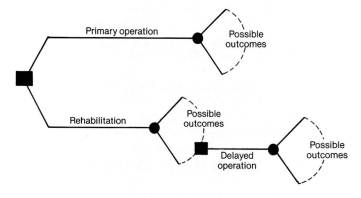

Figure 13–8. Consideration of the logical structure of the decision problem permits some generalizations.

we could agree about what further data are needed and how to obtain them. Is it that we place different values on the possible outcomes? If so, perhaps we should just admit that to our patients and ourselves and carry on. After all, if we are not working toward the same ends, there is no reason to suppose that we should necessarily employ the same means. Is it instead that we have not adequately thought through the logical structure of the decision problem? If so, this is perhaps where our debate should begin rather than end.

B. ANALYSIS OF A DECISION HAVING MORE THAN TWO POSSIBLE OUTCOMES—THE EFFECT OF VALUE JUDGMENTS ON THE UTILITY OF THE DECISION

As was shown in part A, whenever the possible outcomes of decisions can be classified as desired or undesired, decision analysis is greatly facilitated. Choosing an optimal strategy, i.e., making the best decision or decisions, then becomes a relatively simple matter of maximizing the probability of obtaining the desired result (or minimizing the probability of obtaining the undesired result).

Most clinical decisions, however, have more than two possible outcomes. Also, the possible outcomes often have multiple attributes. For example, in part A the suggested ideal outcome for the treatment of ankle sprains had the following attributes: a return to the sport, no functional impairment, no complications of treatment, a minimal risk of re-injury, no long-term sequelae, no mechanical instability, a minimal downtime, and a minimal cost.

In that example, had the preliminary analysis shown an apparent advantage in primary operation, i.e., that functional stability would more likely be achieved by operating primarily than not, it would have been necessary to analyze the decision further. We should then have had to take into account how we valued the various attributes and what benefit-versus-cost trade-offs we might be willing to make.

Whenever more than two final outcomes are possible, the decision maker needs to consider explicitly the strength of preferences among the possible outcomes.[22] The formal process of determining an optimal strategy under these conditions is called *utility analysis*. As is shown later, the concept of a decision's utility takes into account both the relative values assigned to the possible outcomes and the probabilities of obtaining those outcomes.*

To illustrate, let us consider the problem of an athlete's decision to use or not to use some supposed ergogenic aid. Aside from any ethical and legal questions, there are at least two clinical uncertainties: (1) Will the athlete's performance be enhanced? (2) Will the athlete suffer any untoward side effect or side effects? In terms of decision analysis, the possible outcomes of the decision have at least two *attributes*: (1) performance enhancement or not and (2) an occurrence of a side effect or side effects or not. We can also delineate four possible *outcomes*: (1) performance enhancement, no side effect or side effects; (2) performance enhancement, a side effect or side effects; (3) no performance enhancement, no side effect or side effects; and (4) no perfor- mance enhancement, a side effect or side effects. The logical structure of this decision problem can be represented schematically as shown in Figure 13–9.

Determining an optimal strategy, i.e., deciding whether to use the ergo- genic aid, depends not only on the estimated probabilities of obtaining the various possible outcomes but also on the value placed on each of the possible outcomes. Clearly, outcome number 1 is best, and outcome number 4 worst. The relative values of outcome numbers 2 and 3, however, depend on the extent of performance enhancement, the type and severity of the side effect or side effects, and the *value judgments* of the decision maker.

To analyze this kind of decision problem further, it would be necessary first to rank all possible outcomes from best to worst and then to quantify the values of the possible outcomes. The numerical values assigned to the possible

---

*A similar epidemiological concept is that of the *injury index*, which takes into account both the severity of injury and the incidence (rate of occurrence) of injury in a population. In contrast, the *injury rate* reflects only the incidence of injury—a broken neck and a sprained ankle would each be counted as one occurrence.

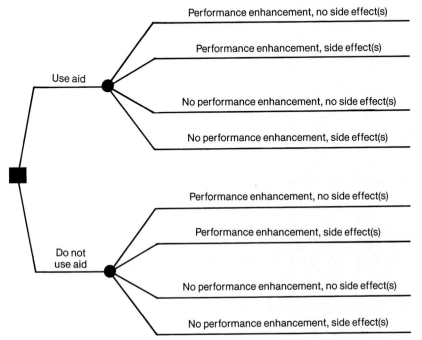

Figure 13–9. Decision tree for considering the strength of preferences among the possible out- comes.

outcomes are called the *utilities* of the outcomes, and the numerical ranking of the possible outcomes, a *utility scale.*

By convention, the utility of an outcome may range from 1 to 0, with the best outcome assigned a value of 1, and the worst, 0. The assignment of numerical values to the intermediate outcomes is somewhat complicated. One approach is to ask the decision maker to compare the certainty of an intermediate outcome with a gamble between the best and worst outcomes.*

Also by convention, the probability of obtaining a possible outcome may range from 1 to 0. A probability of 1 would indicate that its occurrence is certain; a probability of 0, that its occurrence is impossible.

The *utility of a decision* can then be defined as the sum of the products of the utilities of the possible outcomes of the decision times the probabilities of obtaining those outcomes. A perfectly utile decision, one certain to result in the most highly valued outcome, would have a value of 1. A completely inutile decision, one certain to result in the least highly valued outcome, would have a value of 0.

That the utility of the athlete's decision necessarily depends on the values assigned to the possible outcomes of that decision raises a fundamental question: Whose values should be taken into account—those of the athlete, the coach, the governing body of the sport, or the physician?

How might the value judgments of some athletes and physicians differ? In a survey, Yesalis asked high school anabolic steroid users if they would stop taking the drugs "if it was proved beyond doubt that anabolic steroids would greatly increase the risk of cancer, greatly influence the risk of heart attack before age 40, or lead to permanent sterility."[24] About 25% said that they would not. Among "heavy users"—those who had "cycled" on and off the drug or drugs more than five times—40% said they would not.

As a rough approximation, the logical structure of the question posed by Yesalis can also be represented schematically by the decision tree shown in Figure 13–9. It is doubtful that any of the respondents thought about the question in precisely these terms, but the bottom line is that, for some of them, deciding to keep taking the drug had greater utility than deciding to stop taking it. By implication, they ascribed greater utility to performance enhancement than disutility to deleterious effects on their health, and they estimated the probability of their achieving the desired level of performance without pharmacological help to be small.

In sharp contrast, most physicians would find it unconscionable to ascribe *any* utility to *any* outcome in which the athlete's health and well-being were so adversely affected. In terms of decision analysis, the attribute of health versus ill health would be considered completely *value dominant* to the attribute of performance enhancement versus no performance enhancement. Thus for physicians the utility of the decision to continue to take the drug would be 0.

It is encouraging that most of the athletes in the survey came to similar conclusions—that they would find less utility in continuing to take a harmful drug than in not continuing to take it. The fact that the more the athletes had used the drugs, the more likely they were to keep using them is evidence of psychological drug dependence and of a change in value judgments as a result of drug use.

An implication of Yesalis' work for those who might hope to modify

---

*The reader interested in learning more about decision analysis is referred to the introductory text *Clinical Decision Analysis.*[22]

athletes' behavior is that some will be influenced by educational efforts and others will not. For a college freshman football player, the risk of succumbing to a heart attack at the age of 35 years may seem abstract and remote. The risk of having to go out the next Saturday against a steroid-using opponent who is bigger, stronger, crazier, and meaner may be, in contrast, quite real and immediate. The risks of not making the team, not starting, and not being drafted are also very real concerns of many athletes.

The authors did ask their subjects if they would stop taking the drugs "if they were absolutely convinced that their competitors no longer used them." Again, especially among the "heavy users," many reported that they would not. Perhaps more poignant questions to have asked would have been, "Would you stop taking the drug if you knew with certainty that you would be barred from sport if you were caught using it?" and, "Would you stop taking the drug if you knew that you could be arrested and sent to jail if you were caught using it?"

The foregoing was not to debate the dilemma of drug use in sport, but rather to illustrate the effect of value judgments on the utility of a clinical decision. We believe that this effect has several important implications for the sports physician.

If the physician and the athlete value the possible outcomes of a decision differently, it may be quite pointless for the physician to discuss risks just in terms of probabilities. For example, an injured athlete may want to return to a sport before full recovery, even though in doing so there may be risk of re-injury. Depending on the injury, it may be important for the physician to try to convince the athlete that not only the risk (probability) of re-injury but also the *consequences* of re-injury outweigh any advantages of too early return to play.

A decision that is optimal for one athlete/patient may not be for another. Consider, for example, two young adults with anatomically identical knee injuries, one a professional football running back, the other an A-level amateur tennis player. In terms of sports performance the injury may be equally disabling for both. However, in considering the treatment options offered, the young running back may be quite willing to accept odds such as a 50% chance of getting back to his previous level of performance versus a 10% chance of making him substantially worse, and at least 6 months of intensive rehabilitation before getting back to any knee-strenuous activity at all, whereas the individual whose livelihood does not depend on sports may be considerably more "risk averse." Such athletes might rather give up the primary sport altogether than to take any chance of being worse off than they are already or to take a half-year or more out of their lives just to deal with a sports injury.

The primary care physician or team physician who has known the athlete for a long time may very well be in the best position to evaluate the athlete/patient's preferences realistically. Consider, for example, an athlete who has sustained an acute, grade III anterior cruciate ligament sprain with an associated meniscal tear. An orthopedic surgeon to whom the athlete might be referred may axiomatically ascribe utility to any outcome in which meniscal tissue is preserved. Accordingly, the surgeon might, as several authors have,[10, 18] recommend meniscorrhaphy and primary repair/reconstruction of the cruciate ligament to protect the meniscal repair. The athlete, on the other hand, may see little or no inherent value in preservation of meniscal tissue as a matter of principle. However, the athlete might, as would we, ascribe utility to outcomes in which meniscal tissue is preserved, if the athlete were convinced that there is a positive correlation between this and improved functional stability or prevention of long-term sequelae, or both. As in the previous example, the athlete may or may not be willing to trade off such potential benefits against the certainty of prolonged time away from an occupation and a sport and the risk of operative complications. Important responsibilites of the primary care physician are, as accurately as possible, to estimate the patient's preferences, to make appropriate specialty referrals, and to communicate the patient's needs and wants to the specialist.

REFERENCES

1. Balduini FC, Tetzlaff J: Historical perspectives on injuries of the ligaments of the ankle. Clin Sports Med 1:3–12, 1982.
2. Bosien WR, Staples OS, Russell SW: Residual disability following acute ankle sprains. J Bone Joint Surg Am 37:1237–1243, 1955.
3. Brand RL, Black HM, Cox JS: The natural history of inadequately treated ankle sprain. Am J Sports Med 6:248–249, 1977.
4. Broström L: Sprained ankles. I: Anatomic lesions in recent sprains. Acta Chir Scand 128:483–495, 1964.
5. Broström L, Liljedahl SO, Lindvall N: Sprained ankles. II: Arthrographic diagnosis of recent ligament ruptures. Acta Chir Scand 129:485–499, 1965.
6. Broström L: Sprained ankles. III: Clinical observations in recent ligament ruptures. Acta Chir Scand 130:560–569, 1965.
7. Broström L: Sprained ankles. V: Treatment and prognosis in recent ligament ruptures. Acta Chir Scand 132:537–550, 1966.
8. Broström L: Sprained ankles. VI: Surgical treatment of chronic ligament ruptures. Acta Chir Scand 132:551–565, 1966.
9. Cox JS, Brand RL: Evaluation and treatment of lateral ankle sprains. Physician Sportsmed 5:51–55, June 1977.
10. Fetto JF, Marshall JL: The natural history and diagnosis of the anterior cruciate ligament deficient knee. Clin Orthop 147:29–38, 1980.
11. Freeman MAR: Treatment of ruptures of the lateral ligament of the ankle. J Bone Joint Surg Br 47:661–668, 1965.
12. Freeman MAR: Instability of the foot after injuries to the lateral ligament of the ankle. J Bone Joint Surg Br 47:669–677, 1965.
13. Freeman MAR: The etiology and prevention of functional instability of the foot. J Bone Joint Surg Br 47:678–685, 1965.
14. Glick JM et al: The prevention and treatment of ankle injuries. Am J Sports Med 4:136–141, 1976.
15. Howard R: The foundations of decision analysis. IEEE Trans Systems Sci Cybernetics SCC-4:211–219, 1968.
16. Jackson DW, Ashley RL, Powell JW: Ankle sprains in young athletes. Clin Orthop 101:201–215, 1974.
17. Raiffa H: Decision Analysis: Introductory Lectures on Choices Under Uncertainty. Reading, Mass, Addison-Wesley, 1968.
18. Sherman MF, Bonamo JR: Primary repair of the anterior cruciate ligament. Clin Sports Med 7:739–750, 1988.
19. Spencer RH (ed): Roundtable on medical decision making. Prim Care/Emergency Decisions 1:7–12, 1985.
20. Staples OS: Ruptures of the fibular collateral ligaments of the ankle. J Bone Joint Surg Am 57:101–107, 1975.
21. Webb DR, Garrick JG: Analysis of the decision to do primary repair of grade III lateral ankle sprains. Presented to American Academy of Sports Physicians, Annual Meeting, Santa Fe, 1989.
22. Weinstein MC et al: Clinical Decision Analysis. Philadelphia, WB Saunders, 1980.
23. Wolf SL: Clinical Decision Making in Physical Therapy. Philadelphia, FA Davis, 1985.
24. Yesalis CE: Anabolic steroid use: Indications of habituation among adolescents. J Drug Educ 19:103–116, 1989.

Index

Note: Page numbers in *italics* refer to illustrations; page numbers followed by t refer to tables.

417